Biomedical
Diagnostic
Science
and
Technology

Biomedical Diagnostic Science and Technology

edited by

Wai Tak Law
PortaScience, Inc.
Moorestown, New Jersey, U.S.A.

Naim Akmal
The Dow Chemical Company
South Charleston, West Virginia, U.S.A.

Arthur M. Usmani
Altec USA
Indianapolis, Indiana, U.S.A.

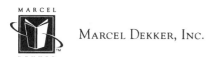

MARCEL DEKKER, INC.   NEW YORK · BASEL

ISBN: 0-8247-0725-7

This book is printed on acid-free paper.

Headquarters
Marcel Dekker, Inc.
270 Madison Avenue, New York, NY 10016
tel: 212–696-9000; fax: 212–685-4540

Eastern Hemisphere Distribution
Marcel Dekker AG
Hutgasse 4, Postfach 812, CH-4001 Basel, Switzerland
tel: 41–61-260–6300; fax: 41–61-260–6333

World Wide Web
http://www.dekker.com

The publisher offers discounts on this book when ordered in bulk quantities. For more information, write to Special Sales/Professional Marketing at the headquarters address above.

Current printing (last digit):
10 9 8 7 6 5 4 3 2 1

PRINTED IN THE UNITED STATES OF AMERICA

Preface

Without medical diagnostic reagents, the practice of medicine would be difficult if not impossible. Medical reagents play an important role in maintaining and improving our wellness. Research in this area will continue unabated, and use of these reagents will ever increase. The gene chip will revolutionize our ability to fight diseases as no method before. The recent development of newer concepts and rapid advances in medical diagnostic reagents encouraged us to bring together the information in this volume.

The book reviews work at the cutting edge in diagnostics, immunodiagnostics, and biosensors. Noninvasive methods, new signals for analyte detection, newer diagnostic polymers and coatings, and enzyme stabilization and immobilization methods are comprehensively discussed. Gene chip, or biochip, and related technologies are also discussed.

This book is organized into five sections: electrochemical biosensing systems; optical biosensing systems; newer detection systems; diabetes and cholesterol: systems and management; and polymeric materials, immobilization, and biocompatibility.

Although we will see more advances in medical diagnostics and biosensors in the future, we believe this comprehensive and authoritative treatise will continue to serve the intended users for many years.

Chemists (bioorganic, physical, polymer), biochemists, engineers (biomedical, chemical, coatings), biotechnologists, and physicians (research and endocrinologists) will find this book useful, as will graduate students working in diagnostics and biosensors. It will serve as a textbook for schools offering graduate courses in biosensors.

With the help of leading scientists, we are most pleased to bring this authoritative book to the readership.

Wai Tak Law
Naim Akmal
Arthur M. Usmani

Contents

Preface   iii
Contributors   ix

Electrochemical Biosensing Systems

1. Electrochemical Biosensors   1
    Charles A. Wijayawardhana and William R. Heineman

2. Improved-Accuracy Biosensor Strip for Accu-Chek™ Advantage®   29
    David W. Burke and Nigel A. Surridge

3. Redox Monomers and Polymers for Biosensors   63
    Naim Akmal and Arthur M. Usmani

4. Amperometric Microcells for Diagnostic Enzyme Activity
    Measurements   81
    *Robert E. Gyurcsányi, Géza Nagy, Livia Nagy, Alessandra Cristalli,
    Michael R. Neuman, Ernö Lindner, Richard P. Buck, H. Troy Nagle,
    and Stefan Ufer*

5. Flow-Through Immunoassay System for Rapid Clinical
    Diagnostics   93
    *Ihab Abdel-Hamid, Plamen Atanasov, Dmitri Ivnitski,
    and Ebtisam Wilkins*

Optical Biosensing Systems

 6. Optical Sensor Arrays for Medical Diagnostics   121
    Keith J. Albert, Caroline L. Schauer, and David R. Walt

 7. Optochemical Nanosensors for Noninvasive Cellular Analysis   139
    Susan L. R. Barker, Heather A. Clark, and Raoul Kopelman

 8. Ultrasensitive and Specific Optical Biosensors Inspired by Nature   165
    Xuedong Song and Basil I. Swanson

 9. Evanescent-Wave Biosensors   187
    Brent A. Burdick

10. Glow-Discharge-Treated Quartz Crystal Microbalance
    as Immunosensor   203
    Selma Mutlu, M. Hadi Zareie, Erhan Pişkin, and Mehmet Mutlu

11. Diagnostic Polymer Reagents Carrying DNA   215
    *Mizuo Maeda, Takeshi Mori, Daisuke Umeno,
    and Yoshiki Katayama*

12. Electrochemical Gene Sensors   227
    *Toshihiro Ihara, Masamichi Nakayama, Koji Nakano,
    and Mizuo Maeda*

13. Sensing of Second Messengers Using Oligopeptides   243
    *Yoshiki Katayama, Yuya Ohuchi, Mizuo Maeda,
    Hideyoshi Higashi, and Yoshihisa Kudo*

14. Recombinant Photoproteins in the Design of Binding Assays   259
    Jennifer C. Lewis, Agatha J. Feltus, and Sylvia Daunert

Newer Detection Systems

15. Particle Valency Strip Assays   271
    Judith Fitzpatrick, Michael Munzar, and Regina B. Lenda

16. "Smart" Materials for Colorimetric Detection of Pathogenic Agents   291
    Quan Cheng and Raymond C. Stevens

17. Reagentless Diagnostics: Near-IR Raman Spectroscopy   307
    *Irving Itzkan, Tae-Woong Koo, Michael S. Feld,
    Andrew J. Berger, and Gary L. Horowitz*

Diabetes and Cholesterol: Systems and Management

18. Noninstrumented Quantitative Devices Using Detection Film Built
on Woven Fabric 323
Wai Tak Law

19. A Survey of Structural and Nonreactive Components Used in the
Research, Development, and Manufacture of Solid-Phase Medical
Diagnostic Reagents 331
Myron C. Rapkin

20. Current Status and Future Prospects of Dry Chemistries
and Diagnostic Reagents 343
Richard Kordal, Naim Akmal, and Arthur M. Usmani

Polymeric Materials, Immobilization, and Biocompatibility

21. Water-Soluble Phospholipid Polymers as a Novel Synthetic
Blocking Reagent in an Immunoassay System 353
*Shujirou Sakaki, Yasuhiko Iwasaki, Nobuo Nakabayashi,
and Kazuhiko Ishihara*

22. Biocompatible Phospholipid Polymers for Prevention of
Unfavorable Bioreactions on the Surface of Medical Devices 367
*Kazuhiko Ishihara, Yasuhiko Iwasaki, Nobuo Nakabayashi,
Michiharu Sakakida, and Motoaki Shichiri*

23. Site-Directed Immobilization of Proteins on Surfaces:
Genetic Approaches 381
Jianquan Wang, Dibakar Bhattacharyya, and Leonidas G. Bachas

24. Polymeric Microspheres and Related Materials for Medical
Diagnostics 393
*Stanislaw Slomkowski, Beata Miksa, Dorota Kowalczyk,
Teresa Basinska, Mohamed M. Chehimi, and Michel Delamar*

Index 413

Contributors

Ihab Abdel-Hamid, Ph.D.   Senior Research Engineer, MesoSystems Technology, Inc., Albuquerque, New Mexico, U.S.A.

Naim Akmal, Ph.D.   Analytical Specialist, Research and Development, The Dow Chemical Company, South Charleston, West Virginia, U.S.A.

Keith J. Albert, Ph.D.   Research Assistant, Department of Chemistry, Tufts University, Medford, Massachusetts, U.S.A.

Plamen Atanasov, Ph.D.   Assistant Professor, Department of Chemical and Nuclear Engineering, University of New Mexico, Albuquerque, New Mexico, U.S.A.

Leonidas G. Bachas, Ph.D.   Professor, Department of Chemistry, University of Kentucky, Lexington, Kentucky, U.S.A.

Susan L. R. Barker, Ph.D.   Senior Scientist, Systems Division, Veridian, Charlottesville, Virginia, U.S.A.

Teresa Basinka, Ph.D.   Department of Polymer Chemistry, Center of Molecular and Macromolecular Studies, Polish Academy of Sciences, Lodz, Poland

Andrew J. Berger, Ph.D.   Assistant Professor, Institute of Optics, University of Rochester, Rochester, New York, U.S.A.

Dibakar Bhattacharyya, Ph.D.   Professor, Department of Chemical and Materials Engineering, University of Kentucky, Lexington, Kentucky, U.S.A.

Richard P. Buck, Ph.D.*   Professor, Department of Chemistry, University of North Carolina, Chapel Hill, North Carolina, U.S.A.

Brent A. Burdick, Ph.D.   Licensing and Intellectual Property Management, Sandia National Laboratories, Albuquerque, New Mexico, U.S.A.

David W. Burke, B.A.   Principal Scientist, Test Development, Roche Diagnostics Corporation, Indianapolis, Indiana, U.S.A.

Mohamed M. Chehimi, Ph.D.   Research Director, Department of Chemistry, University of Paris, Paris, France

Quan Cheng, Ph.D.   Assistant Professor, Department of Chemistry, University of California, Riverside, Riverside, California, U.S.A.

Heather A. Clark, Ph.D.   Postdoctoral Fellow, Center for Biomedical Imaging Technology, University of Connecticut Health Center, Farmington, Connecticut, U.S.A.

Alessandra Cristalli   Engineer, Novel GmbH, München, Germany

Sylvia Daunert, Ph.D.   Professor, Department of Chemistry, University of Kentucky, Lexington, Kentucky, U.S.A.

Michel Delamar, D.Sc.   Professor, Department of Chemistry, University of Paris, Paris, France

Michael S. Feld, Ph.D.   Director and Professor of Physics, G. H. Harrison Spectroscopy Laboratory, Massachusetts Institute of Technology, Cambridge, Massachusetts, U.S.A.

Agatha J. Feltus, Ph.D.   Department of Chemistry, University of Kentucky, Lexington, Kentucky, U.S.A.

Judith Fitzpatrick   Serex, Inc., Maywood, New Jersey, U.S.A.

Robert E. Gyurcsányi, Ph.D.   Postdoctoral Fellow, Institute of General and Analytical Chemistry, Budapest University of Technology and Economics, Budapest, Hungary

---

*Retired.

William R. Heineman, Ph.D.   Professor, Department of Chemistry, University of Cincinnati, Cincinnati, Ohio, U.S.A.

Hideyoshi Higashi, Ph.D.   Senior Researcher, Mitsubishi Kagaku Institute for Life Sciences, Tokyo, Japan

Gary L. Horowitz, M.D.   Director of Clinical Chemistry, Department of Clinical Pathology, Beth Israel Deaconess Medical Center, Boston, Massachusetts, U.S.A.

Toshihiro Ihara, Ph.D.   Associate Professor, Department of Applied Chemistry and Biochemistry, Faculty of Engineering, Kumamoto University, Kumamoto, Japan

Kazuhiko Ishihara, Ph.D.   Professor, Department of Materials Engineering, The University of Tokyo, Tokyo, Japan

Irving Itzkan, Ph.D.   Senior Scientist, Spectroscopy Laboratory, Massachusetts Institute of Technology, Cambridge, Massachusetts, U.S.A.

Dmitri Ivnitski, Ph.D.   Research Professor, Department of Chemical Engineering, New Mexico Technical University, Socorro, New Mexico, U.S.A.

Yasuhiko Iwasaki, Ph.D.   Associate Professor, Institute of Biomaterials and Bioengineering, Tokyo Medical and Dental University, Tokyo, Japan

Yoshiki Katayama, Ph.D.   Associate Professor, Department of Applied Chemistry, Faculty of Engineering, Kyushu University, Fukuoka, Japan

Tae-Woong Koo, Ph.D.   Research Scientist, Department of Research, Intel Corporation, Santa Clara, California, U.S.A.

Raoul Kopelman, Ph.D.   Professor, Departments of Chemistry, Physics, and Applied Physics, University of Michigan, Ann Arbor, Michigan, U.S.A.

Richard Kordal, Ph.D.   Director, Intellectual Property Office, University of Cincinnati, Cincinnati, Ohio, U.S.A.

Dorota Kowalczyk, Ph.D.   Department of Polymer Chemistry, Center of Molecular and Macromolecular Studies, Polish Academy of Sciences, Lodz, Poland

Yoshihisa Kudo, Ph.D.   Professor, Department of Cellular Neurobiology, School of Life, Tokyo University of Pharmacy and Life Science, Tokyo, Japan

Wai Tak Law, Ph.D.   President, PortaScience, Inc., Moorestown, New Jersey, U.S.A.

Regina B. Lenda   Serex Inc., Maywood, New Jersey, U.S.A.

Jennifer C. Lewis, Ph.D.   Department of Chemistry, University of Kentucky, Lexington, Kentucky, U.S.A.

Ernö Lindner, Ph.D.   Associate Professor, Department of Biomedical Engineering, The University of Memphis, Memphis, Tennessee, U.S.A.

Mizuo Maeda, Ph.D.   Professor, Department of Applied Chemistry, Faculty of Engineering, Kyushu University, Fukuoka, Japan

Beata Miksa, MSc   Engineer, Department of Polymer Chemistry, Center for Molecular and Macromolecular Studies, Polish Academy of Sciences, Lodz, Poland

Takeshi Mori, Ph.D.   Department of Applied Chemistry, Kyushu University, Fukuoka, Japan

Mehmet Mutlu, Ph.D.   Professor, Department of Food Engineering, Hacettepe University, Ankara, Turkey

Selma Mutlu, Ph.D.   Associate Professor, Department of Chemical Engineering, Hacettepe University, Ankara, Turkey

Michael Munzar, M.D.   Medical Director, Nymox Corporation, Maywood, New Jersey, U.S.A.

H. Troy Nagle, Ph.D., M.D.   Professor, Department of Electrical and Computer Engineering, North Carolina State University, Raleigh, North Carolina, U.S.A.

Géza Nagy, Ph.D.   Professor, Department of General and Physical Chemistry, University of Pécs, Pécs, Hungary

Livia Nagy, Ph.D.   Senior Scientist, Department of General and Physical Chemistry, University of Pécs, Pécs, Hungary

Nobuo Nakabayashi, Ph.D.   Professor Emeritus, Tokyo Medical and Dental University, Tokyo, Japan

Koji Nakano, Ph.D. Associate Professor, Department of Applied Chemistry, Faculty of Engineering, Kyushu University, Fukuoka, Japan

Masamichi Nakayama, Ph.D. Department of Materials and Physics, Faculty of Engineering, Kyushu University, Fukuoka, Japan

Michael R. Neuman, Ph.D., M.D. Professor and Chair, Department of Biomedical Engineering, The University of Memphis, Memphis, Tennessee, U.S.A.

Yuya Ohuchi, Ph.D. Department of Applied Chemistry, Faculty of Engineering, Kyushu University, Fukuoka, Japan

Erhan Pişkin, Ph.D. Professor, Department of Chemical Engineering, Hacettepe University, Ankara, Turkey

Myron C. Rapkin, M.S. UriDynamics, Inc., Indianapolis, Indiana, U.S.A.

Shujiro Sakaki Institute of Biomaterials and Bioengineering, Tokyo Medical and Dental University, Tokyo, Japan

Michiharu Sakakida, M.D., Ph.D. Assistant Professor, Department of Metabolic Medicine, Kumamoto University School of Medicine, Kumamoto, Japan

Caroline L. Schauer, Ph.D. Research Scientist, Department of Chemistry, Tufts University, Medford, Massachusetts, U.S.A.

Motoaki Shichiri, M.D., Ph.D. Medical Adviser, Kikuchi Medical Doctor's Association Hospital, Kumamoto, Japan

Stanislaw Slomkowski, Ph.D., D.Sc. Professor, Department of Polymer Chemistry, Center of Molecular and Macromolecular Studies, Polish Academy of Sciences, Lodz, Poland

Xuedong Song, Ph.D. Senior Research Scientist, Department of Corporate Emerging Technologies, Kimberly-Clark Corporation, Roswell, Georgia, U.S.A.

Raymond C. Stevens, Ph.D. Professor, Departments of Molecular Biology and Chemistry, The Scripps Research Institute, La Jolla, California, U.S.A.

Nigel A. Surridge, Ph.D. Director of Research and Development, Roche Diagnostics Corporation, Indianapolis, Indiana, U.S.A.

Basil I. Swanson, Ph.D. Laboratory Fellow, Bioscience Division, Los Alamos National Laboratory, Los Alamos, New Mexico, U.S.A.

Stefan Ufer, M.Sc. Research Associate, Department of Electrical and Computer Engineering, North Carolina State University, Raleigh, North Carolina, U.S.A.

Daisuke Umeno, Ph.D. Department of Applied Chemistry, Kyushu University, Fukuoka, Japan

Arthur M. Usmani, Ph.D. Chief Scientific Officer, Research and Development, Altec USA, Indianapolis, Indiana, U.S.A.

David R. Walt, Ph.D. Professor, Department of Chemistry, Tufts University, Medford, Massachusetts, U.S.A.

Jianquan Wang, Ph.D. Senior Research Associate, Department of Chemistry, University of Kentucky, Lexington, Kentucky, U.S.A.

Charles A. Wijayawardhana, Ph.D. Scientific Assistant – C1, Department of Chemistry, University of Oldenburg, Oldenburg, Germany

Ebtisam Wilkins Department of Chemical and Nuclear Engineering, University of New Mexico, Albuquerque, New Mexico, U.S.A.

M. Hadi Zareie, Ph.D. Research Assistant, Department of Chemical Engineering, Hacettepe University, Ankara, Turkey

Biomedical
Diagnostic
Science
and
Technology

1
Electrochemical Biosensors

Charles A. Wijayawardhana
University of Oldenburg, Oldenburg, Germany

William R. Heineman
University of Cincinnati, Cincinnati, Ohio, U.S.A.

I. INTRODUCTION

Since the development of the first electrochemical biosensor, the glucose electrode, in 1962, electrochemical biosensors have represented a thriving area of research in both academia and industry. It is fueled by an ever-growing need in biomedical, industrial, and environmental testing for improved sensors that allow early detection for taking timely remedial steps. The success in biosensors is owed as much to the fundamental research in finding novel biorecognition mechanisms as to a number of rapidly evolving technologies, such as the microfabrication of sensors and the production and immobilization of enhanced biorecognition elements. The area of electrochemical biosensors has also greatly benefited from the remarkable advances made in microelectronics over the last two decades to give powerful and reliable instrumentation. The articles that follow in the first section of the book represent some of the exciting new developments in electrochemical biosensors. The purpose of this introductory chapter is to present the fundamentals of electrochemical biosensors so that the reader can better appreciate these articles. In keeping with the theme of the book, emphasis is given to biomedical applications of electrochemical biosensors. The reader is also referred to the biannual review of chemical and biosensors in the journal *Analytical Chemistry* [1] and several books that deal with biosensors in general but that also have a significant part dedicated to electrochemical biosensors [2–7].

What is an electrochemical biosensor? An electrochemical biosensor is commonly defined as a sensor consisting of a biological sensing element immobilized onto an electrode (transducer) wired to a signal processor that gives a visually observable or recordable response to a biorecognition event or events. The basic layout of an electrochemical biosensor thus defined is illustrated in Figure 1. In going from the sensor–sample interface, the components are first the layer of the pertinent biological sensing element, second the electrode, and third the signal processor that gives the output signal. Though this definition is generally well accepted, it could also be the source of considerable confusion. According to this definition, an electrochemical biosensor does not necessarily have to be a sensor for detecting an analyte of biological origin, though it often is. Nor does detection of a biological analyte or an analyte in a biological matrix alone make a sensor an electrochemical biosensor. For example, some of the electrodes used in blood analysis, including oxygen- and ion-selective electrodes, are not true biosensors, in that they lack a biological sensing element.

As with any kind of sensor, the quality of an electrochemical sensor is determined by several factors, including (1) selectivity, (2) signal-to-noise (S/N) ratio and detection limit, (3) sensitivity, (4) response time, (5) concentration range of linear response, and (6) ability to monitor dynamic fluctuations in real time. The selectivity of a biosensor is achieved primarily at the sensor–sample

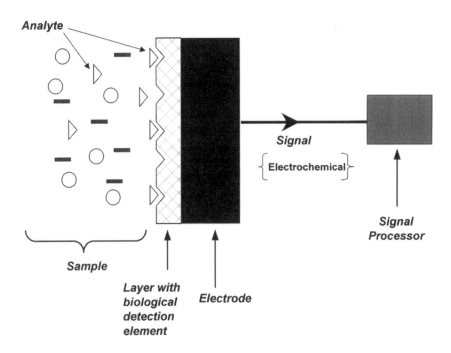

Figure 1 Schematic representation of an electrochemical biosensor.

interface by the natural specificity of the biological sensing element. Another level of selectivity is also available to most electrochemical biosensors by virtue of being able to select the electrode potential so that as few interferents are co-oxidized or reduced as possible. This second level of selectivity alone, however, is usually inadequate for most biosensor applications. The response time of a biosensor, is largely determined at the sensor–sample interface, depending on how efficiently the analyte is transported to the sensor surface and, once captured there, on how fast the electroactive product signaling analyte binding is brought to a detectable level. This last parameter can be very important where the electroactive product is produced enzymatically, as indeed it is for a majority of biosensors, because fairly long substrate incubations may be necessary to get a detectable concentration of product when dealing with a small concentration of analyte. A common practice to speed up the response time is to force hydrodynamic conditions on the sample that generally enhance the analyte capture efficiency as well as the detection sensitivity.

The ultimate success of any biosensor depends on its marketability, and this calls for many practical considerations, such as production cost, user-friendliness, ruggedness, and minimization of additional reagents. With regard to ruggedness, it is important that the proteins in the biomembrane not denature during storage or use. For example, most enzymes and antibodies tend to lose their activity when exposed to high or fluctuating temperatures. Also, a successful biosensor should be easily reusable, unless it is sufficiently cheap to be disposable. Renewing a biosensor might involve lengthy procedures that limit its utility even when the response time for a single analysis may be fast.

In the following sections we first discuss the commonly used biosensing elements and then describe the three general categories of electrochemical biosensors (potentiometric, amperometric, and conductimetric). We conclude by noting some current and possible future trends in the area.

II. BIOLOGICAL SENSING ELEMENTS (BIOELEMENTS)

Five different classes of bioelements have received considerable attention for use in electrochemical biosensors. They are enzymes, cells, tissues, antibodies, receptors and nucleic acid ligands. In this section we present only the basic properties of these bioelements, leaving examples of their applications to other sections.

A. Enzymes

Enzymes are by far the most widely used bioelement in electrochemical biosensors. This is due to the excellent catalytic properties and the high selectivity for a specific substrate or a class of substrates associated with enzymes. In enzyme-based biosensors, the substrate or a cofactor involved in the enzymatic reaction represents the analyte, and detection is done in one of three ways. In the simplest scheme, one of the reactants or products directly involved in the enzymatic reaction is measured to obtain the rate of reaction. As long as this is done below substrate saturation conditions, the rate of reaction is directly proportional to the concentration of analyte, and the analyte can be quantified from a previously established calibration curve. Many electrochemical biosensors work on this principle, as discussed in Secs. III.A.2 and III.B.1.a. In the second scheme, the turnover rate of a mediator or a cofactor involved in an enzymatic reaction is detected to give an indirect measure of the amount of the analyte. Biosensors based on this detection scheme, also often referred to as second-generation biosensors, are discussed in Sec. III.B.1.b. The third detection scheme is based on the direct oxidation or reduction of enzyme at the electrode, as discussed in Sec. III.B.1.c.

B. Cells and Tissues

Cells and tissues can be convenient and cost-effective sources of enzyme. Being in their natural surroundings, where all the enzymatic pathways and cofactors are present, the enzymes are in stable and optimal activity. For biosensor applications, cells and tissues are usually entrapped over the electrode with a semipermeable membrane. The main limiting factor of cell- and tissue-based sensors is the high resistance to diffusion within cell walls, which can delay the sensor response time considerably. Also, the various constituents present in cells make these biosensors generally less selective than those that use purified enzymes. Although long recovery times (3–4 hr) can also be a problem, these sensors can be cheap enough to be disposable. Various biosensors based on microorganisms (i.e., bacteria), mammalian systems, and plant-tissue matter have been developed. A good example is the "banana electrode" for detecting dopamine, made by applying a banana slice on an oxygen electrode [8]. Certain enzymes in the banana paste catalyze the oxidation of dopamine, and the "banana electrode" can detect dopamine by measuring the loss of O_2 during enzyme catalysis. Other examples of cell- and tissue-based biosensors are given in Table 1, in Sec. III.A.

C. Antibodies

Antibodies, one of nature's most selective and versatile reagents, provide the basis for the highly successful bioanalytical method *immunoassay* [9]. Antibodies bind to their target antigen (analyte) with high selectivity, and the associated binding (affinity) constants can be as high as 10^6–10^{12}. Antibodies are readily available for many compounds of biomedical and environmental importance, such as drugs, toxins, metabolites, and pesticides. Antibodies have traditionally been obtained as polyclonal antibodies in the antisera of animals immunized with the analyte (antigen) of interest. The polyclonal antibodies target different sites or epitopes of the analyte. Monoclonal antibodies have been developed to avoid the inconsistency in the antisera between batches from different animals or even the same animal [10]. Monoclonal antibodies are harvested from cell cultures grown from antibodies retrieved from an immunized animal and selected for producing the desired antibody. In the future, recombinant antibodies produced with molecular engineering methods are also likely to be widely used in biosensors, because they can be produced inexpensively and tailored for improved or novel specificities [11]. Because antibodies and antigens lack catalytic properties, they are often labeled for biosensor applications.

D.   Receptors

Receptors are proteins found at the surface of cell membranes, whose main function is to transmit signals across the lipid bilayers surrounding cells. In the body, receptors react to the binding of certain ligands by triggering various physiological responses, such as hormone regulation and neural transmission. Unlike antibodies, a receptor binds to several structurally similar ligands, and although the number of ligands (analytes) that can be detected by receptors is limited, they represent an important group of analytes. Receptors have excellent affinities for steroids, neurotransmitters, protein hormones, and a number of metabolites and drugs. For biosensor applications, receptors can be used either in their intact form as found in membranes or in isolated form. Incorporating receptors into a sensor without losing their special properties, however, has proven to be very difficult.

E.   Nucleic Acid Ligands

The high specificity involved in the interchain base pairing of DNA and RNA is the basis for a relatively new and exciting group of biosensors called *nucleic acid probes* [12,13]. These biosensors hold great promise for early detection of genetic defects that can cause disease or even death. In developing electrochemical DNA probes, a strand complementary to the base sequence of the analyte is synthesized and immobilized on the electrode. DNA strands are very robust and, because of their amenability to covalent attachments, can be easily coupled to surfaces. Also, DNA probes can be regenerated for multiple assays by changing the ionic strength of the buffer to denature and detach the bound protein.

III.   ELECTROCHEMICAL TRANSDUCTION METHODS

The transducers in electrochemical biosensors fall into one of three types: potentiometric, amperometric, or conductimetric. The first two involve the measurement of reactions at the electrode surface or at a membrane, while the third involves the measurement of changes in conductivity in the bulk medium between two electrodes. We begin each of the three categories with a brief discussion of the underlying principles of electrochemistry. For more information, the reader is referred to two books on fundamentals and applications of electrochemistry [14,15].

A. Potentiometric Sensors

1. Potentiometry

Measurements of the difference in potential between the two electrodes of an electrochemical cell under the condition of zero current are described by the term *potentiometry*. Since no current passes through the cell while the potential is measured, potentiometry is an equilibrium method. Potentiometric techniques are important because they can provide accurate measurements of (1) activities, concentrations, and/or activity coefficients of many solution species and (2) free-energy changes and equilibrium constants of many solution reactions.

Typical apparatus for potentiometry is shown in Figure 2. The potential difference between the two electrodes immersed in solution is usually measured with a pH/mV meter. One electrode, the *indicator electrode*, is chosen so that its half-cell potential responds to the activity of a particular species in solution whose activity or concentration is to be measured. The other electrode is a reference electrode whose half-cell potential is invariant. The most commonly used reference electrodes for potentiometry are the saturated calomel electrode (SCE) and the silver–silver chloride electrode (Ag/AgCl). The potential of the electrochemical cell, E_{cell}, is given by $E_{cell} = E_{ind} - E_{ref} + E_{lj}$ where E_{ind} is the half-cell potential of the indicator electrode, E_{ref} is the half-cell potential of the reference electrode, and E_{lj} is the liquid-junction potential. Liquid-junction potentials develop at the interface between two electrolytes because of the differences in the migration rates of charged species across the interface. In potentiometric cells such as in Figure 2, E_{lj} is typically found at the junction of the solution in the cell with the reference electrode.

The indicator electrode is of paramount importance in analytical potentiometry. This electrode should interact with the species of interest so that E_{ind} reflects the activity of this species in solution and not any other compounds in the sample. The importance of having indicator electrodes that selectively respond to numerous ionic and gaseous species of analytical significance has stimulated the development of many types of indicator electrodes. An electrode that responds to a specific ion in solution is called an ion-selective electrode (ISE); one that responds to a gas is called a gas-sensing electrode. However, a gas-sensing electrode is in essence an adaptation of an ISE, because what is measured is an ionic species in solution involved in an equilibrium reaction with

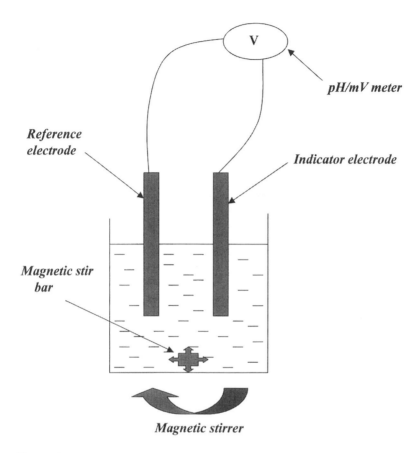

Figure 2 Schematic diagram of apparatus for potentiometry.

the gaseous species as it dissolves in solution. The relationship between E_{ind} and the concentration of the ion X in an ISE is given by the Nernst equation,

$$E_{ind} = k \pm \left(\frac{RT}{zF} \right) \log [X]$$

where k is a constant, R the gas constant, T the temperature, F the Faraday constant, and z the charge on the ion being sensed.

2. Potentiometric Enzyme Biosensors

Potentiometric biosensors, as shown in Figure 3, have an ISE or a gas-sensing electrode in contact with a thin layer of biocatalytic material (enzyme). The

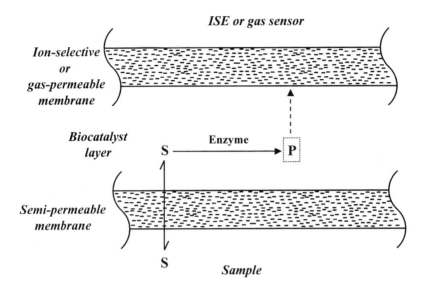

Figure 3 Schematic diagram of a biocatalytic (enzymatic) membrane assembly and the chemical reactions in a potentiometric biosensor.

enzyme converts the substrate (the analyte) into a product that is detectable at the electrode. The biocatalytic layer consists of an immobilized enzyme chosen for its catalytic selectivity toward the analyte. Immobilized bacterial particles, a tissue slice that contains an enzyme, or perhaps several enzymes that catalyze a sequence of reactions leading to a detectable product can also be used.

The first type of potentiometric biocatalytical membrane electrode was based on the immobilization of an enzyme on the surface of an ISE. A classic example is the first potentiometric biosensor, the urea biosensor developed by Guilbault and Montalvo in 1969 [16]. In their work, the enzyme urease in a polyacrylamide gel was immobilized at the end of a glass ISE for NH_4^+. Urease catalyzes the hydrolysis of urea to NH_4^+ and CO_3^{2-}. When the biosensor is immersed in a solution containing urea, urea diffuses into the enzyme layer and the enzymatic product NH_4^+ is detected at the ISE. The concentration of NH_4^+ detected is proportional to the concentration of urea in the sample.

Intact bacterial particles and thin slices of tissue can also be applied to ISE electrodes in making potentiometric biosensors. The advantages of using cells and tissues as biosensor elements have already been discussed. One cited advantage was the presence of various enzymatic pathways and cofactors. An early yet good example of this is a biosensor for detecting nitrilotriacetric acid (NTA), which consisted of an NH_3-sensitive electrode coated with *Pseudomonas* bacterial cells [17]. The detection of NTA, as shown in the following scheme, depended on the presence of several components in the bacterial cells.

$$NTA + NADH + O_2 \xrightarrow[\text{monooxygenase}]{\text{NTA}} (\alpha - \text{hydroxyl NTA})$$
$$+ \text{iminodiacetate}$$
$$+ \text{glyoxylate}$$

$$\text{iminodiacetate} \longrightarrow \text{glycine} + \text{glyoxylate}$$

$$\text{glycine} \xrightarrow[\text{decarboxylase}]{\text{glycine}} \text{serine} + O_2$$

$$\text{serine} \longrightarrow \text{hydroxy pyruvate} + NH_3$$

Potentiometric biosensors based on numerous enzymes have been reported, some of which are listed in Table 1.

3.   Enzyme Field-Effect Transistors (ENFETs)

Miniaturized biosensors, as discussed in more detail later, are fast becoming an important area of biosensor research and development because of a host of advantages they hold over large, conventional biosensors. With regard to potentiometric biosensors, field-effect transistors (FETs) have received considerable attention for miniaturized biosensors. A schematic of an enzyme-based FET (ENFET), the most common adaptation of FETs in biosensor application, is shown in Figure 4. The enzyme layer is attached to the top of the sensor and exposed to solution. Below the enzyme layer are a Si_3N_4 layer and a SiO_2 insulator followed by a p-Si semiconductor. Incorporated at the top corners of the p-Si semiconductor are two n-Si semiconductors called the *source* and the *drain*. The drain is kept at a constant positive potential from the base of the p-Si and the source. This causes a reverse bias at the p-Si–drain interface. However, if there is an increasing positive charge in the enzyme layer due to the formation of positively charged species, it attracts electrons to the top end of the p-Si semiconductor, resulting in a conduction band for electrons to move from the source to the drain. The function of the variable potential is to cancel this effect by applying a positive potential to the base of the p-Si that opposes the movement of electrons to the top of p-Si. Thus the potential needed to maintain null-current conditions, as measured relative to the reference electrode, becomes an indirect measure of the potential increase in the enzyme layer: the more positively charged product formed in the layer, the greater the potential needed to maintain the null-current condition. As with the potentiometric enzyme biosensors, the ability to measure potential changes in the enzyme layer is the basis for using ENFETs as electrochemical biosensors.

Table 1   Representative Biocatalyst Membrane Electrodes

Biocatalyst category	Substrate	Biocatalyst	Detected substance
Enzyme	Urea	Urease	NH_4^+, NH_3, CO_2, or H^+
	Glucose	Glucose oxidase and peroxidase	I^-
		Glucose oxidase	H^+
		Glucose oxidase	F^-
	Amygdalin	β-glucosidase	CN^-
	Pencillin	Pencillinase	H^+
	L-Phenylalanine	L-Amino acid oxidase	I^- or NH_4^+
		Horseradish peroxidase	I^-
		Phenylalanine ammonia lyase	NH_3
		Phenylalanine decarboxylase	CO_2
	Uric acid	Uricase	CO_2
	Acetylcholine	Acetylcholinesterase	H^+
	D-Gluconate	Gluconate kinase and 6-phospho-D-gluconate dehydrogenase	CO_2
	Acetaldehyde	Aldehyde dehydrogenase	H^+
	Oxalate	Oxalate decarboxylase	CO_2
	Flavin adenine dinucleotide	Alkaline phosphatase and adenosine deaminase	NH_3
	Methotrexate	Dihydrofolate reductase and 6-phophogluconic dehydrogenase	CO_2
	Aspartane	L-Aspartase	NH_3
	Creatinine	Creatinase	NH_3
	Salicylate	Salicylate hydroxylase	CO_2
Bacterial particle	L-Arginine	*Streptococcus faecium*	NH_3
	L-Aspartate	*Bacterium cadaveris*	NH_3
	L-Glutamine	*Sarcina flava*	NH_3
	NAD+	*Escherichia coli/NADase*	NH_3
	Nitrilotriacetate acid	*Pseudomonas* sp.	NH_3
	L-Tyrosine	*Aeromonas phenologenes*	NH_3
	L-Histodine	*Pseudomonas* sp.	NH_3
	L-Serine	*Clostridium acidiurici*	NH_3
	Nitrate	*Azotobacter vinelandii*	NH_3
	Uric acid	*Pichia membranaefaciens*	CO_2
	L-Glutamic acid	*Escherichia coli*	CO_2
	Pyruvate	*Streptococcus faecium*	CO_2
	L-Cysteine	*Proteus morganii*	H_2S
	Sugars	Bacteria from human dental plaque	H^+

(*continued*)

Table 1 Continued

Biocatalyst category	Substrate	Biocatalyst	Detected substance
Tissue	Glucosamine	Porcine kidney tissue	NH_3
	Adenosine	Mouse small intestine mucosal cells	NH_3
	Adenosine 5'-monophosphate	Rabbit muscle	NH_3
	L-Glutamate	Yellow squash	CO_2
	Glutamine	Porcine kidney cortex	NH_3
	Guanine	Rabbit liver	NH_3

Source: Adapted from Ref. 17A.

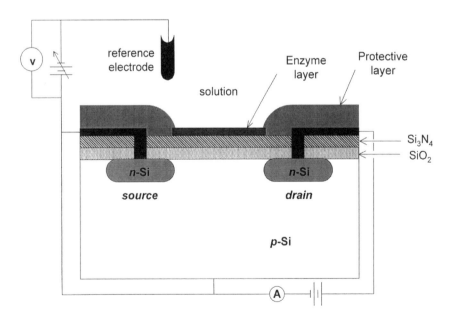

Figure 4 Schematic representation of an enzyme field-effect transistor (ENFET).

In spite of their attractive feature of a simple detection scheme in a miniaturized test platform, the use of FETs in biosensors has been hampered by their sensitivity to pH changes as well as the nonspecific binding of substances [18]. These problems would have to be solved before FETs can be widely used for biosensor applications.

B. Voltammetric (Amperometric) Biosensors

1. Voltammetry

Voltammetry is the measurement of the current–potential (I–E) relationship in an electrochemical cell. A variety of voltammetric techniques, in which a potential is applied to an electrochemical cell and the resulting current is measured, have been developed. Since the potential applied to the electrochemical cell can force the oxidation or reduction of species at the electrode surface, voltammetry is an active technique. Potentiometric techniques, on the other hand, are passive techniques, since they simply respond to the activity of an analyte in solution without measurably disturbing it.

The basic concept of applying a potential E to an electrochemical cell and measuring the current resulting from electrolysis can be implemented in numerous ways depending on the experimental conditions. Some of these are:

1. The solution may be moving or stationary with respect to the electrode.
2. The waveform of the applied potential (i.e., how the applied potential varies with time) may be varied.
3. The timing sequence of the current-measurement process with respect to the waveform of the excitation signal may be varied.
4. Numerous electrode and cell geometries, which affect the current response, can be used.

All of these factors can dramatically influence the shape of the current–time response. Consequently, numerous voltammetric techniques in which the specific parameters of the measurement differ have been developed, both theoretically and experimentally. Although the output signals and the practical applications of these techniques are quite varied, they all share the common basis of applying E and measuring I or a parameter derived from I, such as charge Q. Out of the many different voltammetric techniques available, amperometry is by far the most widely used in electrochemical biosensors.

In amperometry, the electrode is held at a constant potential to detect the pertinent electroactive species by oxidation or reduction. Amperometry, when applied to a convective solution, is often called *hydrodynamic chronoamperometry* to distinguish it from amperometry in stationary solution, but we do not make this distinction here. The optimum potential for detection in amperometry is chosen after obtaining the current response of the analyte as a function of electrode potential. The typical current response for an analyte has three distinctive regions of behavior, as shown in Figure 5 for an electrode in stirred solution: (1) a region where the analyte is electroinactive and the current is negligible; (2) a region of rising current defined by the Nernst equation; and (3) a current plateau independent of the potential and limited by the rate of mass transport of analyte. The detection potential is best kept in the third region, where changes in the electrode potential have a negligible affect on the current measurement. This plateau current is given by the equation $I = nFADC^o/d$, where I is the diffusion-controlled current, n the number of electrons involved in the reaction, F the Faradaic constant, A the electrode surface area, D the diffusion coefficient, C^o the bulk analyte concentration, and d the thickness of the diffusion layer. According to this equation, the current I is linearly proportional to C^o; this relationship established in a previous calibration curve can be used to quantify the analyte. It should be noted, however, that D and d depend on the viscosity and the efficiency of stirring, respectively, and these variables should be maintained constant to make meaningful current-to-analyte-concentration relationships. In general, it is desirable to have a high degree of forced convection in the solution to facilitate mass transport of analyte to the sensor and also decrease d for enhanced sensi-

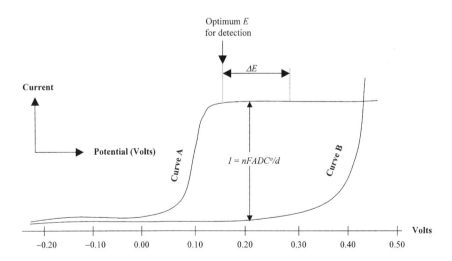

Figure 5 Hypothetical hydrodynamic (stirred solution) voltammogram for an analyte (Curve A) and an interferent (Curve B). The plateau current is given by $I = nFADC^o/d$ (see Sec. III.B.1 for more details).

tivity. Another critical factor in amperometry is minimizing the deleterious effects on the detection limit arising from background noise and the interference from extraneous electroactive species in sample. Both effects increase with increasing magnitude of electrode potential. As shown in Figure 5, the plateau current region may extend over a large potential range, but in the presence of an electroactive interferent, the potential window for detection ΔE may be reduced significantly. The choice of electrode potential alone, however, often cannot remove the effects of interferents, and, as discussed shortly, physical barriers such as membranes are often necessary to keep out interferents.

2.   Amperometric Enzyme Electrodes

Amperometric biosensors have been the most successful of all biosensors. It is beyond the scope of this chapter to discuss in great detail all the various amperometric biosensors and their applications. Hence we shall limit our focus primarily to the class of amperometric biosensors that has been by far the most important, glucose biosensors.

   Glucose Electrode.   The detection of blood glucose has been at the forefront of electrochemical biosensor research ever since the development in 1962 of the first electrochemical biosensor by Leland Clark, the glucose electrode. Although there have been many different glucose sensors since, the glucose sensor based on the original design and marketed by Yellow Springs Instruments continues to be widely used and often serves as the benchmark glucose sensor. The basic design of this glucose biosensor is illustrated in Figure 6. As shown, glucose oxidase (GO), which serves as the enzyme, is applied as a thin layer and held between two membranes. When the electrode is immersed in sample solution, glucose diffuses through the outer membrane into the enzyme layer, where it is catalytically oxidized. The reaction product H_2O_2 diffuses through the inner membrane to the electrode, where it is detected via the electrode oxidation reaction

$$H_2O_2 + 2OH^- \rightarrow H_2O + O_2 + 2e$$

at +0.7 V versus the Ag/AgCl reference electrode. Since the amount of H_2O_2 generated is proportional to the concentration of glucose in the sample, a calibration plot can be constructed by measuring the limiting anodic current for oxidation of H_2O_2 as a function of glucose concentration in standard solutions. Alternately, the concentration of glucose can be measured by monitoring the depletion of O_2 via the electrode reduction reaction

$$O_2 + 2e^- + 2H^+ \rightarrow H_2O_2$$

at −0.7 V versus Ag/AgCl.

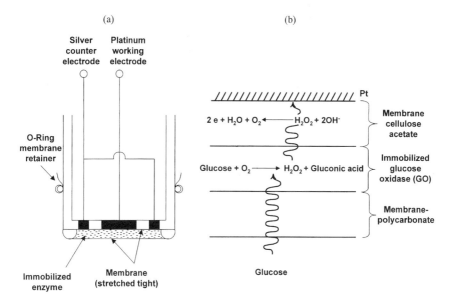

Figure 6 Amperometric glucose sensor. (a) Cross section of electrode; (b) membrane assembly and chemical reactions.

    The selectivity of the glucose electrode is determined by the specificity of the enzyme for glucose and the permeability of the membranes to species that would interfere. The outer membrane (polycarbonate) traps the thin layer of glucose oxidase and serves as a barrier to large molecules, such as proteins. The inner membrane (cellulose acetate) is permeable only to very small molecules, such as H_2O_2. It keeps both GO and electroactive components in the sample, such as uric acid, ascorbic acid, and acetaminophen from the electrode surface.

    One of the drawbacks of a glucose sensor, as in Figure 6, is its susceptibility to signal fluctuations from changes in the ambient partial pressure of oxygen (pO_2). Also, at high glucose concentrations, oxygen can kinetically limit the reaction rate, leading to nonlinearity of signal. These variables can be removed by prediluting the sample to ensure that there is adequate O_2, as indeed is done in the Yellow Springs blood glucose sensors. But there has been much interest in developing glucose sensors that are insensitive to O_2, require no sample dilution, and can be applied directly on the sample. There is also the impetus to avoid membranes, which are cumbersome to work with and are generally not completely leach-proof. These goals are at the heart of the so-called second- and third-generation biosensors.

Mediators (Second-Generation Biosensors).   Mediators were developed primarily for use as oxygen substitutes in biosensors that would otherwise depend on ambient O_2 for one or more of its enzymatic reactions. Much of the work in the area has focused on mediators for GO in the detection of glucose. The general mediator-based glucose detection scheme is illustrated in Figure 7a. As shown,

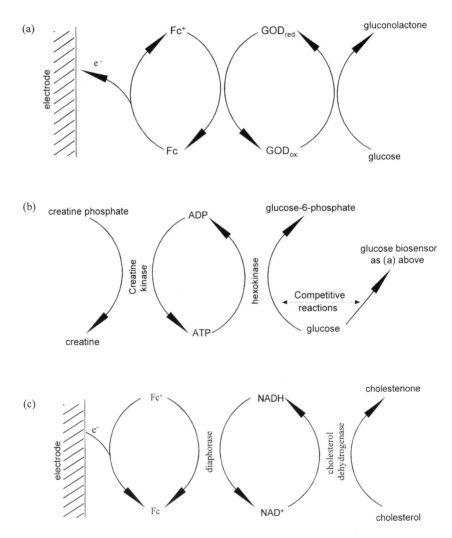

Figure 7   Mediator-based amperometric biosensors for (a) glucose, (b) creatine kinase based on glucose detection, and (c) cholesterol.

the mediator is first in its oxidized form, M_{ox}; following the reaction with the reduced form of the enzyme (GO_{red}), it is reconverted to M_{ox} at the electrode and the catalytic cycle is repeated. The amperometric current is directly proportional to the concentration of glucose because of a concurrent increase in the number of catalytic cycles that causes an increased flux of M_{red} to the electrode. But for the mediator to work effectively, it should have the following properties: (1) exhibit reversible electron transfer kinetics, (2) react rapidly with the enzyme, (3) have a low redox potential, (4) be unreactive toward O_2 or any species other than the enzyme, (5) be stable at all possible pH's, and (6) be nontoxic. For GO, ferrocene and a number of its derivatives have proven to be excellent mediators (see Figure 7a). The redox potential of ferrocene/ferrocenium ion is 220 mV versus Ag/AgCl, a 400-mV improvement over the oxidation potential of H_2O_2 without compromising the rate of electron transfer reactions. Furthermore, ferrocene can be immobilized on the electrode along with the enzyme and, because of its low solubility, remain largely confined to the electrode, thus making it unnecessary to add ferrocene to solution or to entrap it over the electrode. These properties have indeed been successfully exploited in several commercial glucose sensors [4]. These sensors, made by coimmobilizing glucose oxidase with ferrocene on screen-printed electrodes, are used conveniently in home-based glucose detection by applying a microdrop of blood obtained by "fingersticking." The competition of ambient O_2 in oxidizing GO does not pose a serious interference to the detection scheme. In addition to ferrocene, benzoquinone, ferricyanides, N-methylphenazinium (NMP^+), and 2,6-dichlorophenolindophenol can be used as mediators for GO.

Being the most advanced of biosensors, glucose sensors are also a good choice for adapting to other biosensor applications. A good example of this is a biosensor developed for creatine kinase, a major component of soluble proteins in muscles whose presence in blood is a marker of several forms of muscle damage, including myocardial infarction [19]. As shown in Figure 7b, creatine kinase can be detected by incorporating it into an enzymatic reaction that competes with GO for the substrate glucose. When the other reagents are kept at a known optimized concentration, a high concentration of creatine kinase relates to a decreased signal from the glucose, because less glucose enters the GO enzymatic pathway. The practical value of this type of biosensor, however, can be limited by the complexity of having to use more reagents than would be required in a direct sensor.

Another very useful mediator in biosensors is nicotinamide adenine dinucleotide (NAD^+), a cofactor found in over 250 reactions involving dehydrogenases (DH). The basic detection scheme can be represented as follows:

Enzyme reaction:

$$SH_2 + NAD^+ \xrightarrow{\text{DH}} S + NADH + H^+$$

Detection scheme1:

$$\text{NADH} \xrightarrow{\text{electrode}} \text{NAD}^+ + \text{H}^+ + 2e$$

Detection scheme2:

$$\text{NADH} + \text{X} \xrightarrow{\text{2nd enzyme}} \text{NAD}^+ + \text{XH}$$

$$\text{XH} \xrightarrow{\text{electrode}} \text{X} + \text{H}^+ + e$$

Because of the high oxidation potential of the enzymatic product NADH, it is common to couple it to a another mediator X to give XH that can be detected at a lower potential, as just illustrated in detection scheme 2. The specific case for cholesterol detection is shown in Figure 7c, where a three-cycle relay involving the second enzyme, diaphorase, and the mediator ferrocene convert cholesterol to cholestenone. Methyl viologen is another common mediator for diaphorase. Although such a detection scheme can in principle be used to detect any one of the numerous dehydrogenases or their substrates, the high cost of NAD^+ limits its use. Furthermore, unlike ferrocene, NAD^+ is highly soluble and thus not as easily immobilized for making solid-state sensors.

Nondiffusing Mediators (Third-Generation Biosensors). The development of reagentless biosensors has long been pursued because of their ease of use and, more importantly, the promise of use as implantable sensors in humans. In making implantable sensors, it is critical to ensure that the components of the sensor do not leach out in any way. Leaching would cause degradation of the sensor and, moreover, release potentially toxic substances into the body. The ideal situation of perfectly immobilized enzymes with direct electrical contact between the redox centers of the enzyme and the electrode has unfortunately been difficult to achieve. Enzymes generally tend to denature at surfaces of electrodes, and even when successfully immobilized, the protein shell around the redox centers of the enzyme keeps the redox centers too far from the electrode to allow facile transfer of electrons. The approach taken in overcoming this limitation therefore has been to introduce a nonleachable and nondiffusing mediator that could act as a conduction path between the redox centers and the electrode. The search for such a mediator has indeed become an important and active area of research over the past decade, and a few key accomplishments can be identified.

One successful approach for third generation biosensors has been to use electrodes with built-in conducting organic salts that act as charge-transfer complexes to make an electrical bridge [20,21]. For flavo-enzymes, which include GO, the tetracyanoquinodimethane$^-$—tetrathiafulvalene$^+$ (TCNQ^-—TTF^+) complex has been particularly effective in making this electrical bridge. For dehydrogenases involving the natural cofactor NAD^+, the $TNCQ^-$—NMP^+ complex has been successful.

More recently, Heller and coworkers pioneered the use of enzyme-tethered redox active functional groups such as ferrocenium to act as electron relays between the electrode and the redox centers of the enzyme [22]. However, an enzyme like GO can accommodate only about 12 relays, and unless the modified enzyme molecules are held within a membrane that allows their free tumbling, not even all of these relays are effective. A more successful approach has been to use an electrode-bound redox polymer first to electrostatically bind the enzyme and then to penetrate the crevices of the enzyme. In this way, parts of the redox polymer get close enough to the enzyme redox centers to allow electron transfer via electron tunneling [23]. Enzyme-modified electrodes of this type are often referred to as "wired enzyme" electrodes. The rate of electron transfer to the natural electron acceptor oxygen in these biosensors was shown to be slow enough not to pose a serious competition for electron transfer across the "wire." For GO, polymers substituted with osmium-polypyridine and ferrocene have been particularly effective. Although these biosensors are characterized by an electron "diffusion coefficient" that is two orders of magnitude lower than for second-generation biosensors, the gain of a completely reagentless, nonleaching system is a considerable advantage for novel biosensor applications. Furthermore, it is likely that the electron diffusion coefficient in the polymer can be improved by at least one order of magnitude by changing polymer properties, such as flexibility and hydrophilicity [24]. Examples of wired enzymes in immunosensors and subcutaneous glucose sensors are given later.

Yet another way to wire enzymes was proposed recently where the redox centers were first extracted from the enzyme via suitable protein unfolding protocols, then tethered to an electron relay already bound to an electrode, and finally reconstituted with the apo-enzyme. For example, the redox centers of GO, flavine adenine dinucleotide (FAD), can be tethered in this way to ferrocene and pyrroloquinoline quinone (PQQ) relays [25]. The same approach has been applied to heme-containing enzymes by attaching the excluded electroactive heme groups to self-assembled thiol monolayers on gold electrodes via carbodiimide coupling [26].

3. Implantable Glucose Sensors

Since the introduction of the first commercial glucose sensor by Yellow Springs Instruments in the mid-1970s, several glucose sensors have been introduced to the market, some of which we have already noted. Unlike the Yellow Springs sensors, which are dedicated to use in clinics and hospitals, the new sensors are sold to diabetics for home-based monitoring of blood glucose levels. Although they are easily applied with painless "fingersticking" to draw small amounts of blood for analysis, testing must be done frequently; even then, it is impossible to know fluctuations in glucose levels between tests. A more ambitious idea in detecting blood glucose has been to use implantable sensors for continuous monitoring. These sensors would be free of uncertainties associated with sensors that make discrete measurements [27,28]. Furthermore, an alarm attached to the sensor could be used to warn of hyperglycemic (too much glucose) or hypoglycemic (too little) conditions.

Two approaches have been taken to develop implantable biosensors: one, to use sensors fully implanted in the body, and the other, to use needlelike sensors applied through the skin (percutaneous). For success in either case, a number of challenges have to be overcome, and because they are meant for use in humans, the sensors must necessarily be judged with extreme scrutiny. It is critical to ensure that the sensor materials do not in any way leach into the body. Thus the second-generation type of biosensors is not easily adaptable for implantable sensors. Another problem is that the immune system seeing the sensor as "nonself" could respond by forming a capsule around it, causing a partial or complete barrier to the transport of glucose to the sensor. With needle-like sensors, the risk of infection could mitigate the practical conveniences of self-application, an often-cited advantage over fully implantable sensors, which have to be placed and removed surgically.

As daunting as the foregoing challenges might appear, there have recently been some very promising results with implantable sensors in both test animals and human volunteers that suggest the routine use of implantable sensors in humans may indeed become a reality. With regard to percutaneous sensors, this success is best exemplified in the glucose sensors developed independently first by Wilson [30] and later by Heller [31,32]. Both types share a similar design in that a wire-type electrode of approximately 300-μm diameter shielded along its length with a polymeric material for insulation and biocompatibility serves as the transducer. The main difference is in how the enzyme is applied. In the sensors developed by Wilson's group, GO is used for the enzyme and is applied as a thin layer inside a small cavity formed by extending the polymeric shield slightly beyond the edge of the electrode. A composite membrane of Nafion and cellulose acetate is used to both contain the enzyme and keep out possible interferents. Detection is based on measuring the H_2O_2 produced in the enzymatic reaction in much the same way as in the first glucose sensor. Blood glucose levels of 5–15 mM have been detected this way, and even though the response time lagged by 10–15 minutes when the glucose level was increasing, detection was virtually instantaneous when decreasing. In the sensors developed by Heller, GO was "wired" to the electrode for glucose sensing as described earlier.

Fully implantable glucose sensors too have come a long way, and sensors tested subcutaneously and in blood vessels have retained activity for over 100 days [33]. Unlike in percutaneous sensors, a power source, control electronics, and a signal transmitter have to be incorporated into a fully implantable biosensor. In this regard, the rapidly growing area of micro-total analysis systems (μTAS) [34], where the goal is chemical analysis in a "lab-on-a-chip" platform, holds much promise. Progress in microfabrication methods continues at a remarkable pace, and it is envisioned that this will lead to μTAS small enough for implantation in humans.

4. Amperometric Immunosensors

As noted earlier, immunoassay is a bioanalytical technique based on antibody–antigen interactions for selectivity. The development of immunoassay is one of the great success stories of bioanalytical chemistry. Millions of immunoassays are done annually in clinics, hospitals, laboratories, and field tests to detect a wide range of analytes, including drugs, metabolites, and pollutants and pathogens in the environment and food [35]. Although immunoassay with optical detection is currently the most popular type of immunoassay, the recent advances in immunoassay with electrochemical detection (ECI) are making ECI more attractive than it had been [36–38]. Some of the most sensitive assays have been reported with ECI, and, being insensitive to the color and to a large degree the turbidity of the sample, ECI is particularly suitable for direct application to samples. For example, analysis in whole blood, a difficult task for assays with optical detection because of spectral interferences, can be successfully accomplished with ECI [39]. The feasibility of multianalyte detection on a single sensor platform has also been successfully demonstrated with ECI [40–42].

Detection in ECI has been based on a variety of markers, including electroactive functional groups and metal labels. But the greatest success has come with using enzyme labels that catalyze the production of electroactive product. The chemical amplification associated with enzyme catalysis makes enzyme immunoassay the most sensitive type of immunoassay. These assays typically use antibody-coated micro-titer wells to carry out the assay reactions, including the final enzyme substrate incubation, and the enzymatic product is detected usually by transferring the solution to an external electrochemical cell. Since the electrode and the immunoreactive surface are separated in space, these systems are not true biosensors. However, there has been a great deal of interest in adapting ECI in less complicated systems called immunosensors where the antibodies are attached directly to the electrode. Although immunosensors generally do not have the same high throughput capacity that the standard assay formats do, they are better suited for situations that require "on-the-spot" analysis, such as in field-testing of environmental samples and the development of home-based diagnostic kits. This section focuses only on electrochemical immunosensors that are true biosensors; the reader is referred to a few key review articles for information on nonbiosensor ECI formats [36–38].

A challenge to overcome in developing electrochemical immunosensors is to apply the antibody on the electrode without causing either the denaturation of antibody or the passivation of the electrode. Furthermore, where cost prohibits the use of immunosensors in a disposable manner, it is necessary to renew the immunosensors for multiple assays. Although the sensor surface can in principle be renewed by cleaving the antibody–antigen bonds in acidic media, it is tedious to do and often results in the loss of antibody activity. A number of immunsensor designs have been used to overcome these challenges. One of these has been to bind the antibodies to a membrane, which is then placed over the electrode [43]. Detection in these immunosensors is based on a competitive assay format, as illustrated in Figure 8. Here, an aliquot of enzyme-labeled analyte (Ag*) of known concentration is added to the sample for competitive binding to the antibody. The higher the concentration of analyte in sample, the less the Ag* that binds to the antibody, and vice versa. The membrane allows the free passage of the enzymatic product to the electrode. The immunsensor signal is inversely proportional to the analyte concentration because of the competitive assay format, and a previously established calibration curve is used to quantitate the analyte. Membrane immunosensors, however, are rather cumbersome to use because membranes have to be replaced between assays. Therefore, the general trend now is to develop disposable immunsensors. To be disposable, immunosensors must be inexpensive and made in large numbers. In this regard, the development of screen-printed electrodes (SPEs) using thick-film technology has been particularly important [44]. In SPE immunosensors a graphite-based ink is printed on a polystyrene surface to serve as the electrode material and adapted for immunosensors by the passive adsorption of antibodies. They have been used in a number of applications, including the detection of herbicides, atmospheric pollutants, and hormones [38,45]. Another material for making disposable immunosensors is pencil lead, which can be adapted for immunosensors by dip-coating with antibody.

Most of immunosensors developed thus far rely on a heterogeneous assay format, in which the excess Ag* in the bulk solution is rinsed away to avoid the false signal that could otherwise result. A heterogeneous assay format is

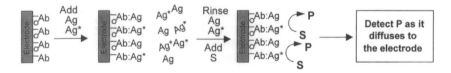

Figure 8   Schematic showing the principle of competitive electrochemical enzyme immunoassay.

clearly incompatible with the ideal "on-the-spot" and reagent-free immuno-sensors for a single-step analysis. To the best of our knowledge, the ideal re-agent-free electrochemical immunosensor has not yet been developed. However, the "separation-free" immunosensors that have appeared in the literature come a step closer to this goal. Although these immunosensors require additional re-agents, they do not require the removal of excess Ag*. A number of different approaches have been taken in developing "separation-free" immunosensors. In one, a reagent that acts as a scavenger of the electroactive enzymatic substrate is chosen such that it reacts selectively with the enzymatic product in the bulk [46]. The product formed by Ag* at the surface of the immunosensor surface undergoes oxidation at the electrode before the scavenger can take effect. An-other approach has been to use a microporous immunosensor surface so that the enzymatic substrate is introduced from the backside; because of proximity and flow effects, only the enzymatic product formed by the surface-bound Ag* is detected [47]. A very promising "separation-free" immunosensor type has used the concept of enzyme-channeling immunoassay [48]. Here, a second enzyme that catalyzes the formation of the substrate for Ag* is coimmobilized with the antibody on the electrode surface in making the immunosensor. Because of the diffusion distances involved, the product generated at the second enzyme is channeled in effect only to the Ag* at the immunosensor surface, thus avoiding the effects of Ag* in the bulk [49,50].

Electrochemical immunosensors is a very active area of research. The same attractive features of electrochemical biosensors in general, such as ease of miniaturization and insensitivity to color and to a large degree the turbidity of the sample, make electrochemical immunosensors more attractive than other types of immunosensors for many applications. The remarkable advances made in the recent past give hope for realizing the ultimate one-step, reagent-free, and "on-the-spot" immunosensor.

C. Conductimetric Sensors

Conductimetry stands in contrast to the preceding two methods, which involve the measurement of changes in interfacial redox reactions or membrane poten-tials at an indicator or working electrode. Conductance, by contrast, is a nonspe-cific property of electrolytes that has been useful in the measurement of concen-trations of ionic species, in elucidating the extent to which ionogenic substances dissociate in solvents, and in the development of electrolyte solution theory. Its application to biosensors is envisioned to be one in which a measurable change in conductivity in the vicinity of the biosensor surface is caused by either a reaction or a change in the double-layer capacitance following analyte capture. Hence, the detection scheme of a conductimetric sensor is less complicated than in an amperometric or a potentiometric sensor. Also, conductimetric sensors do not require a reference electrode, which is a considerable advantage, since making robust and reliable reference electrodes for chemical sensors has proven to be difficult. Despite such promise and the seemingly simple and elegant detection scheme, the development of conductimetric biosensors has been very slow. The main reason for this is the inherently nonselective nature of conductimetric sensors: The signal reflects the total change in conductivity and not any one of its contributory changes, one of which might be due to the analyte. Conductimetric biosensors with enzymes as the selective biocomponent have been reported. For example the enzyme urease catalyzes the hydrolysis of urea to ammonium, carbonate and hydroxide ions, which cause an increase in conductance [53]. Conductimetric immunosensors have also been demonstrated [54].

IV. A FUTURE OUTLOOK

Electrochemical biosensors have come a long way since the development of the first biosensor in 1962. It is an area of research that is truly multidisciplinary and continues to depend on advances in both fundamental and applied science. It is also an area of research that throughout its evolution has been guided by a very clear set of goals. Of these, the ultimate goal has been the electrochemical biosensor that continuously monitors the relevant analyte and triggers a feedback system to deliver the required dosage of medication when abnormal levels of analyte are detected. The artificial pancreas to regulate blood glucose has been a widely discussed topic. From a practical point of view, such a sensor also has to be small in size and noninvasive or nontoxic for implantation. Although this has not been realized, much progress has been made in the right direction, especially in connection with percutaneous and subcutaneous sensors, such as the glucose sensors discussed earlier.

Many current trends in biosensor research are likely to play a key role in the future. Likely to enter the arsenal of widely used biorecognition elements are DNA probes and, perhaps, molecular imprinted polymers (MIPs) [51]. DNA probes will extend the range of biosensor applications to encompass the detection of genetic defects or mutations that might allow early disease prevention measures. Such promise has stimulated a $500 million-per-year market for nucleic acid probes, with an estimated 25% annual growth over the next few years [52]. Use of MIPs, which are synthetic polymer-based mimics of catalysts, might become very important where exceptionally rugged bioelements are required. The rapidly growing areas of micro-and nano-technologies, including μTAS, will also play a critical role in developing miniaturized biosensors that might someday result in extremely small biosensors to be implanted in the human body for monitoring a host of different physiological conditions. The following chapters should give the reader not only an idea of what has been accomplished in electrochemical biosensors, but also a sense of what can be achieved in the future.

REFERENCES

1. The June 15 issue of *Analytical Chemistry* of every even-numbered year reviews the recent progress in chemical and biosensors.
2. D. Diamond, ed. Principles of Chemical and Biological Sensors. Wiley, New York, 1998.
3. A. P. F. Turner, I. Karube, G. S. Wilson, eds. Biosensors: Fundamentals and Applications. Oxford University Press, New York, 1987.
4. G. Ramsay, ed. Commercial Biosensors. Wiley, New York, 1998.
5. A. J. Cunningham. Introduction to Bioanalytical Sensors. Wiley, New York, 1998.
6. B. Eggins. Biosensors: An Introduction. Wiley-Teubner, New York, 1996.
7. F. W. Scheller, F. Schubert, J. Fedrowitz , eds. Frontiers in Biosensorics 1 & 11. Birkhäuser Verlag, Basel, 1997.
8. J. S. Sidwell, G. A. Rechnitz. Biotechnol. Lett. 7:419, 1985.
9. C. P. Price, D. J. Newman, eds. Principles and Practices of Immunoassay. 2nd ed. Macmillan Reference, London, 1997.
10. G. Kohler, C. Milstein. Nature 256:495, 1975.
11. G. Winter, C. Milstein. Nature 349:293, 1991.
12. L. B. McGown, M. J. Joseph, J. B. Pitner, G. P. Vonk, C. P. Linn. Anal. Chem. 67:663A, 1995.
13. F. F. Bier, J. P. Fürste. In: Frontiers in Biosensorics 1: Fundamental Aspects (F. W. Scheller, F. Schubert, J. Fedrowitz, eds.). Birkhäuser-Verlag, Boston, 1997, pp. 97–120.
14. A. J. Bard, L. R. Faulkner. Electrochemical Methods. 2nd ed. Wiley, New York, 2001.
15. W. R. Heineman, P. T. Kissinger, eds. Laboratory Techniques in Electroanalytical Chemistry. 2nd ed. Marcel Dekker, New York, 1996.
16. G. G. Guilbault, J. Montalvo. J. Am. Chem. Soc. 91:2164, 1969.
17. R. K. Krobs, H. Y. Pyon. Biotechnol. Bioeng. 23:627, 1981.
17A. C. E. Lunte, W. R. Heineman. Electrochemical Techniques in Bioanalysis. In: Topics in Current Chemistry. Vol. 143 (E. Stehkhan, ed.). Springer-Verlag, Berlin, 1988.
18. C. L. Morgan, D. J. Newman, C. P. Price. Clin. Chem. 42:193, 1996.
19. M. J. Green, G. Davis, H. A. O. Hill. J. Biomed. Eng. 6:176, 1984.
20. W. J. Albery, P. N. Bartlett, A. E. G. Cass. Phil. Trans. R. Soc. Lond. B 316:107, 1987.
21. W. J. Albery, D. H. Cranston. In: Biosensors: Fundamentals and Applications (A. P. F. Turner, I. Karube, G. S. Wilson, eds.). Oxford University Press, New York, 1987, pp. 180–210.

22. A. Heller. Acc. Chem. Res. 23:128, 1990.
23. Y. Degani, A. Heller. J. Am. Chem. Soc. 111:2357, 1989.
24. I. Katakis, A. Heller. In: Frontiers in Biosensorics 1 (F. W. Scheller, F. Schubert, J. Fedrowitz, eds.). Birkhäuser Verlag, New York, 1996.
25. E. Katz, V. Heleg-Shabtai, B. Willner, I. Willner, A. F. Buckmann. Bioelectrochem. Bioenerg. 42:95, 1997.
26. L. Gorton, A. Lindgren, T. Larsson, F. D. Munteanu, T. Ruzgas, I. Gazaryan. Anal. Chim. Acta 400:91, 1999.
27. C. Henry. Anal. Chem. 70:594A, 1998.
28. G. Reach, G. S. Wilson. Anal. Chem. 64:381A, 1992.
29. B. Aussedat, V. Thomé-Duret, G. Reach, F. Lemmonier, J. C. Klein, Y. Hu, G. S. Wilson. Biosens. Bioelectron. 12:1061, 1997.
30. V. Thomé-Duret, G. Reach, M. N. Gangnerau, F. Lemonnier, J. C. Klein, Y. Zhang, Y. Hu, G. S. Wilson. Anal. Chem. 68:3822, 1996.
31. E. Csoregi, D. W. Schmidtke, A. Heller. Anal. Chem. 67:1240, 1995.
32. J. G. Wagner, D. W. Schmidtke, C. P. Quinn, T. F. Fleming, B. Bernacky, A. Heller. Proc. Natl. Acad. Sci. USA 95:6379, 1998.
33. J. C. Armour, J. Y. Lucisano, B. D. McKean, D. A. Gough. Diabetes 39:1519, 1990.
34. A. van der Berg, P. Bergveld, eds. Micro-Total Analysis Systems. Kluwer Academic Press, Boston, 1995.
35. A review of immunoassays appears biannually in the journal *Analytical Chemistry*. The most recent is: D. S. Hage. Anal. Chem. 71:294R, 1999.
36. C. A. Wijayawardhana, H. B. Halsall, W. R. Heineman. In: Encyclopedia of Electrochemistry (A. J. Bard, M. Stratmann, eds.). Vol. 9 (G. S. Wilson, ed.). Wiley-VCH, New York, 2002 .
37. C. P. Price, D. J. Newman, eds. Principles and Practices of Immunoassay. 2nd ed. Macmillan Reference., London, 1997.
38. W. R. Heineman, H. B. Halsall. Anal. Chem. 57:1321A, 1985.
39. H. Yao, H. B. Halsall, W. R. Heineman, S. H. Jenkins. Clin. Chem. 41:591, 1995.
40. Y. Ding, L. Zhou, H. B. Halsall, W. R. Heineman. J. Pharm. Biomed. Anal. 19: 153, 1999.
41. C. A. Wijayawardhana, G. Wittstock, H. B. Halsall, W. R. Heineman. Anal. Chem. 72:339, 2000.
42. D. J. Pritchard, H. Morgan, J. M. Cooper. Anal. Chem. 67:251, 1995.
43. M. Aizawa, A. Morioka, S. Suzuki, Y. Nagamura. Anal. Biochem. 94:22, 1979.
44. H. D. Goldberg, R. B. Brown, D. P. Liu, M. E. Meyerhoff. Sens. Actuators (B) 21: 171, 1994.
45. P. Skládal. Electroanalysis 9:737, 1997.
46. R. W. Keay, C. J. McNeil. Biosens. Bioelectron. 13:963, 1998.
47. M. W. Ducey Jr., A. M. Smith, X. Guo, M. E. Meyerhoff. Anal. Chim. Acta 357: 5, 1997.
48. D. J. Litman, T. M. Hanlon, E. F. Ullman. Anal. Biochem. 106:223, 1980.
49. J. Rishpon, D. Ivnitski. Biosens. Bioelectron. 12:195, 1997.

50. C. N. Campbell, T. de Lumley-Woodyear, A. Heller. Fresenius J. Anal. Chem. 364: 165, 1999.
51. D. Kriz, O. Ramstrom, K. Mosbach. Anal. Chem. 69:345A, 1997.
52. A. M. Thayer. Chem. Engineer. News 8:19–28, 1999.
53. A. M. Gallordo Soto, S. A. Jaffari, S. Bone. Biosens. Bioelectron. 16:23, 2001.
54. S. C. Pak, W. Penrose, P. J. Hesketh. Biosens. Bioelectron. 16:371, 2001.

2

Improved-Accuracy Biosensor Strip for Accu-Chek™ Advantage®

David W. Burke and Nigel A. Surridge
Roche Diagnostics Corporation, Indianapolis, Indiana, U.S.A.

I. INTRODUCTION

The use of handheld blood glucose meters is now widespread in developed countries and occurs not only within the diabetic population in the home environment, but also in a variety of professional health care settings. Although there is certainly controversy concerning the use of these devices with critically ill patients [1,2], it is apparent that penetration into these settings is increasing. Critical care and neonatal settings are even more sensitive to clinical accuracy than the outpatient and doctor's office professional segments, where these devices already see a high level of acceptance and use.

With this trend in mind, it is important that successive generations of blood glucose meters and strips address the increasing need for clinical accuracy in all settings and with multiple sample types, such as venous, capillary, neonatal, and arterial blood.

In this product arena, the last five years has seen an increase in the use of biosensor-type systems where the blood glucose is determined by an electrochemical measurement rather than photometric. Bayer and Medisense (Abbott Laboratories) both continue to concentrate on their core electrochemical technology for new product offerings, and recently LifeScan also made the jump from photometric systems with the launch of their FastTake glucose system. All three of these major manufacturers rely on screen printing technology and carbon-containing inks to create the electrodes that ultimately determine glucose. Another, smaller company, Therasense, has also recently received FDA approval to market an electrochemically based glucose system requiring remarkably small sample volumes of approximately 0.5 µL.

The electrochemical systems from Roche Diagnostics Corp. are characterized by the use of noble metals as the electrodes and by the use of a glucose dehydrogenase (GDH) enzyme for conversion of glucose to measurable redox equivalents. This enzyme has some advantages in electrochemical systems over the more widely used glucose oxidase, which is sensitive to the variation in oxygen content of the blood sample. Indeed, the Therasense system recognizes the need to remove this source of clinical inaccuracy by incorporating the dehydrogenase enzyme.

In addition to the variation in oxygen tension of blood samples, the volume percentage of red blood cells ("hematocrit," or %HCT) in a given blood sample is another major influence on the accuracy of the glucose result reported by electrochemical test strips. In addition to Roche Diagnostics Corp., other major manufacturers go to some length to reduce the effect of %HCT on the glucose result [3]. This source of error is particularly worthy of attention due to the wide and common variation in %HCT values that are regularly seen in the populations using these products; the importance of this intrinsic variation is highlighted in an upcoming publication [4], particularly as it affects clinical accuracy.

Comfort Curve®, which is the most recent biosensor strip offering [5] from Roche Diagnostics, is the subject of this study; it has also been described more generally in a previous publication [6]. We will focus here on efforts and studies to ensure that the %HCT sensitivity is minimized, and we will compare the product with other state-of-the-art glucose test strips.

II. DESCRIPTION

A depiction of a Comfort Curve® test strip is shown in Figure 1. Essentially, two identical palladium electrodes are sealed between two thin sheets of plastic, with cutouts for meter contacts and for placement of the glucose-specific reagent. Palladium is used in the sensor for its resistance to surface oxidation and to maintain a well-characterized electrochemical surface over long periods of time. During manufacture, small amounts of liquid reagent containing the GDH enzyme and ferricyanide mediator are dispensed into the appropriate window and dried. Following this, the capillary roof and top covering (label) are applied. The "capillary roof" is a specially formulated coating that is able to maintain a high surface energy for very long times, even in the presence of silicones, fluoropolymers, and other hydrophobic contaminants. The final strip forms a capillary chamber of internal volume ~5 µL that can be filled from the edge of the strip. The "curve" in the side of the strip aids in tactile location of the capillary entrance for users of limited visual acuity; it also allows small amounts of blood to be "scraped" into the capillary channel even if the sample has

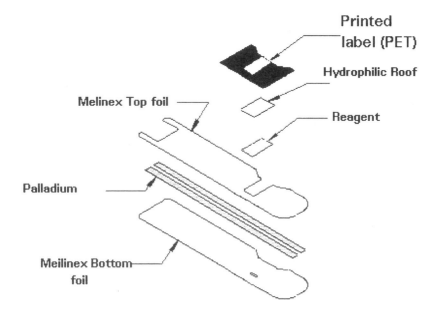

Figure 1 Comfort Curve® strip showing exploded view of the Melinex plastic strip body, Pd electrodes, reagent, hydrophilic roof, and polyester label.

smeared over the skin surface. The actual volume required in the chamber for an accurate result is only 4 μL, for partial coverage of the second electrode in the channel has little or no effect on the measured current response.

III. MEASUREMENT PRINCIPLE

The measurement principle is chronoamperometry, by which the meter detects the entry of blood into the capillary and enters into a fixed incubation time determined by parameters contained in a ROM key supplied with each container of strips and placed by the user into the meter. After this period, which allows the GDH-glucose-ferricyanide reaction to produce ferrocyanide, a potential difference is applied between the electrodes, and current readings are collected for another fixed period of time. The form of the current decay during the measurement time when potential is applied is nominally described by the Cottrell equation, according to normal diffusion-limited current assumptions [7], shown in Eq. 1:

$$i_d(t) = \frac{nFAD^{1/2}C^{1/2}}{\pi^{1/2}t^{1/2}} \tag{1}$$

In reality, blood samples show deviation from this ideal behavior to various degrees. This can be due partly to rheology; certainly the deviation varies according to %HCT. The apparent diffusion constant of the species being oxidized (ferrocyanide) is also matrix dependent and is convoluted with the concentration, C, that is desired from the measurement. The intrinsic temperature dependency of the apparent diffusion constant is generally compensated for to some extent by thermistor-based measurements of the ambient temperature around the meter. In the case of very small blood samples such as used in Comfort Curve®, the thermal equilibration of the sample itself with the strip body is quite fast, and the outside surface of the strip is exposed to the ambient environment.

We can see from this situation, that it is highly desirable to provide a reagent matrix that essentially allows the physical properties of the measurement matrix to be accurately controlled and to vary little with sample variations.

IV. VARIATION OF HEMATOCRIT

Given the possible effect of %HCT on the nature of the sample matrix, it is useful to know what variations these devices are exposed to in the field. During standard clinical trials of the Comfort Curve® strip, the product was used in six different clinical sites, mostly professional and hospital settings in the United States. The types of samples studied were capillary, fresh venous, arterial (surgical, critical care units), and neonatal blood. In all these cases the %HCT value was collected alongside the glucose readings from the same sample. Figure 2 is a summary of the frequency distribution by %HCT bin of blood samples regularly encountered in normal medical practice. A total of 1033 samples were collected.

It is readily apparent from a clinician's perspective that glucose strips used in hospitals should be relatively unaffected by %HCT values between 20% and 70%. This is particularly true in the case of neonatal units where the first evaluation of a baby's blood glucose level is obtained mostly by means of a handheld meter. In Figure 2, neonatal samples were responsible for >95% of all the %HCT readings falling in the 60% and above bins. Additionally, hemodialysis patients, critical care patients, and patients suffering from acute blood loss in emergency room settings can frequently exhibit %HCT values in the lowermost bins.

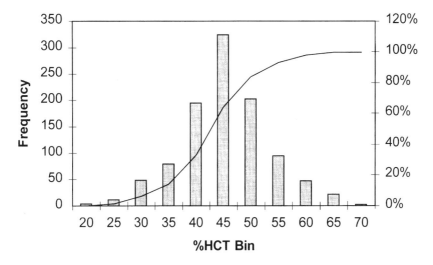

Figure 2 Frequency Distribution of hematocrit values encountered during clinical trials of Comfort Curve.

V. CONSIDERATIONS OF HEMATOCRIT DEPENDENCY

We have already mentioned some of the sources of dependency of the glucose reading on %HCT in electrochemical sensors. In general, for any test strip relying on an enzymatic reaction with glucose to provide the measured species, kinetic factors may also influence the result. Microscopic diffusion and, hence, collision frequencies could potentially be affected by the amount of erythrocytes in the sample. Also, commercial test strips are based on dry reagents that must be dissolved or hydrated by the blood sample in order to react. The rate of this dissolution could play an important part in determining the extent of reaction in a given time period, thus affecting the apparent glucose concentration.

In the case of optical test-strip systems based on a slowly dissolving or nondissolving membrane, it is possible to reduce the effect of these matrix variations by excluding the erythrocytes from the reaction matrix to some extent. Figure 3 demonstrates how it may be possible to use the reaction layer itself to filter the cellular components and to help ensure that the reaction inside the layer proceeds in an environment characterized more by the plasma components of the sample. In this case, the diffusional matrix may be more controlled, but total test time may also be dependent on a relatively slow hydration time.

Figure 4 shows an approach that can be used in electrochemical sensors to compromise between fast test times and lower sensitivity to cellular variations

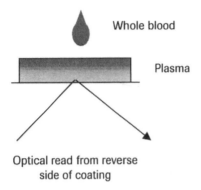

Whole blood

Plasma

Optical read from reverse
side of coating

Figure 3 Optical test strip with insoluble reaction layer.

of the sample matrix. To the extent that a film-forming additive (right-hand panel) can be incorporated into the reaction matrix, it is possible to reduce the influence of the blood cells on the physical characteristics of the film and to reduce the ultimate sensitivity of the glucose result. The left-hand panel represents a very rapidly dissolving matrix, which perhaps can help the reaction come to completion faster but which will be maximally sensitive to sample variation.

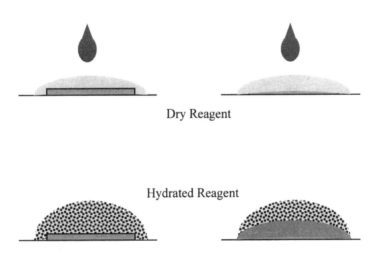

Dry Reagent

Hydrated Reagent

Figure 4 Electrochemical biosensor with rapidly dissolving reaction matrix (left) and rapidly hydrating film-forming matrix (right).

VI. COMFORT CURVE® FORMULATION

This approach has been used in the formulation of the Comfort Curve® strips using polyethylene oxide (PEO) as the film former, as described in Table 1. Because these strips are filled essentially by capillary action, it is important that the reaction matrix not only control dissolution but that it remain hydrophilic throughout the product lifetime. PEO is very effective in both these roles and does not adversely affect the enzyme or mediator stability. Other capillary-fill glucose strips also make use of the hydrophilic nature of PEO [9].

VII. SYSTEM SENSITIVITY TO HEMATOCRIT LEVEL AND TEMPERATURE

Given that effective diffusion constants can be both hematocrit and temperature dependent, it is of clinical significance to characterize the test strips with this in mind. Consequently we have carried out a covariance study using four handeld glucose systems that employ electrochemical measurements: Accu-Chek™ Comfort Curve®, FastTake from LifeScan, Precision G from Abbott Laboratories, and Glucometer Elite from Bayer.

Five levels of glucose were covaried with five contrived %HCT levels, and five test temperatures for all systems in a full-factorial experimental design ($n = 8$ test strips at each combination). The manufacturer's meters were used as well as commercial lots of unexpired strips. Venous blood samples drawn on Li heparin were used in all cases and glycolized for 12 hours to obtain low endogenous glucose levels. Care was taken to allow sufficient time to obtain pO_2 satu-

Table 1 The Composition of the Comfort Curve® Formulation

Component	Composition (wt%)	Includes	Details
Enzyme	1.2%	GDH	Glucose dehydrogenase recombinent from *E. Coli*
Mediator	43.7%	$K_3Fe(CN)_6$	Oxidized electron transfer mediator
Stabilizer*	19.4%	Trehalose	Stabilizes GDH for better highend glucose stability under adverse conditions
Nonreactive components	11.0%	PEO	Effective film former that controls diffusion layer and is compatible with sample matrix

*See Ref. 8.

ration of the blood to avoid aliasing results with oxygen dependency. Data at each temperature was collected during a separate session at a commercial environmental test facility, so the blood samples were collected the day before each respective session. On the day of testing, the blood pool was separated into plasma and cells, which were then then recombined in various ratios and with varying amounts of added dextrose to achieve 5×5 levels of %HCT and glucose. The targeted values of the three variables were as follows:

Temperature (°C): 10, 16 [10], 23, 30, 40
Hematocrit (%HCT): 20, 30, 45, 60, 70
[Glucose] (mg/dL): 50, 100, 150, 300, 450/500 [11]

Of course local variations of %HCT and [glucose] occurred in each combination, and the data graphs shown later indicate the actual values determined by HCT measurements at the time of test and reference glucose values obtained using a Hitachi clinical chemistry analyzer (PCA-HK method).

It is believed that all meter systems use some type of ambient temperature estimation to partially correct the results for temperature variation. For the Fast-Take system, an additional lock-out feature prevented any data from being gathered at 10° or 40°C.

VIII. RESULTS AND DISCUSSION

The meter responses from all systems are plotted in the following figures at all temperatures and %HCT levels. Each manufacturer claims a slightly different range of use for their systems with resect to the tested variables. Therefore the data in each of Figures 5, 6, 7, and 8 are divided into categories where the temperature/%HCT combination falls within the manufacturer's acceptable use range and those that fall outside the published limits. The reason for collecting data outside "acceptable use" will become apparent in the following section, dealing with modeling of the sensor responses.

The data plotted in Figures 5–8 have been overlaid on a modified "Clarke error grid" [12]. For the purposes of interpreting this data, we will define desirable performance based on this grid analysis with the following criteria. If a given point falls within the region labeled A, the response is clinically accurate. If a given point falls within the region labeled B, the response is erroneous but clinically benign, since it leads to the same treatment as an accurate response. If a given point falls within the region labeled C, the error can be sufficient to lead to treatment where none is required. If a given point falls within the region labeled D, the error will mislead patients into believing they are within glycemic control when, in fact, they are not. This leads to no treatment when treatment is appropriate. If a given point falls within the region labeled E, the error can

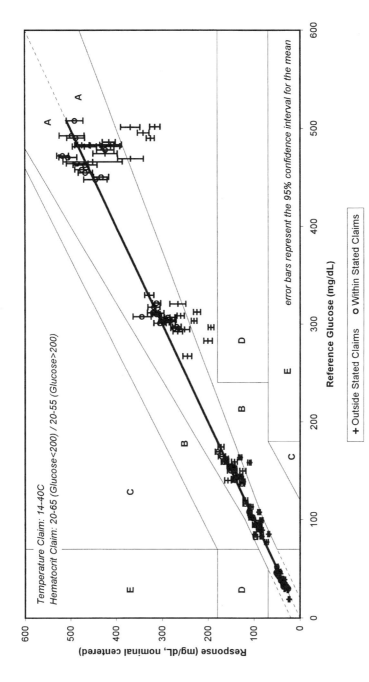

Figure 5 Error grid analysis for Comfort Curve®.

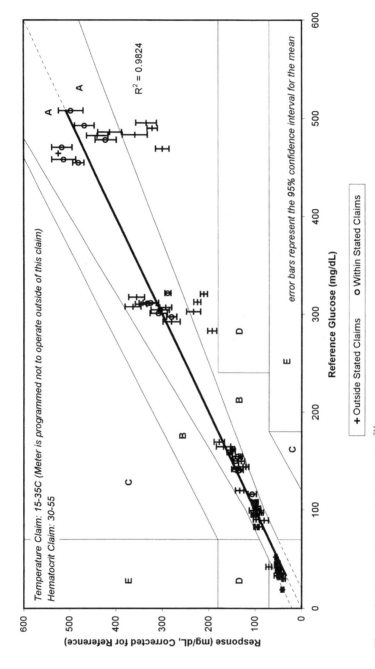

Figure 6 Error grid analysis for Fast*Take*™.

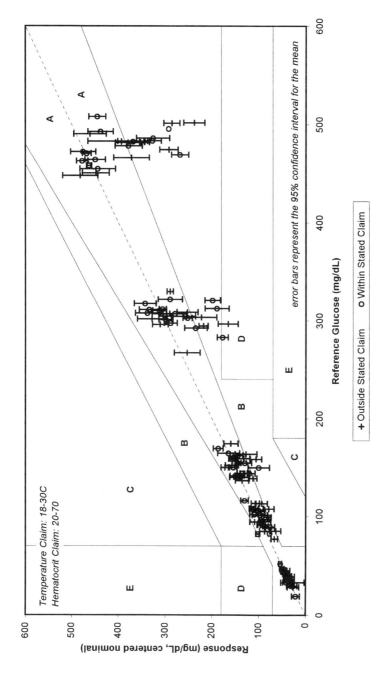

Figure 7   Error grid analysis for Precision G™.

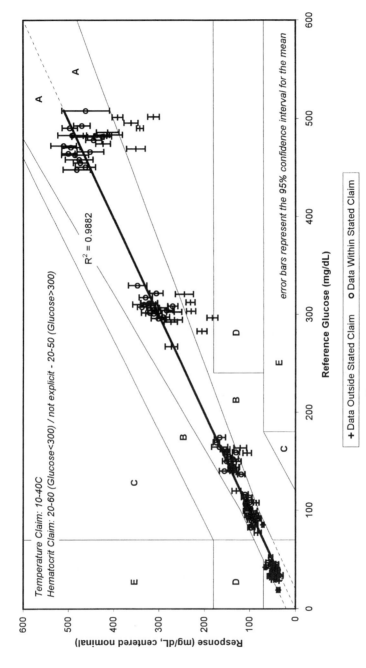

Figure 8 Error grid analysis for Glucometer Elite®.

result in a treatment opposite to that which is necessary, i.e., treatment for hypo-glycemia when the patient is hyperglycemic, or the reverse.

Although no points outside of the A region can be regarded as desirable, data within the E region represents the strongest risk to the health of the patient. The outcome of such mistreatment can certainly result in the death of the patient. Data within the C and D regions are less likely to lead to fatality but may, nonetheless, lead to complications.

Clarke's error grid is a standard reference method; however, as shown in Figures 5–8, the boundaries of the normal glucose range are at 70–180 mg/dL. Presently, the ranges in use by most physicians are 70–120 or 70–140 mg/dL. If the more up-to-date ranges are employed, the C and D regions should contract somewhat. Also, Clarke's error grid makes no decisions about accuracy or precision at glucose levels below 70 mg/dL [13]. It has, however, been our experience that accuracy in this region is of special interest where neonatal claims are in place. For this reason, I have included dashed lines that would extend Clarke's ±20-mg/dL criteria through to the origin of the plot; for our purposes, this will be the lower definition of the A region, since treatment decisions for neonates are different than for adults.

With respect to response vs. reference glucose, the reference method we used is whole blood PCA-HK. This method is approximately 10% biased relative to plasma reference, which is the reference method used for many systems in the United States (though not in Europe). Additionally, although pO_2 effects will have been standardized across all systems, this effect may still have caused an increase or decrease in response slope, depending on the system. For these reasons, as well as any inherent Hitachi reference analyzer error, we have normalized the responses by removing the baseline slope and intercept in a linear fashion across the range. This was done by using only the nominal data falling within the claimed range, to center the data set about the center axis. This is the reason the reader will not see systematic biases vs. the reference in Figures 5–8. Given that this study specifically addresses HCT and temperature effects, we felt this was a way to present unbiased results [14].

In each of Figures 5–8, the error bars represent 95% of the confidence interval (2 SD), and the ranges of acceptable use with respect to temperature and %HCT are quoted where, and to the extent that, they can be determined from packaging accompanying the product.

In general, it can be seen that the majority of responses outside the A region occur above 300 mg/dL of glucose. In addition, the blood samples giving rise to *all* of these deviations have %HCT of 60 or 70. With the exception of Precision G, all samples with %HCT of 20–45 fell within the A region at all temperatures, even outside the manufacturer's claim, as indicated in each of the figures. Also, with the exception of Precision G, it was found that for the remaining systems, all data falling below the A region were in the temperature range of 10–23°C. This general trend of low-biased response at low temperature and high %HCT is consistent with diffusional control of the electrochemical processes and activated processes involved in the enzyme reaction pathway. Precision G was the only system that exhibited significant data points outside the A region that still fell within the claimed range of usage. Both Precision G and Elite gave some responses in the D region, although for Elite these points were *all* outside the claimed range. Only FastTake and Comfort Curve displayed results where all the claimed readings were within the A region.

A. Modeling

Although the data that has been collected is thorough in representing the entire spectrum of combinations of glucose, temperature, and hematocrit, it is by no means complete. To assist in the interpretation of this data, the mean responses of Figures 5–8 have been regressed across the temperature, glucose, and hematocrit dimensions using a third-order polynomial regression to predict where the mean response will fall given any combination of glucose, temperature, and hematocrit. The essential equation used to develop the model is shown in Eq. (2), used to predict actual response, R, at all glucose concentrations, G, and %HCT values:

$$R = (\alpha_0 + \alpha_1 G + \alpha_2 G^2 + \alpha_3 G^3)[\beta_0 + \beta_1(HCT)$$
$$+ \beta_2(HCT)^2 + \beta_3(HCT)^3] \qquad (2)$$

After regressing the actual responses, the model response was compared to the observed response for every system. Figure 9 shows one example of the correlation, for Glucometer Elite in this case. The correlation parameters for all systems are shown in Table 2, where it can be seen that the model is well suited to all the systems responses.

With the predictive model it is then possible to calculate the response at all combinations of variables. However, in order to compare all systems, which use different reference methods and are calibrated independently, we will not display the results of the model prediction in absolute terms. Rather, we use the model to calculate differences between the response at a nominal %HCT of 45 vs. the %HCT of interest at any given glucose concentration. This difference or bias can then be expressed as follows:

If reference glucose value < 100mg/dL:

$$\text{Bias} = R(HCT) - R(45) \qquad (3a)$$

If reference glucose value > 100mg/dL:

$$\text{Bias} = \frac{100[R(HCT) - R(45)]}{R(45)} \qquad (3b)$$

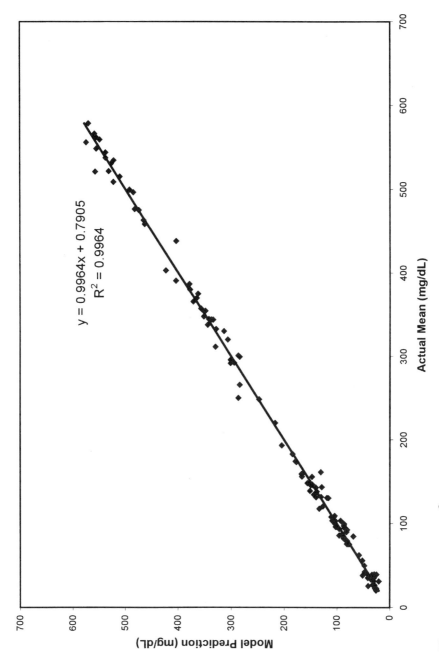

$$y = 0.9964x + 0.7905$$
$$R^2 = 0.9964$$

Figure 9 Glucometer Elite®: comparison of actual response *vs.* model.

Table 2 Comparison of Actual Responses to Predicted Responses

System	Slope	Intercept	R^2
Comfort Curve	0.9957	0.6875	0.9961
FastTake	0.9953	0.8496	0.9956
Precision G	0.9941	1.1608	0.9938
Elite	0.9964	0.7905	0.9964

where bias above 100 mg/dL glucose is in percentage, while that below 100 mg/dL is in mg/dL. This is a common formulation in systems where the SD of the response increases proportionately with the nominal response. The result of this predicted bias at room temperature across the varying dimensions of glucose and %HCT are shown in Figures 11, 14, 17, and 20 for the Comfort Curve, FastTake, Precision G, and Elite systems, respectively. The information is shown as contour plots where the central four intervals, which are not filled in the diagrams, span the response bias region of −10% to +10% (or mg/dL in the low-glucose region).

The model can also be applied to the data sets at different temperatures to predict absolute responses at varying glucose and %HCT. This was done, and predicted biases were calculated from the same nominal baseline case of %HCT = 45 at room temperature. The bias calculated this way then includes bias due to %HCT and temperature variations in an independent, additive manner from the room-temperature 45% HCT nominal condition. The response surface of this calculated bias is shown for all systems in Figures 10, 12, 13, 15, 16, 18, 19, and 21 for all systems. These high and low temperatures were selected from all those tested using the published claims limits for each system; i.e., the lowest and highest temperatures shown for each system are the temperatures we tested that are closest to the lower and upper claim limits for that particular system. In this way we begin to see the underlying sensitivity to both parameters of interest for all systems, without aliasing of reference and calibration errors. It is likely that all systems are nominally calibrated for close to room temperature.

B. Detailed Discussion of Tested Systems

1. Comfort Curve

Comfort Curve® has a claimed temperature range of 14°C–40°C, with the system functioning over a range of 5°C–50°C but with a warning icon to alert the user to potentially biased results. The %HCT claim is split, depending on the

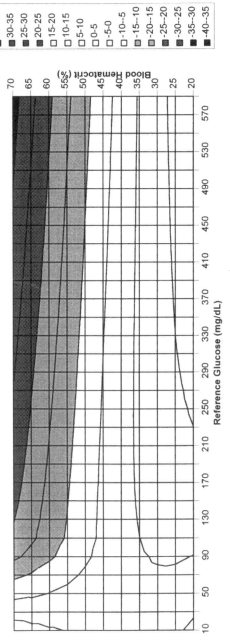

Figure 10 Comfort Curve®: predicted bias at 14°C.

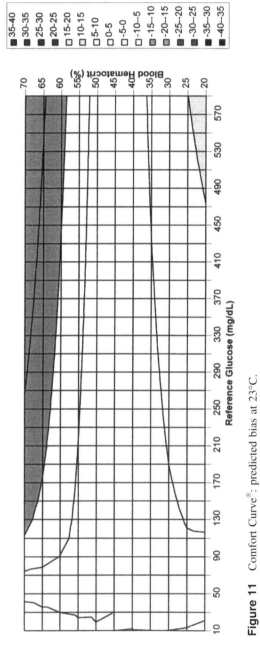

Figure 11   Comfort Curve®: predicted bias at 23°C.

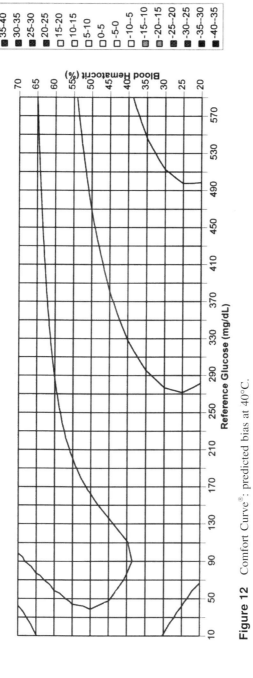

Figure 12 Comfort Curve®: predicted bias at 40°C.

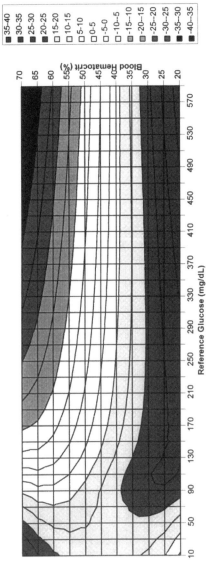

Figure 13   Fast*Take*™: predicted bias at 16°C.

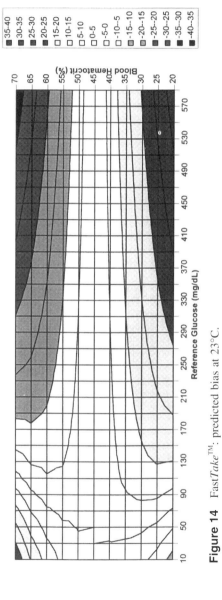

Figure 14 Fast*Take*™: predicted bias at 23°C.

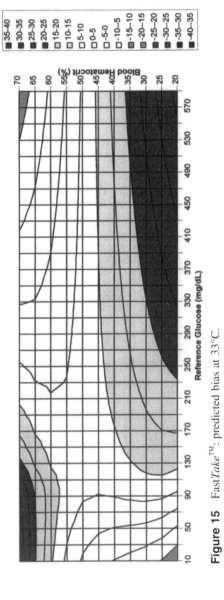

Figure 15 Fast*Take*™: predicted bias at 33°C.

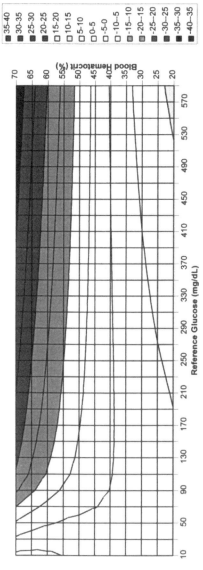

Figure 16   Precision G™: predicted bias at 18°C.

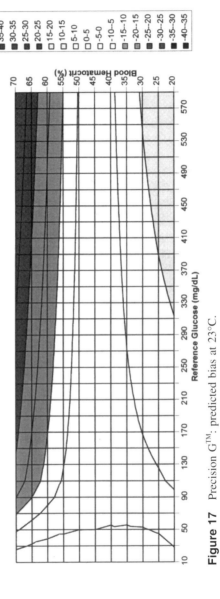

Figure 17 Precision G™: predicted bias at 23°C.

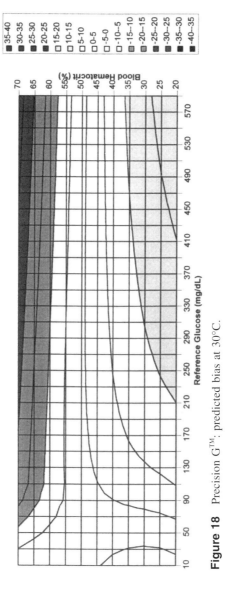

Figure 18 Precision G™: predicted bias at 30°C.

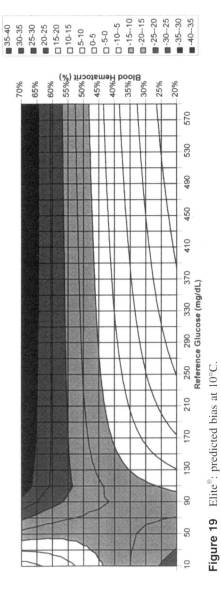

Figure 19 Elite®: predicted bias at 10°C.

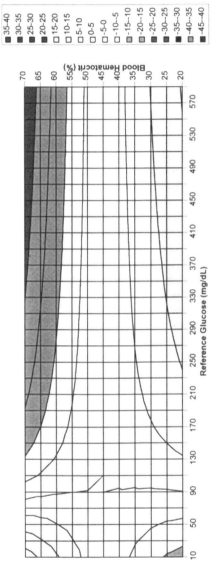

Figure 20 Elite®: predicted bias at 23°C.

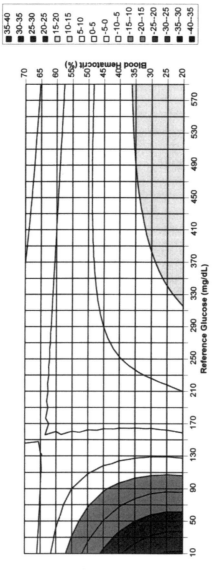

Figure 21 Elite®: predicted bias at 40°C.

glucose concentration, with claimed limits of 20–65% HCT for glucose below 200, and 20–55% HCT at glucose greater than 200 mg/dL.

As can be seen in Figure 5, the data that falls within the system claims shows acceptable accuracy and precision. Performance of the system outside the stated claims shows that, with the combination of high hematocrit and low temperatures, a progressive negative bias begins to manifest above 100 mg/dL. Essentially, the slope of the system is sensitive to temperature and hematocrit, with the most extreme depression in slope being where the two effects combine, so that larger negative bias is observed at high glucose and high %HCT at the lower temperature of Figure 10. Conversely, the system becomes hyperrobust at the high end of the temperature range (Fig. 12), where bias is within ±10% at all combinations.

From Figures 10 and 12, we can see that the split %HCT claim with a more conservative maximum acceptable %HCT of 55 is necessary above 200 mg/dL of glucose. This helps to alert patients and clinicians that results could be unacceptably biased at high %HCT and helps to avoid any data falling in the D region when the system is used at or beyond the limits of the claim.

2. FastTake

FastTake claims an operating temperature range of 15°C through 35°C and a hematocrit range of 30–55%; it uses a system lockout feature to prevent testing outside of the claimed temperature range.

After normalizing the data to remove any error not related to temperature or hematocrit, such as calibration differences, the form of the sensitivity profiles for FastTake are seen to be very similar to those of Comfort Curve. Indeed, all data within the claimed range is acceptable. However, it is important to note that the underlying sensitivity to %HCT is much stronger, leading to pronounced positive bias predicted at high glucose and low %HCT, and pronounced negative bias predicted at high glucose and high %HCT (Figs. 13 and 14). It is also interesting to note, however, that like Elite, a pronounced sensitivity of the dose response intercept to %HCT is also seen, just discernable in Figure 6 in the very-low-glucose region. This results in an increased sensitivity for FastTake to hematocrit variation at low glucoses, which shows as positive predicted bias in the upper left corner of Figures 14 and 15.

When comparing Figures 13–15 it becomes clear that the temperature compensation methods used on the FastTake system are not optimal, and shifts in bias may be attributable to over-or undercompensation. Thus there is a clear interaction between the sensitivity of the system to hematocrit and the temperature at which the system is operating. It should be noted, however, that the tight hematocrit and temperature claims should be more than sufficient to avoid the D region entirely. Additionally, the temperature lockout will prevent testing below 16°C where inaccuracy becomes critical.

3. Precision G

Precision G claims an operating temperature range of 18°C through 30°C and a hematocrit range of 20–70%. It should be noted that this system does not disclaim testing outside of these conditions, but indicates ranges "for best results" instead. This makes the claim much softer and less effective in limiting liability.

As can be seen in Figure 7, the actual response vs. whole blood reference for Precision G saw reasonable accuracy for a subset of the claimed data. However, the same figure shows that the appropriateness of the accuracy claims across the combined temperature and %HCT range is in serious doubt, with an r-squared value of 0.9059 across all claimed responses. In addition to the inaccuracy, the precision of Precision G was the worst of the four systems reported here.

After normalizing the data, the sensitivity profiles for Precision G can be seen in Figures 16–18. Unlike the other systems, it was also noted that at high hematocrits, a high incidence of false strip errors were seen, and most tests at 60+% hematocrit saw a delay in sample recognition, which was most pronounced at lower temperatures. By examining the contour plots, it is clear that the mean response is predicted not to fall within ±10% bias across very large proportions of the claimed hematocrit range at any temperature. Using similar criteria applied for ComfortCurve, the claims for hematocrit would instead be 20–55%. No split point is practical, since the negative bias at low hematocrits covers most of the glucose range.

Temperature compensation over the claimed range for Precision G is good, with no evidence of significant over-or undercompensation, and the degree of overall sensitivity to %HCT is less than that of FastTake. It is also interesting to note that the sensitivity to hematocrit varies much less significantly as the temperature varies. This may be due to a fundamental difference between Precision G reagent and that used by other electrochemical systems. Precision G uses a ferrocene mediator, while the other 3 systems use ferricyanide.

4. Elite

Elite claims an operating temperature range of 10°C through 40°C and a hematocrit range of 20–60%. They have a split in their claim at 300 mg/dL, with hematocrits above 55% being contraindicated.

Again, after normalizing the data to remove calibration or reference-induced inaccuracy (see Fig. 8), the overall accuracy for Elite can be seen to be very similar that for Comfort Curve. It is interesting to note, however, that unlike with ComfortCurve, a pronounced sensitivity in the dose response intercept is also seen, observed as positively biased data near the intercept of Figure 8. This results in an increased sensitivity for Elite to hematocrit variation at low glucoses (see the left-hand side of Figs. 19–21). This behavior is shared by FastTake.

As can be seen when comparing Figure 20 to Figure 11, the sensitivity of Elite at higher glucoses is similar to, though more pronounced than, that observed with ComfortCurve®. The increased sensitivity at low glucoses, however, is not. This sensitivity, where higher hematocrits have positively biased the intercept, would be problematic for any desired neonatal claims, where high hematocrit, high bilirubin, a positive interferent, and low glucose are combined. The only significant problem region for Elite, as with the other sensor products, is where low temperature and high hematocrit combine near the corner of the D region at 240 mg/dL. Although the exposure of Elite to D region responses is similar to that of the ComfortCurve sensors, the disclaimer for high hematocrits occurs at 300 mg/dL instead of 200 mg/dL, which would be more appropriate. This places a larger proportion of the data in the wider claim of 20–60%. Additionally, the lower-claimed temperature for Elite is 10°C, further compounding the problem.

When comparing the bias as temperature varies (Figs. 19–21), the Elite system is not predicted to perform as well at low temperatures as it does at high temperatures. The upper limit of the hematocrit claim, 60%, is predicted to fall outside of the A region at glucoses above 90 mg/dL. The convolution of temperature and hematocrit effects also results in greater negative biases for hematocrits within the normal range, 40–50%.

C. Overall Comparison and Conclusions

To make the most valid comparisons possible with respect to temperature and hematocrit sensitivity, we disregard the system claims with respect to hematocrit in this section. The criteria by which claims are established and validated obviously vary widely between companies and products, as can be seen from the preceding section.

In the analysis that follows, the mean responses for all available data were analyzed using a common method. Normalized biases, "NBias," are calculated for all responses relative to the nominal test conditions and reference glucose as in Eqs. (3a) and (3b). These biases are used to calculate the system error, "SErr," which is the absolute value of the sum of the normalized biases plus twice the standard deviation of the biases. We use this statistic internally, since it does not mask problems near the intercept, as is the case with more standard statistics, such as the root mean square error.

In Table 3, the system error has been calculated across all hematocrits and glucoses for each of the temperatures for which all systems are represented: 18°C, 23°C, and 33°C. Table 3 is organized in order of increasing system error from top to bottom. It should be noted that while the system errors in Table 3

Table 3 System Error

System	SErr at 18°C	SErr at 23°C	SErr at 33°C	Combined SErr
Comfort Curve	31.9%	16.9%	11.2%	20.0%
Elite	29.5%	22.2%	19.2%	23.6%
FastTake	34.4%	34.0%	21.8%	30.1%
Precision G	40.6%	35.7%	24.4%	33.6%

can be compared in a relative sense, the absolute numbers are derived from a fairly nonideal set of data. Specifically, the blood samples used to obtain such a large range of %HCT and glucose concentrations were, by necessity, heavily manipulated. As such, the samples are not the "fresh venous" blood normally used in clinical settings.

In summary, all the electrochemical systems studied display sensitivity to the %HCT level of blood samples. These sensitivities are both glucose dependent and, to varying extents, temperature dependent. From a theoretical perspective, both variables are likely to interact with the electrochemically determined glucose signal; therefore it is of value to users and manufacturers alike to understand the nature of covariance in system performance. Generally little information on this variation is included in product packaging, and with reason. In recent years, pressure on industry to simplify packaging information to levels far below the current level of sophistication has increased, and it is not possible to see how such complex relationships could be expressed easily to the end user. In addition, there currently exist no established criteria or methodologies by which these interactions can be established, within either industries or regulatory bodies. Nonetheless, the type of covariance studies attempted here can aid in the characterization of future blood glucose systems, and indeed it appears that well-designed electrochemical glucose systems are capable of delivering accurate results over wide ranges of %HCT and temperature. In addition, these systems also are able to meet the user need for faster test times, such as exhibited by FastTake, and measurement times of less than 15 seconds can be hard to achieve with complete filtering of blood samples to remove the effect of %HCT.

Until commonly understood and presumably more regulated criteria can be applied to setting performance limitations, physicians and health care professionals should certainly be aware of the limits of handheld glucose systems operating near the limits of their claims. These considerations should also be made in light of the tremendous benefit to users of these products in terms of convenience and rapid access to the clinically important information.

ACKNOWLEDGMENTS

The authors would like to recognize the significant efforts of Sarion Adams, Anna Afshar, Kyra Armold, Michelle Baker, Kim Brackin, Mary Brown, Stacia Earl, Kerwin Kaufman, Joel Kavanaugh, Eric Overdorf, Angel Schaefer, and Harpreet Singh, all of Roche Diagnostics, in gathering the large amounts of data for this extensive study.

REFERENCES AND NOTES

1. Maser, RE; Butler, MA; DeCherney, GS. Use of arterial blood with bedside glucose reflectance meters in an intensive care unit: are they accurate? Crit Care Med. 1994; 22, 595–599.
2. Walker, EA; Paduano, DJ; Shamoon, H. Quality assurance for blood glucose monitoring in health care facilities. Diabetes Care. 1991, 14, 1043–1049.
3. Nankai, S; Kawaguri, M; Ohtani, M; Iijima, T. Biosensor and a Process for Preparation Thereof. June 9, 1992, US Patent 5,120,420.
4. Tang, Z; Lee, JH; Louie, RF; Kost, GJ. Effects of different hematocrits on glucose measurements with handheld glucose meters for point-of-care testing. Arch Pathol Lab Med. 2000, manuscript accepted for publication.
5. Crismore, WF; Surridge, NA; McMinn, DR; Bodensteiner, RJ; Diebold, ER; Delk, RD; Burke, DW; Ho, JJ; Earl, RK; Heald, BA. Electrochemical Biosensor Test Strip. Dec. 7, 1999, US Patent 5,997,817.
6. Kuhn, L. Biosensors: blockbuster or bomb? Interface. 1998, 7(4), 26–31.
7. Bard, AJ; Faulkner, LR. Electrochemical Methods. Wiley, New York 1980, Ch 5.
8. Roser, BJ. Protection of Proteins and the Like. Jan. 2, 1990, US Patent 4,891,319.
9. Charlton, SC; Johnson, LD; Musho, MK. Electrochemical Biosensor. Aug. 25, 1998, US Patent 5,798,031.
10. For the FastTake strips this temperature category was set at 18°C to avoid excessive meter-generated errors due to low temperature.
11. Due to the limitations of reportable range of the handheld systems, target [glucose] was 450 mg/dL for 20% and 30% HCT samples and 500 mg/dL for other samples.
12. Clarke WL, et. al. Evaluating clinical accuracy of systems for self-monitoring of blood glucose. Diabetes Care. 1987, 10, 622–628.
13. Gough DA, Botvinick, EL. Reservations on the use of error grid analysis for the validation of blood glucose assays. Diabetes Care. 1997, 20, 1034–1035.
14. The exception to this normalization was Precision G, where the spread between data even within the claimed % HCT/temperature range was so large that we had to use only the room-temperature 45% HCT data to normalize the whole data set.

3

Redox Monomers and Polymers for Biosensors

Naim Akmal
The Dow Chemical Company, South Charleston, West Virginia, U.S.A.

Arthur M. Usmani
Altec USA, Indianapolis, Indiana, U.S.A.

I. INTRODUCTION

Biosensors are relatively new to the field of diagnostic reagents. Despite advances in biosensors, dry chemistry dominates and may continue to dominate as the primary choice for analyte detection in body fluids, e.g., blood. The main reason is economics. Dry reagents are much less expensive than biosensors, both in developmental and manufacturing costs. Essentially, a biosensor is a device that incorporates a bioactive substance, e.g., an enzyme or antibody that specifically recognizes an analyte, in contact with a transduction system.

In the early 1960s, a promising approach to glucose monitoring was developed in the form of an enzyme electrode that used oxidation of glucose by the enzyme glucose oxidase (GOD)[1]. At that time, it was anticipated that the enzyme electrode would replace dry reagent for blood glucose determination. Dry chemistry was in its infancy at that time. The approach was incorporated into a few clinical analyzers for blood glucose determination.

In this work we report scale-up of a redox polymer known by its common name, Polymer 6/1, as well as synthesis of Os-containing redox monomers useful for fourth-generation biosensors. We will also discuss useful backbones for attachment of Os. Additionally, we report biosensor coatings from redox monomers and why they act much like the polymer coatings. Enzymes are polymeric in nature but are not film formers. A polymer is essential to make the biosensor coating that can be applied onto a working electrode.

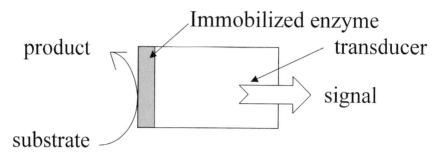

Figure 1   Schematic of a biosensor.

II. HISTORICAL AND BIOSENSOR TYPES

The schematic of a basic biosensor is shown in Figure 1. Tranducers, ranked in order of importance are electrochemical, optical, mass (piezoelectric), electrochemical/optical combination, and calometric (enzyme thermistor). Electrochemical biosensors are of the amperometric, conductometric, and impedimetric types. Commercially, the amperometric type is by far the most important. Fluorescence, absorbance, SPR, evanescent wave, diffraction grating, and ellipsometry methods are important concepts in optical biosensors. Electrochemiluminescence and light addressable potentiometrics are examples of electrochemical and optical combination transduction.

Applications of biosensors are in the medical and clinical, industrial, defense, environmental, agricultural, and remote-sensing areas. The estimated 1998 worldwide sales for biosensors are given in Table 1.

Table 1   Estimated 1998 Market for Biosensors

Application	Sales in $M
Medical/clinical	300
Industrial	350
Defense	150
Environmental	175
Agricultural	50
Remote-Sensing	15
Others	20
Total	1060

Gene probe and gene chip technology should grow at a quantum pace in the near future. In 1998, this market was $125 million; the current market is projected to be around $600 million and is expected to jump to about $2.7 billion by 2005.

III. CHEMISTRY

In 1962, Clark devised the first glucose sensor based on an oxygen electrode [1]:

$$\text{Glucose} + O_2 \xrightleftharpoons{\text{Glucose oxidase}} \text{Gluconic acid} + H_2O_2$$

$$O_2 + 2H_2O_2 + 4e^- \xrightarrow[-0.65\ V]{\text{Pt cathode}} 4OH^-$$

Subsequently, in 1970, Clark developed the second-generation biosensor, based on peroxide measurement. This is the basis of the YSI glucose analyzer:

$$H_2O_2 \xrightarrow[+0.6\ V]{\text{Pt anode}} 2H^+ + O_2 + 4e^-$$

The limitation of Clark's biosensors is interference from other elecroactive species present in blood at high applied overpotentials. In 1984, Hill described the third-generation glucose biosensor, utilizing a synthetic mediator. This is the basis of the Medisense ExacTech and QID glucose monitors:

$$\text{GOD-FAD} + \text{Glucose} \rightleftharpoons \text{GOD-FAD}_2 + \text{Gluconic acid}$$

$$\text{GOD-FAD}_2 + \text{Med}_{(oxidized)} \rightleftharpoons \text{GOD-FAD} + \text{Med}_{(reduced)}$$

$$\text{Med}_{(reduced)} \rightleftharpoons \text{Med}_{(oxidized)} + e^-$$

The fourth-generation biosensors are based on redox polymers and associated redox monomers. The current fourth-generation biosensor takes advantage of the fact that the biochemical reaction takes place in two steps. The GOD enzyme is reduced by glucose, and then the reduced enzyme is oxidized by an electron acceptor, i.e., a mediator, for example, a redox polymer. Direct electron transfer between GOD, an insulator polymer, and the electrode occurs extremely slowly. Therefore an electron acceptor mediator is required to make the electrochemical reaction rapid and effective [2].

The detection methods just described for glucose biosensors are summarized in Figure 2.

Buck of the University of North Carolina at Chapel Hill has used thin films and photolithographic techniques to microfabricate arrays of ISE on flexi-

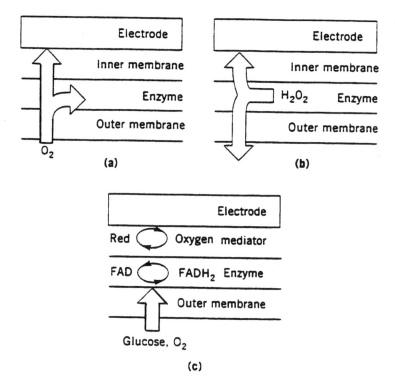

Figure 2 Detection methods for glucose biosensors based on (a) oxygen, (b) hydrogen peroxide, and (c) a mediator.

bile substrate, e.g., Kapton (polyimide). Researchers are now applying technique, e.g., photolithography and silicon micromachining, used in the integrated circuit (IC) industry to develop miniature biosensors. An example of a silicon-based biosensor is i-STAT. This is a handheld clinical analyzer that uses disposable cartridges based on biosensor technology. The six-parameter disposable cartridge contains a mixed multianalyte sensor array fabricated on two separate silicon chips (4×7 and 4×4 mm). It performs six simultaneous assays in less than 120 sec.

IV. REDOX POLYMERIC SYSTEMS

Some exploratory and developmental work has been done on redox polymers that can rapidly and effectively shuttle the electrons. Okamoto and coworkers, at Polytech University developed a family of redox polymers based on flexible polysiloxanes to which they attached mediators, e.g., ferrocene [3,4]. Okamoto's redox polymers provide excellent communication between GOD's redox centers and the electrode. Furthermore, these redox polymers are stable and nondiffusing.

Heller and coworkers at the University of Texas at Austin were successful in attaching an enzyme to the electrode using a long-chain polymer having a dense array of electron relays. The polymer that penetrates and binds the enzyme is also bound to the electrode.

Heller et al. worked on osmium-containing polymers. A number of such polymers were experimented and evaluated [5,6]. A stable and reproducible redox polymer of this kind is a poly(4-vinyl pyridine) (PVP) to which Os(bpy) 2Cl$_2$ (where bpy = 2,2'-bipyridine) has been attached to one-sixth of the pendant groups. The resultant redox polymer is water insoluble and is made biologically compatible by partial quaternization of the remaining pyridine groups using 2-bromoethyl amine. This redox polymer is called Polymer 6/1 (Fig. 3). The quaternized amine groups can react with a water-soluble epoxy, e.g., polyethylene glycol diglycidyl ether, and GOD to produce a cross-linked biosensor coating film. Such biosensor coating films produce high current densities and a linear response to glucose up to 600 mg/dL. The use of water-soluble epoxy in biosensor coatings is not necessary, as demonstrated by Usmani [7].

Usmani et al. scaled up and refined the synthesis and application of osmium polymers. Osmium monomers that also shuttle electrons much like the polymer have been made by Usmani [7]. Such osmium monomers can associate with carboxylated polymers to give stability and nondiffusing characteristics. A

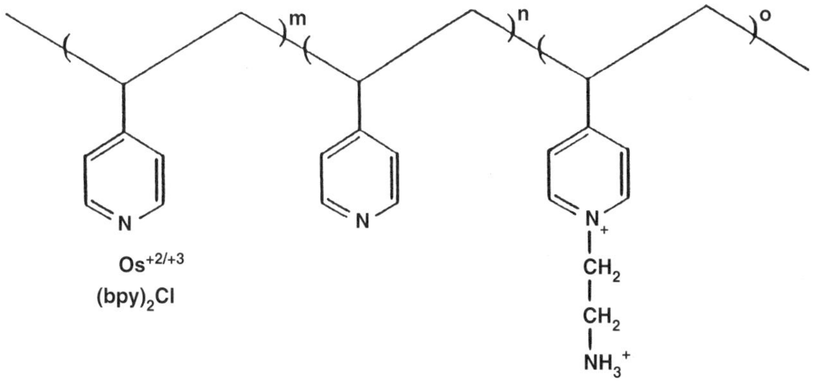

Figure 3 Structure of osmium-containing Polymer 6/1.

schematic of the Os polymer-GOD or Os monomer-carboxylated polymer-GOD hydrogel films is shown in Figure 4 [8].

V. SYNTHETIC STEPS IN POLYMER AND MONOMER SYNTHESIS AND SCALE-UP

Osmium-containing polymers, e.g., Polymer 6/1, are highly stable and produce high current density and an excellent dynamic range. The structure of Polymer 6/1 is shown in Figure 3.

The polymer or monomer synthesis involves the following steps.

1. Selection of heterocyclic (N) monomer or polymer
2. Preparation of $Os(bpy)_2Cl_2$ or other complexing intermediate
3. Complexation
4. Quaternization
5. Recovery and cleaning

A. Scale-Up of Polymer 6/1

Poly(4-vinyl pyridine) is commercially available as a 20% solution in methanol. The recovery of the solid PVP is shown in Figure 5. Figure 6 presents a flow-sheet for preparation of $Os(bpy)_2Cl_2$. We wish to point out that the intermediate precursor, K_2OsCl_6, is rather expensive and that the workup is also tedious. The flow diagram for the complexation and quaternization is given in Figure 7. Again, the recovery of Polymer 6/1 from its solution in DMF and ethylene glycol takes lots of nonsolvent acetone. Therefore, handling of the precipitation step is cumbersome.

B. Characterization of Polymer 6/1

The characterization of Polymer 6/1 is difficult due to the charges, the functional pendant groups, and the overall complex nature of the polymer's structure. We developed the methods, however [7]. Applicable methods are shown in Table 2.

C. Modified Polymer 6/1

Polymer 6/1 has several shortcomings. The glass transition temperature is high and the biosensor coatings are rather brittle. This brittleness can result in de-bonding of the biosensor coating films from the electrode surface. The brittle-ness and debonding is best solved by internal flexibilization of the polymer backbone. Vinyl pyridine polymer was flexibilized by monomers, e.g., butyl

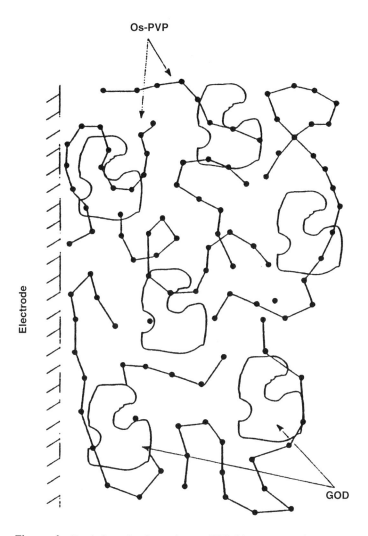

Figure 4   Depiction of redox polymer-GOD biosensor coating.

methacrylate (BMA), 2-hydroxyethyl methacrylate (HEMA), and 2-hydroxye-
thyl acrylate (HEA). In addition to flexibilizing, our objective was to use elec-
tron-donating groups to reduce the relatively high redox potential ($E_{1/2}$) of Polymer 6/1. The $E_{1/2}$ of Polymer 6/1 is about 230 mV. This may result in interference
in blood glucose measurement by interfering substances, e.g., uric acid, ascorbic
acid, etc.

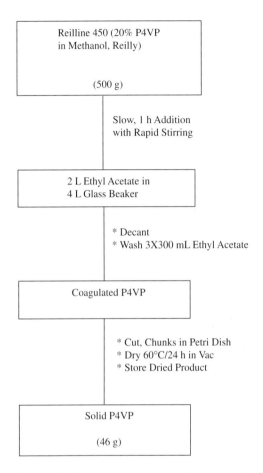

Reilline 450 (20% P4VP
in Methanol, Reilly)

(500 g)

Slow, 1 h Addition
with Rapid Stirring

2 L Ethyl Acetate in
4 L Glass Beaker

* Decant
* Wash 3X300 mL Ethyl Acetate

Coagulated P4VP

* Cut, Chunks in Petri Dish
* Dry 60°C/24 h in Vac
* Store Dried Product

Solid P4VP

(46 g)

Figure 5   Recovery of starting polymer, poly(4-vinyl pyridine) (P4VP).

We made the starting copolymers and the modified Polymer 6/1 therefrom. The results are summarized in Table 3.

We thus find that copolymerizing 4-vinyl pyridine affords wide latitude in the synthesis of redox polymers.

D. Redox Monomer Synthesis

The monomer synthesis involves the same steps as the polymer synthesis. The reaction conditions are less rigorous, however. The synthesis—specifically, cleaning and recovery of the monomer—is much easier. The structure of a typical redox osmium monomer is shown in Figure 8.

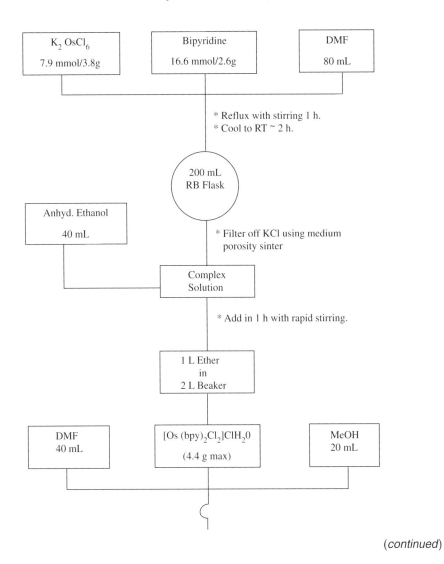

Figure 6 Scale-up of complexing intermediate.

(*continued*)

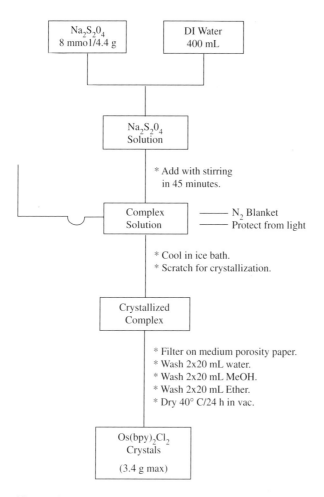

Figure 6 Continued.

During the 1980s, Murray and his students at North Carolina made certain redox compounds. These compounds are an academic curiosity, since they are not suitable to prepare redox coatings for glucose biosensors. The redox monomers that we synthesized are shown in Table 4.

All synthesized redox monomers are saturated except those made with vinyl pyridine (VP) and vinyl imidazole (VIM). Saturated monomers will not polymerize by free radical polymerization. The vinylic redox monomers will be highly resistant to free radical polymerization. Low-temperature initiators, e.g.,

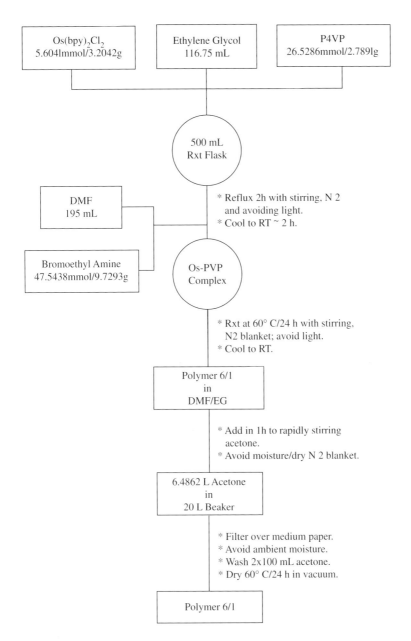

Figure 7 Complexation, quaternization, and recovery of Polymer 6/1.

Table 2 Characterization Methods for Os-Containing Polymers

Parameter[a]	What measured	Primary method	Secondary methods
α_C	% Os	ICP	AA, EDAX, XRD
α_Q	% Amine	NMR	Nonaqueous Titration
Molecular weights	M_n, M_w, d	GPC	

[a]α_C is degree of Os complexation; α_Q is degree of quaternization.

Table 3 Modified Polymer 6/1

Polymer precursor	Performance
4-Vinyl pyridine (VP) (100/0) (Polymer 6/1)	Brittle: biosensor coating may debond
VP/BMA (75/25)	Flexible; biosensor coatings have good adhesion
VP/Styrene (75/25)	Gel-like; intractable; no good
VP/HEMA (75/25)	Flexible; lower $E_{1/2}$
VP/HEA (75/25)	Flexible

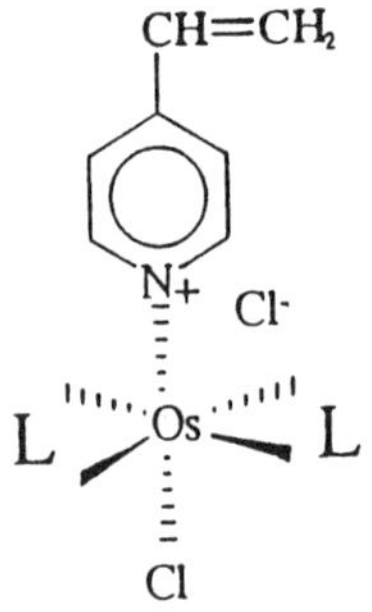

where L = 2,2'-dipyridyl, 1,10-phenanthroline,
4,4'-dimethyl-2,2'-dipyridyl.

Figure 8 Structure of an osmium redox monomer.

Table 4 Typical Os-Containing Redox Monomers

Monomer	Complexing compound	Redox monomer
4-Vinyl pyridine	$Os(bpy)_2Cl_2$	$Os(bpy)_2Cl.VP^+X^-$
Vinyl imidazole (VIM)	$Os(diMebpy)_2Cl_2$	$Os(diMebpy)_2Cl.VIM^+X^-$
VIM	$Os(bpy)_2Cl_2$	$Os(bpy)_2Cl.VIM^+X^-$
Imidazole (IM)	$Os(bpy)_2Cl_2$	$Os(bpy)_2Cl.IM^+X^-$
VIM	$Os(1,10\ Phen)_2Cl_2$	$Os(1,10\ Phen)_2Cl.VIM^+X^-$
2,4,6-Collidine (CLD)	$Os(bpy)_2Cl_2$	$Os(bpy)_2Cl.CLD^+X^-$
3,3-Oxybismethylpyridine (OMP)	$Os(bpy)_2Cl_2$	$Os(bpy)_2Cl.OMP^+X^-$
3,3-Oxybismethylpyridine (OMP)	$Os(diMebpy)_2Cl_2$	$Os(diMebpy)_2Cl.OMP^+X^-$

benzoyl peroxide, will produce incomplete conversion at 120°C. Polymerization maybe driven to completion by a high-temperature initiator, e.g., dicumyl peroxide. These monomers copolymerize with other neutral monomers. Based on our prior work, these vinyl monomers will photopolymerize by UV and electron beam (EB).

Because of the chain transfer, the molecular weight is low, around 5,000. These low-molecular-weight redox polymers can be used to develop biosensor coatings. This is not a good approach, however.

E. Biosensor Coatings from Redox Monomers

The redox monomers are small compounds and will not be nondiffusing unless they are somehow immobilized via a suitable method. The redox monomer is a quaternized base. A polyacid will interact with the base and will immobilize the redox monomer. In a similar vein, the redox polymer, a polyelectrolyte (polybase), will complex with an acidic polymer (polyacid) to give a polyelectrolyte complex. The generalized association of a redox monomer with a polyacid is shown in Figure 9.

F. Advantages of Redox Monomers over Polymers

The are many advantages of redox monomers over polymers in the development of biosensor coatings. Nonvinylic heterocylic monomers can be used to prepare redox monomers. It is easier to make monomers than polymers with higher yields.

Precise loading of Os, at will, is possible with the monomer. There are three cases:

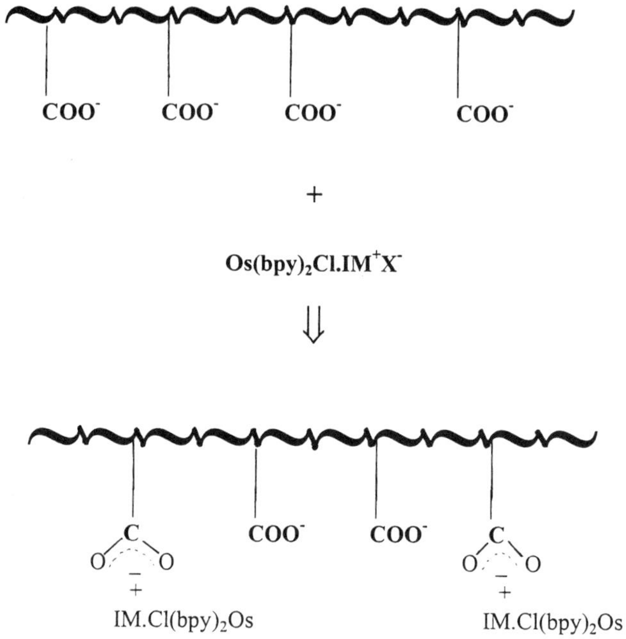

Figure 9 Association of redox monomer with polyacid.

Case 1: $[COO^-] > [N^+]$ Pendant Os spacing
Case 2: $[COO^-] = [N^+]$ 1:1 Salt
Case 3: $[COO^-] < [N+]$ Salt + free monomer

The ionic linkages of association provide high water solubility and therefore better biological compatibility. Furthermore, it is easier to regulate biosensor coating film properties than when a redox polymer is used in the coating. Another advantage is easy manufacture and characterization.

G.   Useful Polyacid Binders

These include vinyl ether/maleic anhydride copolymers, styrene/maleic anhydride (SMA), highly carboxylated acrylic polymers with a degree of neutralization from 0.0 to 1.0, HEMA/methacrylic acid copolymers, and HEA/acrylic acid copolymers.

Table 5 Typical Biosensor Coating Formulation

Polyacid binder	20.0 g
Os monomer	6.0 g
Glucose oxidase	4.0 g

H. Biosensor Coatings

A typical biosensor coating formulation is shown in Table 5.

The dose response curve for an vinyl osmium monomer attached to a vinyl ether/maleic anhydride copolymer is given in Figure 10. In a similar vein, a biosensor coating from vinyl osmium monomer and HEMA/metharylic acid

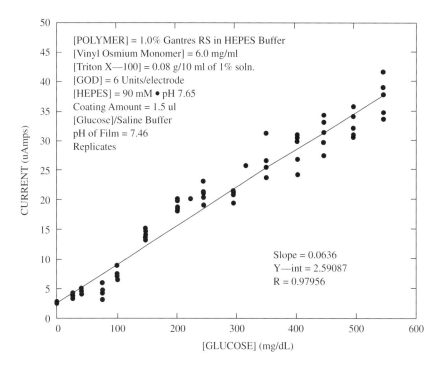

Figure 10 Glucose dose response for Os monomer/(VE/MA) biosensor coating film.

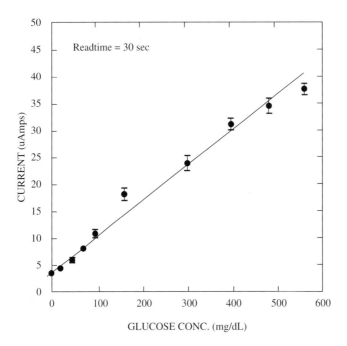

Figure 11 Glucose dose response for Os-monomer/(HEMA/MAA) coating film.

(50/50) with a 0.25 degree of NaOH neutralization was made. The dose response is given in Figure 11.

VI. CONCLUSIONS

We have synthesized a new family of Os-containing redox monomers. Redox monomers from 4-vinyl pyridine, vinyl imidazole (VIM), and imidazole (IM) were made. The redox potential of monomers from IM and VIM was substantially lower; hence, biosensor coatings made from these monomers should not experience interference from substances such as ascorbic acid, uric acid, and Tylenol. The Os monomers are quaternary base and hence associate with polyacids. Useful polyacids are HEMA/methacrylic copolymers and vinyl ether/maleic anhydride copolymers. The associated polymer is too large and hence very stable and nondiffusing. The characterization and manufacture of the redox monomers are much simpler than for the redox polymers.

The use of redox monomers along with polyacids produces biosensor coatings superior to those made from redox polymers.

The novel redox monomers and polymers that we report have not yet found commercial acceptance. The Os precursor to make the redox monomers should be researched for cost reduction. Applications of these monomers and polymers should be investigated not only in medical diagnostic biosensors but in other areas as well.

REFERENCES

1. L. C. Clark and C. Lyons. Ann. N.Y. Acad. Sci. 102, 29 (1962).
2. G. Reach and G. S. Wilson. Anal. Chem. 64, 381A (1992).
3. H. I. Karan, H. L. Lan, and Y. Okamoto. In A. M. Usmani and N. Akmal (eds.). Diagnostic Biosensor Polymers. ACS Books, Washington, DC, 1994.
4. Y. Okamoto et al. Poly. Mater. Sci. Eng. 64, 332 (1991).
5. B. A. Gregg and A. Heller. J. Phy. Chem. 95, 5970 (1991).
6. A. Heller et al. In: A. M. Usmani and N. Akmal (eds.). Diagnostic Biosensor Polymers. ACS Books, Washington, DC, 1994.
7. A. M. Usmani. Biosensor and Sensor Symposium. Orlando American Chemical Society Meeting, 1996.
8. A. M. Usmani. In: Kirk-Othmer Encyclopedia of Chemical Technology, Vol 16. Wiley, New York, 1995.

4

Amperometric Microcells for Diagnostic Enzyme Activity Measurements

Robert E. Gyurcsányi
Budapest University of Technology and Economics, Budapest, Hungary

Géza Nagy and Livia Nagy
University of Pécs, Pécs, Hungary

Alessandra Cristalli
Novel GmbH, Münich, Germany

Michael R. Neuman and Ernö Lindner
The University of Memphis, Memphis, Tennessee, U.S.A.

Richard P. Buck*
University of North Carolina at Chapel Hill, Chapel Hill, North Carolina, U.S.A.

H. Troy Nagle and Stefan Ufer
North Carolina State University, Raleigh, North Carolina, U.S.A.

I. INTRODUCTION

Bacterial vaginosis (BV) is a polymicrobial, primarily anaerobic infection asso-ciated with a high risk of premature rupture of amniotic membrane and preterm birth. It has been postulated as a possible cause of pelvic inflammatory disease, which could result in infertility. Bacterial vaginosis is the most common type of vaginal infection. Up to 20% of women visiting gynecology clinics, about 15% of pregnant women, and 35% of women visiting sexually transmitted dis-ease clinics are found to have BV [1,2]. The most widely accepted clinical

---

*Retired.

criteria for diagnosis include three of the following four criteria: a vaginal pH of greater than 4.5, the presence of clue cells (vaginal epithelial cells that are coated with *Gardnerella vaginalis* or other infective organisms in the vagina) in the vaginal fluid, a milky homogeneous vaginal discharge, and the release of an amine (fishy) odor after the addition of 10% potassium hydroxide to the vaginal fluid [3].

Laboratory tests to detect microbial products in the vaginal fluid of women having bacterial vaginosis include the detection of amines (putrescine, cadaverine, and trimethylamine) [4], the measurement of the relative levels of succinate (metabolic product of anaerobic bacteria) and lactate by gas chromatography [5], and the determination of sialidases [6] in the vaginal fluid [7].

In recent years we have been interested in the simple and cost-effective electrochemical detection of metabolites associated with bacterial vaginosis. A miniature biosensor [8] and a simple flow-injection assay [9] have been developed for the determination of diamines in the vaginal fluid. However, leaking amniotic fluid may interfere with the diamine determination. It contains increased levels of diamine oxidase (E.C.1.4.3.6.) enzyme activity during pregnancy [10,11]. This increased diamine oxidase activity in the vaginal fluid can be used to detect the rupture of fetal membranes in the absence of vaginal bleeding [12]. A microfabricated, amperometric microcell [13] was developed by our group for the putrescine oxidase (PO) assay [14] in samples of a few microliters. Unfortunately, the diamines in the vaginal discharge of BV patients interfere with the PO determination, because the putrescine oxidase enzyme interferes with the diamine determination.

Proline iminopeptidase (PIP) is an enzyme, produced by bacteria, found in the vaginal fluid of women with BV. It catalyzes the hydrolysis of the amide bonds between L-proline and a peptide residue, aminoacid, or other chemicals attached to the proline with amino groups. The PIP activity can be determined by measuring the reactants or the products of the enzyme-catalyzed reaction. In the spectrophotometric PIP assay, L-proline β-naphthylamide (Prol β-NA) (Scheme 1) [18–20], L-proline *p*-nitroanilide (Scheme 2) [21], and L-Pro-4-(phenylazo) phenylamide [22] are used as enzyme substrates. The colorimetric assays of proline iminopeptidase were reported as a sensitive laboratory method for diagnosing BV [15–17]. The large difference in the PIP activity levels for BV-positive and -negative samples makes the method very reliable [17]. However, the products of the enzymatic hydrolysis of the preceding substrates (β-naphthylamine, *p*-nitroaniline, phenylazophenylamine) can also be measured electrochemically.

This chapter is a general presentation of our recent work in the detection of putrescine oxidase and proline iminopeptidase enzyme activity measurements, with an emphasis on the electrochemical assay of the proline iminopeptidase. In this work we describe a cost-effective thick-film technology for the fabrication of the amprometric microcell with screen-printed graphite or platinum electrodes for proline iminopeptidase and putrescine oxidase assays, respectively.

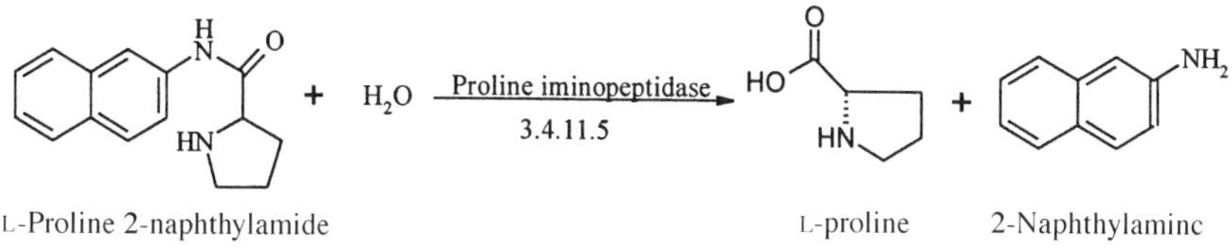

L-Proline 2-naphthylamide   L-proline   2-Naphthylamine

Scheme 1

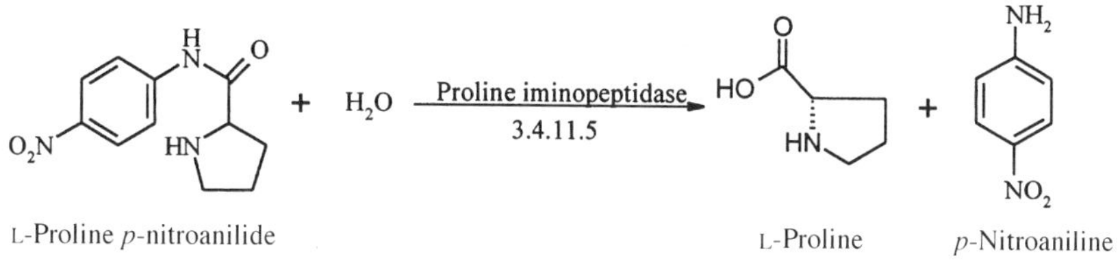

L-Proline *p*-nitroanilide   L-Proline   *p*-Nitroaniline

Scheme 2

II.   EXPERIMENTAL SECTION

A.   Chemicals

Putrescine oxidase (EC 1.4.3.10) from microorganism and Proline iminopeptidase (EC 3.1.11.5) from *Bacillus coagulans* were purchased from Toyobo Co.
Ltd. (Tokyo) and Sigma Chemicals Co. (St. Louis), respectively. L-Proline, β-
naphthylamide hydrochloride, L-proline *p*-nitroanilide trifluoroacetate, β-naphthylamine, *p*-nitroaniline, putrescine dihydrochloride, and bovine serum albumin
(BSA) were all products of Sigma Chemical Co. (St. Louis). The medical-grade
aliphatic polyurethane (Tecoflex SG 85A) was a generous gift of Thermedics
(Woburn, MA). All other chemicals were purchased from Fluka (Buchs, Switzerland) and were of analytical grade. The solutions were prepared with Milli-
Q Gradient A10 system (Millipore Corp, Bedford, MA) water.

B.   Fabrication of the Screen-Printed Electrodes

The sequentially printed layers and the final design of the amperometric microcell are shown in Figure 1. The cells were manufactured on a laser-scribed alumina
substrate (Coors Ceramic, Grand Junction, CO). The 114.3-mm × 114.3-mm-
size, 0.635-mm-thick wafer can accommodate 60 individual cells (9 mm × 22
mm). The single cells were easily separated along the laser-scribed lines. A
model MC810-C (C.W. Price Co., Bloomsbury, NJ) screen printer was used to
deposit the thick film layers through stainless steel wire mesh screens. First the
alumina wafers were cleaned in an ultrasonic bath for 10 minutes in detergent

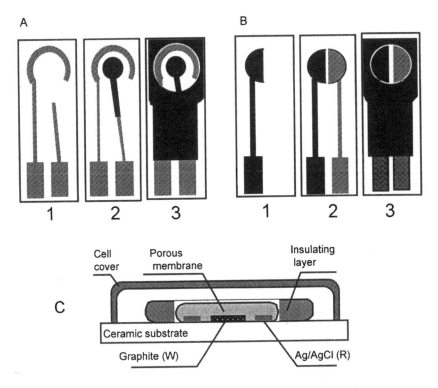

Figure 1 Printed patterns (A and B) and the cross-sectional profile of the amperometric microcell (C). **A:** The printed patterns of the cell with graphite working electrode. (1) silver electrode and connection pads, (2) deposition of the graphite over the silver pattern, (3) final structure with the insulation layer. **B:** The printed patterns of the cell with Pt working (1) platinum electrode; (2) silver electrode, (3) final structure with the insulation layer.

solution, acetone, and methanol, respectively. After each cleaning step, the wafers were rinsed with DI water, acetone, and methanol, respectively.

C. Graphite Electrodes

A silver layer was deposited onto the alumina surface to form the electrical contacts and the internal reference electrode (Fig. 1A1). A Metech 3571 silver ink (Metech, Inc., Elverson, PA) was used in combination with a 325-mesh-count/inch screen (Microcircuit Engineering Corp., Mount Holly, NJ). The silver layer was fired for 9 minutes in a programmable muffle furnace at a peak temperature of 850°C. Next the graphite layer was deposited to form the working electrode surface (Fig. 1A2). A C10903D14 graphite ink (Gwent Electronic Materials Ltd., Pontypool, UK) was screen printed using a 200-mesh-count/inch stainless steel screen and a Fivestar (Autotype Americas, Schaumburg, IL) photodefinable mask. After the printed ink leveled for 10 min at room temperature, the layer was dried in an oven at 80°C for 30 minutes. Finally, up to five layers of a thick-film UV-curable dielectric (type 5018, Dupont, Research Triangle Park, NC) was printed through a 200-mesh screen to form the reaction well and to insulate the conductive paths of the electrodes (Fig. 1A3). Each layer was cured separately under a UV lamp (Model XX-15A, Spectronics Corp., Westbury, NY) for 15 minutes after the ink was allowed to level for 10 minutes at room temperature. The thickness of the layers was determined with a profiler (Alpha-Step 500, KLA-Tencor, San Jose, CA). The thickness of the silver and of the graphite layers was about 10 and 16.6 μm, respectively. The insulating layer thickness (the well depth) was 118.1 ± 8.4 μm ($N = 9$).

D. Platinum Electrodes

First a platinum layer was printed onto the alumina surface using a platinum ink (Heraeus Inc., West Conshohocken, PA) and a 325-mesh-count/inch screen (Fig. 1B1). A single wet printing mode was used. The platinum layer was allowed to level on the alumina substrate for 10 min at room temperature. After drying at 150°C for 10 min, the platinum layer (7.4 μm thick) was fired in a programmable muffle furnace at 1050°C for 12 min. For printing the silver layer, the procedure was identical with the one described for the fabrication of the screen-printed graphite electrodes (Fig. 1B2). Finally, a glass-ceramic insulating layer (type 7600A, Metech, Inc.) was printed through a 200-mesh-count/inch screen using a double wet printing mode (Fig. 1B3). Four layers were deposited before firing. Each layer was allowed to level at room temperature for 10 minutes and then dried in an oven at 150°C for 10 minutes. After deposition of all the layers, the electrodes were fired at a peak temperature of 850°C for 7 minutes.

E. Preparation of the Amperometric Microcell

In both kinds of amperometric microcells (platinum and graphite working electrode) the silver layer was electrochemically chloridized in order to create the Ag/AgCl reference electrodes [23]. To provide size-exclusion-based permselectivity for amperometric hydrogen peroxide detection, an electrochemically formed, thin poly(m-phenylenediamine) film was deposited on the surface of the platinum screen-printed electrodes [9, 24]. The platinum electrodes were placed in 0.01 M phenylenediamine solution in 0.1 M phosphate buffer of pH = 7.2. Cyclic voltammetric scans were made in an 0.2-V to 0.8-V potential range versus Ag/AgCl at a 2-mV/sec scan rate. The electrodes were individually tested in 4 mM potassium hexacyanoferrate (1 M KCl background electrolyte). They were accepted if they exhibited featureless cyclic voltammograms in a potential range of 0–0.6V (max 5% increase in the background current). Finally, a small circular disk (Ø = 5.5 mm) of absorbent paper (Kimwipes EX-L delicate task wiper) was introduced in the well delimited by the insulation layer (Fig. 1C).

F. Measurement Procedure

The procedure for measuring the enzyme activity was the same as described in our earlier paper [13]. All substrate and enzyme solutions were prepared using the following buffer solutions: 0.1 M Tris pH = 7.3, 0.1% BSA for PIP and 0.1 M PBS pH = 7.2, 0.1% BSA, 7g/L NaCl for PO activity measurements. Five to 10 µL of enzyme substrate solution was injected onto the paper disk by a Hamilton micro-syringe, and +0.6 V was applied between the working and the reference electrodes, with simultaneous recording of the current (Model 283 Potentiostat/Galvanostat, EG&G Instruments, Princeton Applied Research, Oak Ridge, TN). The cell was covered with a small vial cap to avoid solution evaporation. After the transient current decayed (~3 minutes), 2–10 µL enzyme solution was added and the current–time curves recorded. The initial slopes of the curves were determined and plotted as a function of the enzyme activity.

III. RESULTS AND DISCUSSION

A. Electrochemical Characterization of the System

Both L-proline β-naphthylamide and L-proline p-nitroanilide can be used as substrates in the PIP-catalyzed enzymatic reaction (Schemes 1 and 2). The cyclic voltammograms of the resulting products, p-nitroaniline and β-naphthylamine, are shown in Figure 2.

The curves were recorded with the screen-printed graphite electrodes in 5 mL 5×10^{-4} M solutions (pH = 7.3 Tris buffer, 0.1% BSA). β-Naphtylamine is oxidized on significantly smaller potential (0.6 V vs Ag/AgCl) on the screen-printed graphite electrode than p-nitroaniline (1 V vs Ag/AgCl)). Also, β-naphthylamine can be determined at higher sensitivity than p-nitroaniline. During their electrochemical oxidation, both substrates form resistive surface films that resulted in the decrease of the oxidation current in consecutive scans. Fortunately the electrode surface can efficiently be restored if β-naphthylamine oxidation is followed by a simple washing step with methanol, as is shown in Figure 3. The enzyme substrates (L-proline β-naphthylamide and L-proline p-nitroanilide) do not show electroactivity on the graphite electrode in this potential win-

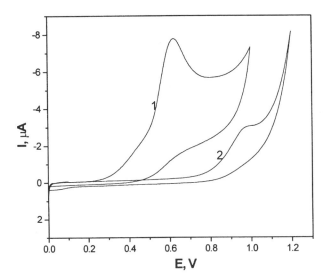

Figure 2 Cyclic voltammograms of 0.5 mM β-naphthylamine (1) and p-nitroaniline (2) in pH = 7.3 Tris buffer solution (0.1% BSA) at 20 mV/sec scan rate. The screen-printed graphite and the electrochemically chloridized Ag/AgCl electrodes were used as working and reference electrodes, respectively.

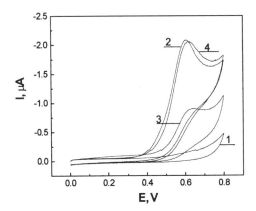

Figure 3 Consecutive scans with the screen-printed graphite electrode in 10^{-4} M β-naphthylamine in 0.1 M, pH = 7.30 Tris buffer (0.1% BSA) solution. (1) background electrolyte; (2) first scan; (3) fifth scan, and (4) scan after cleaning the electrode surface with methanol. Scan rate 20 mV/sec.

dow (not shown). This is an elemental requirement for the selective determination of the products of the enzymatic reaction. Since the oxidation of β-naphthylamine can be made at lower potentials and higher sensitivities than that of the p-nitroaniline and because the electrode surface could easily be renewed after its oxidation, L-prolyl-β-naphthylamide was used as enzyme substrate in the electrochemical PIP assays. However, the calibration curves of β-naphthylamine were linear only in the micromolar range, with a detection limit of 5×10^{-7} M (Fig. 4). At higher concentrations the sensitivity decreased, and no stable steady-state conditions could be established, due to the electrode fouling.

B. Proline Iminopeptidase Activity Measurements

The screen-printed amperometric microcell was tested for PIP enzyme activity determinations in a wide enzyme activity range: 10 mU/mL to 850 mU/mL. Generally, 10 μL of enzyme solution was added to 5 μL of substrate solution of 1 mg/mL concentration. Typical current–time recordings and the calibration curves for three individual microcells are shown in Figure 5. The initial slopes of the transients are proportional with the enzyme activity and were used for the evaluation. Each curve in Figure 5 or each point on a selected calibration curve in the Fig. 5 inset was determined with a new paper disk and a new aliquot of substrate solution; i.e., the porous membrane was replaced and the cell was washed with methanol and distilled water between measurements. The three parallel calibration curves in the Fig. 5 inset were determined with three individual cells. The slopes of the calibration curves (sensitivity) ranged between -0.0195 and -0.0203 $\mu A \cdot mL \cdot mU^{-1} \cdot min^{-1}$ (coefficient of variation = 2.2%).

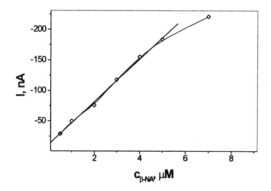

Figure 4   Calibration of β-naphthylamine. Background electrolyte: 0.1 M Tris buffer, pH = 7.3 (0.1% BSA), working electrode potential 0.6 V vs. Ag/AgCl

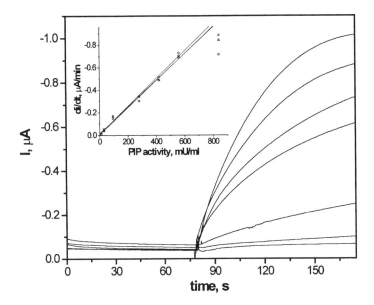

Figure 5 PIP response of the amperometric microcell with screen-printed graphite working electrode at different enzyme activity levels and the resulting calibration curves for 3 individual amperometric microcells (inset). The reaction volume consisted of 5 μL 1 mg/mL Prol-β-NA and 10 μL PIP solution, volume activity range 103–841.5 mU/mL.

The reproducibility of the single measurements depends on the enzyme activity level and the volume of the enzyme solution injected into the microcell. As expected, the scattering of data is larger at low enzyme activities. The coefficient of variation (CV) of parallel measurements in individual cells ($N = 3$) is almost an order of magnitude larger at low enzyme activities (24.1% and 17.1% at enzyme activities of 10.3 and 30.9 mU/mL, respectively) as compared to higher enzyme activities (2.8% and 3.3% at enzyme activities of 421.5 and 561.2 mU/mL, respectively). The use of larger volumes of enzyme solutions improves the coefficient of variation and the sensitivity of the method. The experiments made with 2 μL of enzyme solution show the highest uncertainty. However, there is no difference between the CVs when parallel measurements are made in one amperometric microcell ($N = 5$) or when each measurement was made in a new, separate cell ($N = 5$). Under optimal conditions the CV of the enzyme activity measurement hardly surpasses the CV of peak currents in the electrochemical surface determination.

C. Putrescine Oxidase Activity Measurements

Putrescine oxidase catalyzes the oxidation of diamines according to the following reaction scheme:

$$H_2N\text{-}(CH_2)_4NH_2 + O_2 + H_2O \quad \xrightarrow{\text{Putrescine oxidase}}$$

$$\text{Putrescine} \qquad\qquad H_2N\text{-}(CH_2)_3CHO + NH_3 + H_2O \qquad (3)$$
$$\text{4-Aminobutyraldehyde}$$

The generated hydrogen peroxide was detected amperometrically on the platinum working electrode. Typical current–time response curves following the addition of 10 μL PUO to 5 μL of substrate solution in the low-PUO activity range are shown in Figure 6. In order to avoid the gradual loss of enzymatic activity of the very dilute enzyme solutions, all solutions were freshly prepared from a 140 mU/mL stock solution. A detection limit of 3 mU/mL PO and a sensitivity of $6.2 \cdot 10^{-3}$ nA·mL·sec^{-1}·mU^{-1} could be achieved under the aforementioned experimental conditions. The sensitivity (the slope of the calibration

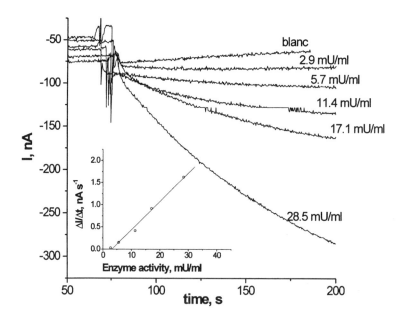

Figure 6   PO current–time response curves at different enzyme activity levels with the screen-printed platinum electrode and the resulting calibration curve. The reaction volume consisted of 5 μL 100 mM putrescine and 10 μL PO solution.

curves) of the putrescine determination with the screen-printed Pt electrodes was about five times larger than our published data with photolithographically prepared thin-film electrodes [14]. The difference in the sensitivity correlated well with the difference in electrochemical surface areas between the two types of electrodes. The detection limits were about the same with the two types of electrodes.

IV. CONCLUSION

The PIP activity in vaginal wash solutions ranges between 25 and 850 mU/mL [17]. The PIP calibrations were done at an even broader PIP activity range, between 10.3 and 841 mU/mL. The small coefficient of variation of the data suggests a reliable discrimination between PIP activities associated with negative (66 ± 41 mU/mL) and positive (704 ± 145 mU/mL) BV samples. Because the enzyme activity evaluation is based on the measurement of the initial slope of the current transients (at low concentration levels of the generated product), the electrode fouling does not significantly affect the reproducibility of the determinations.

ACKNOWLEDGMENTS

This work was supported by NSF/Whitaker Foundation Cost-Reducing Technologies Grant BES-950526 and by OTKA T 030968 grant from Hungary. The authors acknowledge the support of the Varga Jozsef Foundation.

REFERENCES

1. C. A. Spiegel. Clin Microbiol Rev 4:485 (1991).
2. D. A. Eschenbach. Am J Obstet Gynecol 169:441 (1993).
3. R. Amsel, P. A. Totten, C. A. Spiegel, K. C. Chen, D. Eschenbach, K. K. Holmes. Am J Med 74: 14 (1983).
4. K. C. Chen, R. Amsel, D. A. Eschenbach, K. K. Holmes. J Infect Dis 145:337 (1982).
5. C. A. Spiegel, R. Amsel, D. Eschenbach, F. Schoenknecht, K. K. Holmes. N Engl J Med 303:601 (1980).
6. A. M. Briselden, B. J. Moncla, C. E. Stevens, S. L. Hillier. J Clin Microbiol 30: 663 (1992).
7. G. B. Hill. Am J Obstet Gynecol 169:450 (1993).
8. C. X. Xu, S. A. Marzouk, V. V. Cosofret, R. P. Buck, M. R. Neuman, R. H. Sprinkle. Talanta 44:1625 (1997).

9. S. A. Marzouk, C. X. Xu, V. V. Cosofret, R. P. Buck, S. S. M. Hassan, M. R. Neuman, R. H. Sprinkle. Anal. Chim. Acta 363:57 (1998).
10. A. Tornqvist, F. Jonassen, P. Johnson, A. M. Fredholm. Acta Obstet Gynecol Scand 50:79 (1971).
11. N. Tryding, B. Willert. Scand J Clin Lab Invest 22:29 (1968).
12. W. A. Gahl, T. J. Kozina, D. D. Fuhrmann, A. M. Vale. Obstet Gynecol 60:297 (1982).
13. G. Nagy, C. X. Xu, R. P. Buck, E. Lindner, M. R. Neuman. Anal. Chem. 70:2156 (1998).
14. G. Nagy, C. X. Xu, V. V. Cosofret, E. Lindner, R. P. Buck, M. R. Neuman, R. H. Sprinkle. Talanta 47:367 (1998).
15. J. L. Thomason, S. M. Gelbart, P. J. Osypowski, A. K. Walt, P. R. Hamilton. Am J Obstet Gynecol 160:757 (1989).
16. J. L. Thomason, S. M. Gelbart, L. M. Wilcoski, A. K. Peterson, B. J. Jilly, P. R. Hamilton. Obstet Gynecol 71:607 (1988).
17. J. N. Schoonmaker, B. D. Lunt, D. W. Lawellin, J. I. French, S. L. Hillier, J. A. McGregor. Am J Obstet Gynecol 165:737 (1991).
18. S. P. Waters, H. J. Dalling. Plant. Physiol. 73:1048 (1983).
19. K. Ninomiya, K. Kawatani, S. Tanaka, S. Kawata, S. Makisumi. J Biochem (Tokyo) 92:413 (1982).
20. K. K. Makinen, S. A. Syed, P.-L. Makinen, W. J. Loesche. Curr Microbiol 14:341 (1987).
21. S. Fujimura, T. Nakamura, G. Pulverer. Zentralbl Bakteriol Mikrobiol Hyg 260: 175 (1985).
22. K. Senkpiel, H. Mayer. Hoppe-Seyler's Z Physiol Pflanz 166:7 (1974).
23. D. J. G. Ives, G. J. Janz. Reference Electrode. Theory and Practice. Academic Press, New York (1961).
24. S. A. Emr, A. M. Yacynich. Electroanalysis 7:913 (1995).

5

Flow-Through Immunoassay System for Rapid Clinical Diagnostics*

Ihab Abdel-Hamid
MesoSystems Technology Inc., Albuquerque, New Mexico, U.S.A.

Plamen Atanasov and Ebtisam Wilkins
University of New Mexico, Albuquerque, New Mexico, U.S.A.

Dmitri Ivnitski
New Mexico Technical University, Socorro, New Mexico, U.S.A.

I. INTRODUCTION

The range of analyte concentrations encountered in medical diagnostics and clinical chemistry is extremely large. This range has an upper limit greater than 10^{-3} M for analytes such as glucose and cholesterol and a lower limit less than 10^{-9} M for drugs and hormones. It is for the detection of these low-level analytes that the application of immunological techniques, and in particular immunoassays, is essential [1]. Immunoassay is an analytical method based on antigen–antibody interaction. Antibodies are protein molecules (produced by living animals) that recognize (bind to) certain very specific antigens at a molecular level. The ability of antibodies to form complexes with specific antigen molecules is the basis of immunoassays. Immunoassay is a specific and sensitive technique

*Based on a presentation by Ihab Abdel-Hamid at the Medical Diagnostic Reagents Symposium, ACS National Meeting, Boston, Massachusetts, August 23–27, 1998.

due to the high selectivity of antigen recognition and the high affinity of immunointeraction. Contemporary immunological techniques allow production of antibodies against a great number of antigens, and they enable immunoanalysis of
many substances [2]. Immunoassays are now well established as an essential
analytical technique in medical diagnostics, facilitating the measurement of an
increasing number of analytes of clinical significance, and are now routinely
used for the detection of small molecules such as drugs, through peptides, to
large macromolecules such as proteins, including antibodies, and whole cells [3].

Different immunoassay techniques can be categorized based on the principle
used to detect the immunointeraction. Most immunoassay techniques are based
on the separation of free and bound immunospecies. In these techniques, one of
the immunoagents (antigen or antibody) is immobilized on a solid carrier. The
immunointeraction then results in antigen–antibody complex formation on the
surface of the carrier, on a specific sites, when the latter is exposed to the immunoagent solution. Quantification of bound immunocomplex is conducted by using labels covalently bound to the immunoagent with specific properties suitable
for detection. The most common labels are radioactive isotopes, enzymes, or
fluorescent labels [4]. The final stage of immunoassay is the quantitative detection of the label.

Conventional immunoassay techniques have several factors that limit their
applicability, including: complexity of the assay process, lengthy analysis time,
requirement for highly skilled personnel, difficulty of automation of the assay,
and confinement of the assay to laboratory settings. This has resulted in a major
research effort being directed toward the development of alternative assay techniques that avoid these limitations.

A. Immunosensors

Immunosensors offer an attractive approach that attempts to avoid the traditional
limitations of conventional immunoassay techniques. In general, any immunosensor consists of a signal transducer and an interactive system employing principles of biological molecular recognition. Based on the nature of the physical
detection used in the transducer, immunosensing systems can be classified as
optical, gravimetric, and electrochemical.

In *optical* transducers, detection is based on light-sensitive elements. The
optical signal detection can be conducted by spectrophotometric, spectrofluorimet-
ric, chemiluminometric, reflectometric, or other, related techniques. There are
three main principles involved in the design of immunosensors based on optical
detection of the immunointeraction: label-free optical detection of immunointeraction, optical detection of labeled (usually a fluorescent label) immunospecies, optical detection of a product of an enzymatic reaction formed as a result of a
transformation catalyzed by an enzyme label. The most common principle is
based on the optical detection of a fluorescence label. This technique has been

applied to the detection of several substances in medical diagnostics, such as human serum albumin [5], parathion [6], human IgG [7], atrazine [8], human chorionic gonadotropin [9], and botulinum toxin [10].

Gravimetric transducers are based on sensitive detection of mass changes following antigen–antibody complex formation. Piezoelectric detectors (typically piezocrystals) are the usual technical basis for this approach. In piezoelectric-based systems, the change in the oscillation frequency shift of the piezoelectric crystal is related to the mass change on the crystal surface. Therefore, when an immunocomplex is formed on such crystals, the antigen–antibody binding process changes the mass, and hence a frequency shift is observed. The main advantages of this approach lie in the possibility for direct measurement of immunointeractions. In this case, no label is necessary. Piezoelectric immunosensors have been applied to medical diagnostics for the detection of IgM [11], hemoglobin [12], human erythrocytes [13], virus [14], and bacteria [15]. However, these systems suffer from high nonspecific signal and an inability to detect low-molecular-weight substances.

Electrochemical transducers are based on detection of changes in electron transfer caused by the immunointeraction. In particular, this detection is brought about using amperometric, potentiometric, conductometric (at constant voltage), or impedimetric (at alternating voltage) devices. A number of immunoassay systems described in the literature are based on the principle of electrochemical detection of the labeled immunoagent. Electrochemical detection of the label has several advantages compared to other transduction methods. Electrochemical detection in some cases can be more sensitive and does not require transparent properties of reaction media (a requirement for optical-based methods). A larger capacity of the immobilized immunoagents can be achieved mainly by increasing the effective area of the solid support. However, solid supports with large effective area are not transparent and can hardly be used as elements of immunosensors based on optical detection. An electrochemical detector can also be arranged as a microcell, which allows miniaturization of the biosensor. Enzyme-labeled electrochemical immunosensors use the principal of biocatalytic acceleration of chemical reactions. The combination of high enzyme activity and selectivity with the sensitive methods of electrochemical detection provides basis for the development of practical immunosensors. The highly sensitive amperometric detection of enzyme reaction products was applied to the development of immunosensors for analysis of protein A [16], digoxin [17], theophylline [18], *Salmonella* in foods [19], *E. coli* [20], apolipoprotein E [21], IgG [22], and antibiotics [23] determination.

B. Flow-Injection Immunoassays

With the movement toward automation in immunoassays, more research is being conducted with continuous-flow analytical techniques. With respect to immunoassays, flow injection offers an attractive technique with many clear advantages, including: accurate control of reaction times, improvement in accuracy and precision with a sensitivity similar to batch methods, significant decrease in analysis time approaching real-time analysis, easy calibration, flexibility, use of kinetic or differential measurements, the possibility of integration of reaction, separation, and detection processes [24]. Flow injection coupled with immunoassays is rising as a powerful tool for the development of medical diagnostics and the application of flow-injection techniques is expected to contribute greatly to the improvement of both the speed and the quality of the immunoassay [25]. Several flow-injection-based immunoassays coupled with an electrochemical detector have been used for detection of human IgG [26], the steroid drug budesonide [27], thyroid-stimulating hormone (TSH) [28], and blood IgE [29].

II. IMMUNOELECTRODES BASED ON HIGHLY DISPERSED MATERIALS

A novel amperometric immunoassay technique utilizing highly dispersed carbon immunoelectrodes has been proposed [30,31]. This new technique is based on the use of carbon particles with a size of thousands of angstroms, which is comparable to the size of protein molecules. This results in "pseudo-homogeneous" immunointeractions between free (antigen) and immobilized (antibody) immunospecies. The conductivity of carbon materials permits the use of carbon-based immunosorbents as electrode materials for amperometric determination of enzyme labels. Furthermore, the amperometric signal is usually proportional to the electrode surface area. Therefore, using dispersed carbon material as a solid support for immobilization of immunoagents and as an electrode material improves the efficiency of immunointeraction and the sensitivity of electrochemical assay. The use of antibody-modified dispersed carbon material permits the utilization of disposable electrodes.

Figure 1 demonstrates the principle of action of the amperometric immunoassay system based on highly dispersed carbon electrodes. Antigen analysis follows the "sandwich" assay scheme. In this case the dispersed carbon material acts as an antibody immobilization support (immunosorbent) and, at the same time, as an electrode for amperometric determination of the enzyme label. Flow of the analyte-containing solution through the immunosorbent results in the analyte capture by the immobilized antibodies (Fig. 1a). The second stage of the assay is based on the flow of antianalyte antibodies, conjugated with peroxidase (Fig. 1b). This leads to the formation of an antianalyte–analyte–antianalyte antibodies–peroxidase complex. The quantification of this complex is conducted by amperometric detection of iodine, formed by oxidation of iodide catalyzed by peroxidase (Fig. 1c).

The preparation of the antibody-modified dispersed carbon electrodes is based on the use of Woodward's reagent K to chemically modify the carbon particles' surface [30]. The carbon particles treated with Woodward's reagent K

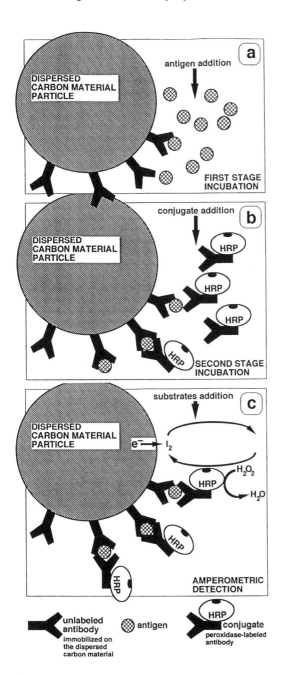

Figure 1 "Sandwich" scheme of immunoassay.

are then suspended in a solution of antibodies that bind to the activated sites on the carbon particle surface. The final step in the immunosorbent preparation is the incubation of the carbon particles in a solution of trypsin inhibitor. Trypsin inhibitor acts a blocking agent and blocks any unoccupied active sites on the carbon particle surface, thus reducing nonspecific analyte/conjugate adsorption. The prepared immunosorbent is stored at 4°C for further use. Scanning electron microscope (SEM) microphotographs of the immunosorbent/immunoelectrode show that the immunoelectrode represents a three-dimensional porous structure with mechanical connections between the particles of the highly dispersed carbon material. These mechanical carbon connections provide conductivity in the immunosorbent layer and result in an overall resistance of 800 Ω/cm [32].

III. IMMUNOASSAY SYSTEM DESIGN

The novel immunoassay technique based on the use of highly dispersed carbon particles, as just described, can be implemented in the form of a flow-injection immunosensor, which in turn can be integrated into a complete immunoassay system. This immunoassay system design combines the advantages of flow-injection immunoassays and the sensitivity of electrochemical measurements.

A. Immunosensor Design

The technical layout of the amperometric flow-through immunoassay system design is presented in Figure 2. The immunocolumn (see Fig. 2), which is the disposable sensing element, consists of a plastic column (1) with a filter membrane at the bottom (2). The immunosorbent (3) is deposited on the filter membrane (by centrifugation), forming the immunoelectrode. A plexiglass column holder (See Fig. 2) is comprised of a supporting electrode assembly: a platinum counter electrode (4) and a Ag/AgCl reference electrode (5) that are placed inside a channel that serves as an outlet for the flow-through immunosensor. The immunocolumn adaptor (see Fig. 2) contains a capillary tube that is inserted and fixed into a hollow carbon rod (6). The capillary tube serves as the inlet to the immunosensor, while the carbon rod serves a current collector for the working electrode (immunoelectrode). The current collector rests on top of the immunoelectrode in order to effectively collect the amperometric output.

Disposability of sensing elements (immunocolumns) is a key principle employed in this work involved. The immunocolumn is represented by a flow-through immunoelectrode and the plastic body of the immunoelectrode. The supporting electrochemical cell consists of a counter electrode and a reference electrode forming the reusable part of the measuring cell. Hence, no regeneration of the immunocolumn between measurements is required.

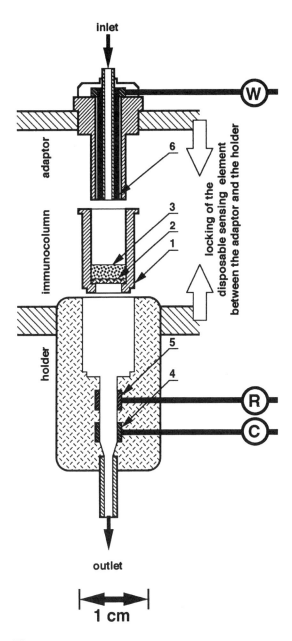

Figure 2 Cross-sectional schematic of the immunosensor: plastic column (1); filter membrane (2); immunosorbent (3); counter electrode (4); reference electrode (5); graphite current collector with capillary inlet tube (6).

B. Integrated Immunoassay System and Laboratory Prototype

The schematic of the complete flow-through immunoassay system is shown in Figure 3. The system has the following main components: the amperometric immunosensor assembly (as shown in Fig. 2), a two-channel peristaltic pump, a six-way valve flow controller, a three-way valve with a mixing chamber, re-agents, and waste vessels, analyte supplier, and an electrochemical/data recorder

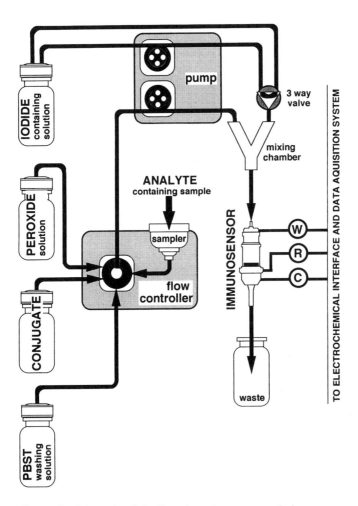

Figure 3   Schematic of the flow-through amperometric immunoassay system setup.

interface. A lever arm is used for moving the holder to lock with the immuno-column and the current collector/inlet adaptor. The analyte supplier and the eluent solution vessels are connected to one of the pump's channels through the flow controller (see Fig. 3). The flow controller determines which solution vessel will be connected to the pump and hence will flow through the sensor. The second pump channel is used for flowing the iodide-containing solution only. A three-way valve is connected to this channel and determines the flow direction of iodide solution. The iodide solution flows through the immunosensor during the electrochemical detection stage; it is recycled back to the storage vessel during all other stages. The two pump channels are connected together by means of a Y-shaped mixing chamber whose outlet is connected to the immunocolumn adaptor of the immunosensor. The Y-shaped chamber is used to mix the hydrogen peroxide and the iodide solutions immediately before the electrochemical detection stage. Separate storage of the peroxidase substrates minimizes nonenzymatic oxidation of iodide by hydrogen peroxide. The electrochemical interface is used to provide the working potential for the immunosensor and to process the output signal.

A photograph of the functioning laboratory prototype of the flow-through immunoassay system is presented in Figure 4. The experiment is started by placing the disposable sensing element into the plexiglass holder (see Fig. 2). The plexiglass holder and sensing element assembly is then manually raised upwards, using a lever arm, until the adaptor is inserted and fixed firmly in the immunocolumn to provide an intimate electrical contact with the immunosorbent. An analyte sample is then injected into the analyte supplier (see Fig. 3). The different solutions are pumped through the immunosensor according to the order described in the immunoassay procedure (following section), and the flow controller is manually adjusted to select the desired solution. The working potential is applied to the immunosensor during the final washing procedure. Immediately before the electrochemical detection stage, the iodide solution is directed to the mixing chamber by switching the three-way valve. Once the output signal is recorded, the working potential and the pump are switched off. The silastic holder/sensing element assembly is then lowered down and the sensing element is removed and disposed of.

C. Sandwich Scheme Immunoassay Procedure

A "sandwich" scheme of detection is employed [31]. The measurement procedure involves the following stages (see Fig. 1):

1. *Prewashing procedure*: flow of a washing solution 0.01 M Na phosphate buffer (pH 7.4) containing 0.15 M NaCl and 0.05% Tween-20 (PBST) through the immunoelectrode

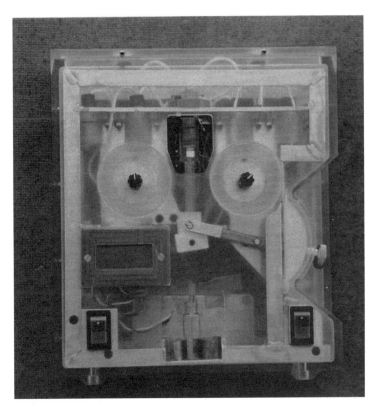

Figure 4 Photograph of the functioning laboratory prototype of the flow-through immunoassay system. The system dimensions are $20 \times 25 \times 8$ cm.

2. *First stage of immunointeraction*: flow of PBST containing the target analyte through the immunocolumn, thereby allowing the target analyte to be bound to the surface of the immunoelectrode that was modified by an immunoagent specific for the target analyte
3. · *First washing procedure*: flow of a washing solution (PBST alone) through the immunoelectrode
4. *Second stage of immunointeraction*: flow of PBST containing peroxidase-labeled antibodies (immunoconjugate) against the target analyte through the immunocolumn, allowing immunoconjugate to form an enzyme-labeled complex on the surface of the immunoelectrode
5. *Second washing procedure*: flow of PBST alone through the immunoelectrode

6. *Amperometric measurement procedure*: flow of an acetate buffer solution (0.1 M, pH 4.5) containing both hydrogen peroxide and iodide (substrates of peroxidase label); allowing oxidation of iodide to occur due to peroxidase label; recording of an amperometric output of the determination of iodine formed as a result of the enzymatic oxidation of the iodide. The polarization of the electrode starts at the beginning of the second washing procedure.

IV. OPTIMIZATION OF THE ELECTROCHEMICAL MEASUREMENT

A. Selection of a Working Potential

The selection of an appropriate working electrode potential is crucial for the amperometric measurement stage. Iodide ions and hydrogen peroxide were selected as substrates of the horse radish peroxidase enzyme label [29]. The iodide ion can be oxidized by peroxidase-forming iodine according to the following reaction:

$$2I^- + H_2O_2 + 2H^+ \xrightarrow{\text{peroxidase}} I_2 + 2H_2O \tag{1}$$

Iodine formed in this reaction can be detected electrochemically:

$$I_2 + 2e^- \xrightarrow{\text{electrode}} 2I^- \tag{2}$$

Electroreduction of iodine on a dispersed carbon material electrode was investigated by cathodic sweep voltammetry [30]. The background voltammogram, obtained in the presence of potassium iodide (concentration 0.1 mM) and H_2O_2 (concentration 10 mM) in the electrolyte solution, shows that electroreduction of H_2O_2 occurs at potentials more negative than 0.07 V. Addition of the horse radish peroxidase enzyme (40 μL of 3 mg/mL water solution) to the system results in formation of iodine (reaction 1). The cathodic sweep voltammogram, obtained in the presence of peroxidase in the system, shows an excess cathodic current, which corresponds to electroreduction of the formed iodine in the system (reaction 2). The maximal difference in the cathodic current in the presence and in the absence of peroxidase is observed at a potential of +0.127 V. This potential was thus selected as an electrode potential for amperometric measurements.

B. Iodide and Peroxide Concentrations

The dependence of the cathodic current on the iodide concentration was investigated [32]. Figure 5 shows the effect of iodide solution concentration (varied from 10^{-5} to 10^{-3} M) on the amperometric signal magnitude for three hydrogen

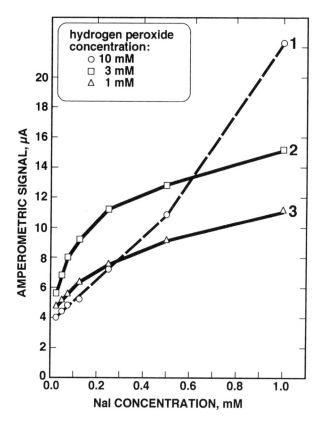

Figure 5 Dependence of flow-through sensor response on the concentration of substrates of peroxidase: NaI and hydrogen peroxide. Conditions: hydrogen peroxide concentration 10 mM (curve 1), 3 mM (curve 2), and 1 mM (curve 3); horseradish peroxidase directly immobilized on the highly dispersed carbon electrode; flow rate is 100 µL/min.

peroxide concentrations (1 mM, 3 mM, and 10 mM). It can be seen that for any hydrogen peroxide concentration, the amperometric signal magnitude increases when increasing iodide concentrations, reaching a maximum value at the highest iodide concentration used (1 mM). It can also be seen that increasing the hydrogen peroxide concentration from 1 mM to 3 mM resulted in an overall increase in the amperometric response. Further increase of the hydrogen peroxide concentration to 10 mM, however, resulted in a change in the character of this dependence: decrease of the amperometric response at low iodide concentrations and higher response at 1 mM NaI. The decrease in the response at low iodide concentrations could be a result of inactivation of the peroxidase enzyme by such a high concentration (10 mM) of hydrogen peroxide. The dramatic increase of the sensor response at 1 mM NaI could be attributed to spontaneous oxidation of iodide by H_2O_2. A hydrogen peroxide concentration of 3 mM has been shown to be an optimal concentration for functioning of horseradish peroxidase–based amperometric sensors [33]. As a result, 1 mM of iodide and 3 mM of hydrogen peroxide were selected as the optimal working range of concentrations for the electrochemical state.

C. Flow Rate of Substrates

The effect of iodide and hydrogen peroxide solutions flow rate on the ampero-metric signal was investigated for the concentrations determined earlier (1 mM iodide and 3 mM hydrogen peroxide) [32]. It was found that increasing the flow rate of the substrates results in an increase in the amperometric signal, reaching saturation at a flow rate of 100 µL/min. Further increase in substrate flow rate did not affect the amperometric signal. Hence, at least 100 µL/min as a mini-mum iodide and hydrogen peroxide flow rate was selected to ensure sufficient sensitivity of the amperometric detection. The investigation of the system behav-ior at higher flow rates provides a basis for the decrease of the overall assay time.

V. OPTIMIZATION OF THE IMMUNOASSAY PROCEDURE

The evaluation of the sensor performance and the optimization of the assay procedure were conducted using rabbit IgG as a model analyte. The dependence of the immunoelectrode response on the duration of flow of both the analyte and the immunoconjugate was investigated for a constant concentration of rabbit IgG (30 nM) [34].

Figure 6a shows the dependence of the immunosensor response to 30 nM IgG on the duration of the first stage of immunointeraction (the flow of antigen). The dependence of the immunoelectrode response on antigen flow duration was investigated for a constant time of immunoconjugate flow (10 minutes). It was demonstrated that the immunoelectrode response increases with increase in the flow duration of the analyte-containing buffer through the immunocolumn. In-creasing the duration of the flow of the analyte beyond 1 minute does not further affect the electrode response (Fig. 6a). This indicates that a duration of flow of at least 1 minute is sufficient for equilibrium antigen–antibody complex forma-tion under the conditions of the experiment. A duration of 2 minutes was chosen for the first stage of the assay procedure in order to reduce the experimental error.

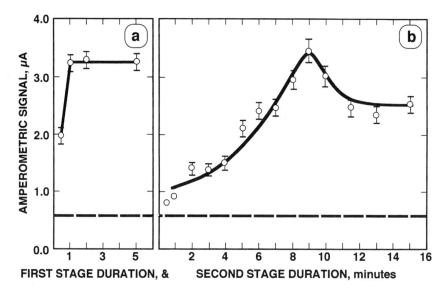

Figure 6 Dependence of flow-through immunosensor response to 30 nM rabbit IgG on the duration of flow of analyte (a) and on the duration of flow of conjugate (b). Conditions: flow rate is 75 µL/min, duration of flow of conjugate is 10 min (a), duration of flow of analyte is 2 min (b). The dashed line represents the background signal.

The dependence of the immunoelectrode response on the duration of the flow of immunoconjugate (second stage of immunointeraction) was investigated for the chosen constant time of analyte flow (2 minutes). Figure 6b presents the dependence of the immunosensor response on the duration of the conjugate flow. This dependence demonstrates a maximum value corresponding to a flow duration of 9 minutes. After 9 minutes of conjugate flow, the electrode response decreases to a steady value (Fig. 6b). The observed decrease in the electrode response may be explained by a hypothesis that this decrease is a result of the immunoagglomeration process of the immunosorbent. It can also be assumed that the analyte bound to the immunosorbent interacts with the flowing immuno-conjugate, forming an unbound analyte–immunoconjugate complex by substitution. This results in a reduction of the amount of bound analyte and leads to a decrease in the sensor signal.

According to the optimization experiments, 2 minutes' duration for the flow of analyte-containing buffer (the first stage) and 9 minutes duration for the flow of immunoconjugate (the second stage) were considered optimum.

VI. ASSAY OF HIGH-MOLECULAR-WEIGHT ANALYTES

A. Immunoglobulin G Assay

Immunoassay system performance evaluation was conducted using IgG as a model analyte [32]. The dependence of the immunoassay system's response on IgG concentration (IgG calibration curves) was investigated for different flow rates and is presented in Figure 7. It can be seen that the highest value of the

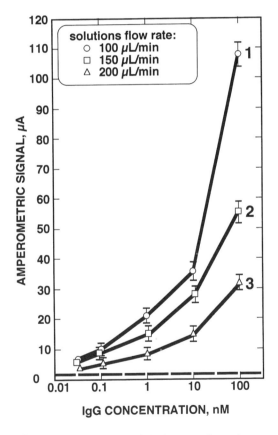

Figure 7 Dependence of the immunoelectrode response on the concentration of rabbit IgG (semilogarithmic plot). Conditions: flow rate of 100 μL/min (curve 1), 150 μL/min (curve 2), and 200 μL/min (curve 3). The dashed line represents the background signal, which is measured in a separate test with no antigen in the sample solution.

response was obtained for a flow rate of 100 µL/min (curve 1), resulting in an overall assay time of 22 min. Increasing the flow rate to 150 µL/min (curve 2) resulted in a 25% decrease in the measured signal (in the nanomolar concentration range) while decreasing the overall assay time to 17 min. Further increase of the flow rate to 200 µL/min (curve 3) resulted in a significant decrease (65% decrease in the same concentration range) in the measured signal while reducing the assay time to 15 min. This observed decrease in the amperometric signal may be explained by the fact that increasing the flow rate decreases the time of immunointeraction, and hence less analyte is bound to the immobilized antibodies. When combined flow rate conditions were used—150 µL/min for the first stage of immunointeraction and 200 µL/min for all other stages—the resulting calibration curves fall between curves 2 and 3 on Figure 7. Such a mixed-flow-rate regime resulted in a 60% decrease in the measured signal and in reduction of the assay time up to 15.5 min.

B. Immunoglobulin M

Fast determination of IgM in human blood plasma is important for medical diagnostics, especially in epidemiological situations. The technology and methods developed using IgG as a model analyte were adapted for application to IgM assay. Figure 8a depicts the dependence of the immunosensor response on the concentration of human IgM [34]. It should be noted that the low detection limit observed for IgM determination is less than 1 nM (8 µg/mL). This detection limit is higher than that obtained for rabbit IgG immunoassay (see earlier and Fig. 7). This is apparently due to a lower affinity of anti-IgM antibodies used in the assay. Figure 8b demonstrates the immunosensor's response to a 16.5 nM (0.015 mg/mL) concentration of IgM in blank PBST and the immunosensor's response to the same concentration of IgM in the presence of excess amount of human IgG. It shows that the large excess of IgG (4.4 mg/mL) does not interfere with the sensor response to human IgM. It can be concluded from this that no cross-immunoreactions occur.

The assay of IgM in the blood plasma samples was demonstrated using this assay technique [34]. Figure 8c represents the sensor's response to a blood sample (1:50 diluted by PBST) and the same after the addition of a standard amount (29 nM) of IgM. The dependence of the immunosensor response on the concentration of human IgM in PBST (Fig. 8a) was used as a calibration curve for a determination of a concentration of IgM in diluted blood plasma (illustrated in Fig. 8c). The concentration of IgM in the diluted blood sample is assumed to be 21 nM (0.019 mg/ml). Thus, the concentration of 29 nM IgM in undiluted blood is equal to 0.95 mg/ml. The standard addition of IgM results in an increased response (Fig. 8c). A concentration of 48 nM IgM can be obtained from this response value using the calibration curve (see Fig. 8a). The concen-

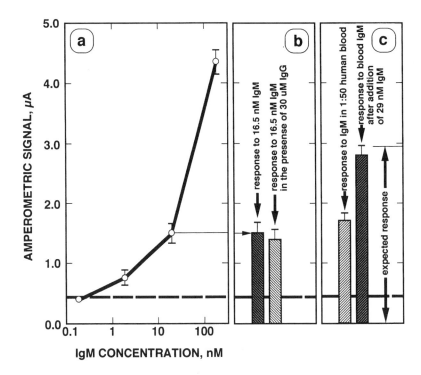

Figure 8 Dependence of the flow-through immunosensor response on the concentration of human IgM (semilogarithmic plot) (a). Immunosensor response to 18 nM IgM concentration alone and in the presence of 3000 nM of human IgG (b). Immunosensor response obtained in 1:50 diluted human blood plasma sample alone and after a standard addition of 29 nM of IgM (c). The dashed line represents the background signal.

tration obtained (48 nM) is very close to that calculated for the sample with the standard addition (21 nM + 29 nM = 50 nM). The measured immunosensor's signal coincides, within experimental error, with the reversed extrapolated signal value, which corresponds to 50 nM (see Fig. 8a). So the discretion of the assay in the nanomolar range is about ±2 nM.

As a result, a fast (22-minute) assay of both normal and hyperphysiological concentrations of IgM in blood can be performed by the flow-through immunosensor using 1:50 diluted blood plasma samples. The sample volume required for the assay is 150 μL. Thus, 3 μL of undiluted blood plasma is required for the quantitative assay.

C. Assay of Hantavirus Infections

A newly discovered hantavirus (family *Bunyaviridae*), sin nombre virus, was identified during a 1993 outbreak of an acute respiratory disease with high mortality in the Four Corners region of the southwestern United States [35]. The human disease, hantavirus pulmonary syndrome (HPS) occurs in man putatively through accidental/incidental inhalation of virus-contaminated excreta of the natural host, the deer mouse (*Peromyscus maniculatus*). Exposure and infection occur in rural areas, often remote from medical centers with sophisticated diagnostic capabilities. Furthermore, the rapidity of the onset of shock after the nondescript viral prodrome demands a rapid diagnostic assay to identify patients who need transport to intensive care before the onset of shock.

The diagnostics of hantavirus infection is based on the determination of antibodies against the virus in human blood serum. The analysis is based on the "sandwich" assay scheme. In this case recombinant protein of hantavirus was immobilized on the surface of the highly dispersed carbon (immunosorbent). The first incubation of immunosorbent with blood plasma results in the formation of the immunocomplex between hantavirus-specific antibodies and recombinant protein of hantavirus immobilized on the surface of immunosorbent. The second incubation of immunosorbent with antihuman antibodies labeled with peroxidase leads to the formation of peroxidase-labeled complex.

Figure 9 demonstrates the sensor response to 1:2 diluted hantavirus-positive (bar 1) and hantavirus-negative (bar 2) blood samples. Background signal— the immunoelectrode current in blank buffer solution—is presented in the same figure (bar 3). It can be seen from this figure that the sensor response to negative blood sample is practically the same as the control background response obtained for buffer solution. However, the hantavirus-positive blood sample demonstrates an electrode response about five times higher than the background sensor response.

Assay of the hantavirus infection was conducted with 2-min incubation time of the first stage of the "sandwich" scheme and 15-min incubation time for the second stage. The amperometric detection was undertaken immediately after the washing procedure and introducing the iodide and peroxide solution. The steady-state current response of the electrode is established within 2–3 minutes. The overall time of the assay (including the washing procedures) is 22 minutes. This is significantly less than the overall assay time for conventional immunoassay of hantavirus performed using a Western Blot procedure with an overall assay time of 24 hours [36].

D. Assay of Proteins

The assay of proteins is of particular interest in many fields, and numerous kits are commercially available for the detection of large numbers of proteins. Pro-

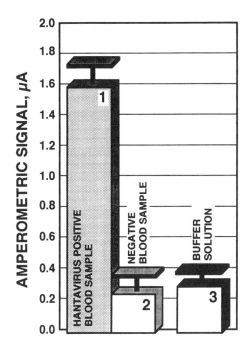

Figure 9   Sensor response to (1) 1:2 diluted hantavirus-antibodies-positive blood sample average of three measurements; (2) hantavirus-negative blood sample average of three measurements; and (3) background response to buffer solution average of three measurements.

tein A was selected as a representative analyte to demonstrate the applicability of the developed system to the detection of proteins [37]. There are two main reasons for this choice. First, there is no commercially available kit for quantitative protein A assay. This makes the development of such an assay of commercial importance. Second, protein A is a membrane protein found in the cell membrane of many bacterial cells, including *Staphylococcus aureus*. The development of assays for *S. aureus* is of paramount importance due to the pathogenity of this bacteria, causing several severe diseases, such as pneumonia, intoxication, and toxic shock syndrome [16]. The determination of protein A expressed by *Staphylococcus* cells is a popular technique for staphylococcus identification.

   A sandwich scheme of assay (described previously) was also employed, and the dependence of the immunoelectrode response on protein A concentration (calibration curve of the immunosensor) obtained under the given conditions is demonstrated in Figure 10. The resulting detection limit of the assay is

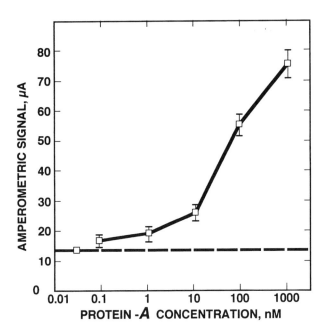

Figure 10 Dependence of the immunoelectrode response on the concentration of protein A (semilogarithmic plot). The dashed line represents the background signal. Conditions: Flow rate is 100 μL/min, duration of flow of analyte: 2 min, duration of flow of conjugate: 90 min.

in the 10^{-11} M range, and the dynamic range of the sensor response is from 10^{-11} M to 10^{-5} M. The overall assay time in this case is 22 minutes.

The performance of the system in detecting protein A was compared to that of the standard ELISA technique, which requires at least 4 hours per assay to reach the same protein A detection range.

VII. ASSAY OF WHOLE BACTERIAL CELLS

Infectious diseases account for nearly 40% of the total 50 million annual estimated deaths worldwide. Microbial diseases still constitute the major causes of death in many developing countries of the world. The effective testing of bacteria requires analytical methods that are rapid, extremely selective, and very sensitive, since the presence of even a single pathogenic organism in the body may be an infectious dose for man. The traditional methods for isolating and identifying bacteria in medical diagnostics rely on the enrichment of liquid samples at $35°-37°C$ for 18–24 hours to increase the bacteria population by culture method to a detectable level. This step is then followed by microscopically counting the colonies or by immunological testing [38,39]. Thus, conventional techniques are not suitable for fast and direct (without pre-enrichment) analyses of bacteria.

A.   *E. coli* O157:H7 Assay

E. coli O157:H7 is one of the most dangerous food-borne pathogens [40]. The O157:H7 is a rare strain of *E. coli* that produces large quantities of a potent toxin that accumulates in the lining of the intestine and causes severe damage to it. The immunoassay system was used for detection of *E. coli* O157:H7; however, the large size of the bacterial cells caused a disruption in the highly dispersed carbon (immunosorbent) layer. This disruption resulted in an increased signal-to-noise ratio and a high nonspecific control signal. Therefore, the highly dispersed immunosorbent part in the immunosensor was replaced with a porous nylon filtration membrane rich in carboxyl groups. This allowed precise control of membrane pore size, which is a critical factor in bacterial cell flow-through immunoassay. Optimization of the parameters affecting the immunoassay, such as selection of appropriate filter membranes, membrane pore size, antibody binding capacity, the concentrations of immunoreagents, and non-specific signals, were investigated [41].

Figure 11 presents calibration curves obtained for increasing *E. coli* O157: H7 (mortalized standard cell suspensions) concentrations in the case of 0.1-mL and 1-mL sample/conjugate volumes [41]. A low sample/conjugate volume (0.1 ml) results in a lower detection limit of 1000 cells/mL and a working range of 1000–4000 cells/mL with an overall analysis of 13 minutes. Increases in the sample/conjugate volume (1 mL) resulted in a shift of the calibration curve toward lower *E. coli* concentrations. In this case, the lower detection limit is 100 cells/mL and the working range is from 100 to 600 cells/mL with an overall analysis time of 30 min. The decrease in the system response at concentrations greater than 600 cells/mL may be attributed to the gradual blocking (clogging) of the membrane pores at higher concentrations of cells.

The results of the amperometric immunoassay system were compared to the results from a standard sandwich ELISA method with spectrophotometric detection. The calibration curves for *E. coli* O157:H7 obtained with the ELISA method demonstrate a lower detection limit of approximately 10^5 cells/mL and a working range from 10^5 to 10^7 cells/mL. Thus, the lower detection limit of the amperometric flow-through immunofiltration system to *E. coli* is 1000-fold greater than that of the standard ELISA assay. Several factors contributed to this amplification. First of all, the porous membranes modified with carboxyl groups offer 100–1000 times more available surface area for immobilization of

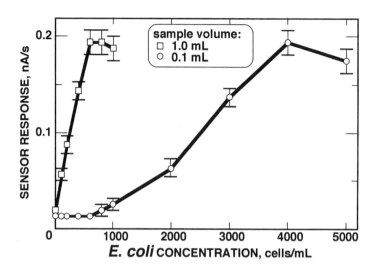

Figure 11 Calibration curves of an enzyme immunofiltration assay for *E. coli* O157:
H7 using a flow-through amperometric biosensor. The volume of the injected sample *E.
coli* and conjugate (1 μg/mL peroxidase-labeled antibody to *E. coli* O157:H7): (1) 1.0
mL sample; (2) 0.1 mL sample.

antibodies than traditional solid wells currently used in ELISA. Secondly, an
acceleration of the diffusion-controlled rate of immunological, enzymatic, and
electrochemical reactions is achieved by using immunofiltration, accumulation
of bacteria and conjugate molecules on the porous membrane surface, and control of the hydrodynamic conditions.

B. Total *E. coli* Assay

The optimized system parameters were used in the flow-through system and
applied to the detection of total *E. coli* (a mixture of O157:H7, O20, O125,
O55, O111 and K12 strains) [42]. Figure 12 presents the calibration curve obtained for increasing concentrations of *E. coli*. The system demonstrated a lower
detection limit of 50 *E. coli* cells/mL, a working range of 50–200 cells/mL, and
an overall analysis time of 35 minutes. The performance of the flow-through
amperometric immunoassay system was compared to that of the standard ELISA
technique. The lower detection limit of the standard ELISA technique is approximately 10^5 cells/mL and the working range is from 10^5 to 10^8 cells/mL. The
sensitivity of the ELISA technique was improved two orders of magnitude by

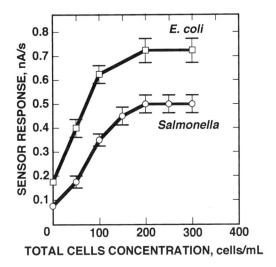

Figure 12 Calibration curves of an enzyme immunofiltration assay for total *E. coli* and total *Salmonella* using the flow-injection system. The volume of the injected sample and conjugate (1 μg/mL peroxidase-labeled antibody to *E. coli* or to *Salmonella*) is 1.0 mL. Other conditions are the same as in Figure 11.

doubling the incubation times (i.e., a 4-hr incubation with the sample and a 2-hr incubation with conjugate), making the overall analysis time 8 hours. In this case the lower detection limit for *E. coli* is approximately 10^3 cells/mL. It can be seen that the sensitivity of the amperometric immunoassay system to *E. coli* is 2000-fold greater than that of the standard ELISA assay. Even with an 8-hour ELISA procedure, the developed system is still 20 times more sensitive and significantly faster (35 minutes).

C. Quantitative *Salmonella* Assay

The same parameters used for the detection of *E. coli* were directly applied for detection of *Salmonella* [42]. Figure 12 presents the calibration curve obtained for increasing concentrations of *Salmonella typhimurium* (used as a representative *Salmonella* strain). The lower detection limit of *S. typhimurium* was 50 cells/mL, the working range was 50–200 cells/mL, and overall analysis time was 35 minutes. The performance of the developed system was also compared to that of the ELISA; the developed immunoassay system was found to be 1000 times more sensitive.

VIII. CONCLUSION

A portable, flow-through amperometric immunoassay system for the detection of a wide range of analytes—of molecular, viral, and bacterial nature—has been developed. One of the variants of the developed system utilizes highly dispersed carbon particles, which act as both a carrier for immobilized antibodies and as a high-surface-area working electrode for detection of immunoglobulins, viral infections, and proteins. Another modification of the system utilizes porous immunofiltration membranes for the detection of whole bacterial cells. A "sandwich" scheme of immunoassay has been used, and iodine formed as a result of the enzymatic oxidation of iodide by peroxidase label has been detected amperometrically. The practical application of the immunoassay system has been demonstrated in the detection and quantification of IgG and of IgM and hanta virus infection in human blood. The system also permits the direct detection of *E. coli* and *Salmonella* cells, with a lower detection limit of 50 cells/mL that is 2000 times more sensitive than the standard spectrophotometric ELISA method using the same immunochemicals. The overall analysis time, including flowing of analyte, flowing of antigen, washing, and detection stages, ranges from 15 to 35 minutes, depending on the analyte. The enhanced sensitivity and short assay time permit the application of the developed system to rapid (near real-time) direct detection of a wide range of analytes in medical diagnostics. The amperometric flow-through immunoassay system may be easily adapted for the detection of other classes of analytes, such as drugs and hormones. Implementation of other immunoassay schemes, such as the displacement analysis and other competitive schemes, is currently in progress.

ACKNOWLEDGMENTS

The financial support of the DoE/Waste Education Research and Management Consortium of New Mexico is gratefully acknowledged.

REFERENCES

1. Foulds, N.C., Frew, J.E., Green, M.J. (1990). Immunoelectrodes. In: Biosensors: A Practical Approach. A.E.G. Cass (Ed.), IRL Press/Oxford University Press, New York, pp. 97–124.
2. Ghindilis, A.L., Atanasov, P., Wilkins, M., Wilkins, E. (1998). Immunosensors: electrochemical sensing and other engineering approaches. Biosensors Bioelectron. 13(1):113–131.
3. Price, C.R. (1998). Progress in immunoassay technology. Clin. Chem. Lab. Med. 36(6):341–347.

4. Miyai, K., and Price, C.P. (1992). Problems for improving performance in immunoassay. JIFCC 4:154–163.

5. Eenink, R.G., de Bruijn, H.E., Kooyman, R.P.H., Greve J. (1990). Fibre-fluorescence immunosensor based on evanescent wave detection. Anal. Chim. Acta. 238: 317–321.

6. Anis, N.A., Wright, J., Rogers, K.R., Thompson, R.G., Valdes, J.J., Valdes, J.J., Eldefrawi, M.E. (1992). A fiber-optic immunosensor for detecting parathion. Anal. Lett. 25:627–635.

7. Lu, B., Lu, C., Wei, Y. (1992). A planar quartz waveguide immunosensor based on TIRF principle. Anal. Lett. 25:1–10.

8. Oroszlan, P., Duveneck, G.L., Ehrat, M., Widmer, H.M. (1993). Fiber-optic atrazine immunosensor. Sensors Actuat. B. 11:301–305.

9. Sloper, A.N., Flanagan, M.T. (1993). Scattering in planar surface waveguide immunosensors. Sensors Actuat. B 11:537–542.

10. Kumar, P., Colston, J.T., Chambers, J.P., Rael, E.D., Valdes, J.J. (1994). Detection of botulinum toxin using an evanescent wave immunosensor. Biosensors Bioelectron. 9:57–63.

11. Suri, C.R., Raje, M., Mishra, G.C. (1994). Determination of immunoglobulin M concentration by piezoelectric crystal immunobiosensor coated with protamine. Biosensors Bioelectron. 9:535–542.

12. Shao, B., Hu, Q., Hu, J. Zhou, X. Zhang, W., Wang, X., Fan X. (1993). Determination of bovine haemoglobin by a piezoelectric crystal immunosensor. Fresenius J. Anal. Chem. 346:1020–1024.

13. Konig, B., Gratzel, M. (1993). Development of a piezoelectric immunosensor for the detection of human erythrocytes. Anal. Chim. Acta 276:323–333.

14. Konig, B., Gratzel, M. (1995). A piezoelectric immunosensor for hepatitis viruses. Anal. Chim. Acta 309:19–25.

15. Bao, L., Deng, L., Nie, L., Yao, S., Wei, W. (1996). Determination of microorganisms with a quartz crystal microbalance sensor. Anal. Chim. Acta 319:97–101.

16. Mirhabibollahi, B., Brooks, J.L., Kroll, R.G. (1990). An improved amperometric immunosensor for the detection and enumeration of protein A-bearing *Staphylococcus aureus*. Lett. Appl. Bacteriol. 11:119–122.

17. Kaneki, N., Xu, Y., Kumari, A., Halsall, H.B., Heineman, W.R., Kissenger, P.T. (1994). Electrochemical enzyme immunoassay using sequential saturation technique in a 20-μL capillary: digoxin as a model analyte. Anal. Chim. Acta 287: 253–258.

18. Palmer, D.A., Edmonds, T.E., Seare, N.J. (1993). Flow injection immunosensor for theophylline. Anal. Lett. 26:1425–1439.

19. Brooks, J.L., Mirhabibollahi, B., Kroll, R.G. (1992). Experimental enzyme-linked amperometric immunosensors for the detection of salmonellas in food. J. Appl. Bacteriol. 73:189–196.

20. Abdel-Hamid, I., Ivnitski, D., Atanasov, P., Wilkins, E. (1998). Fast amperometric immunoassay for *E. coli* O157:H7 using partially immersed immunoelectrodes. Electroanalysis 10:758–763.

21. Meusel, M., Renneberg, R., Spener, F., Schmitz, G. (1995). Development of hetero-

geneous amperometric immunosensor for the determination of apolipoproten E in serum. Biosensors Bioelectron. 10:577–586.

22. Masson, M., Liu, Z., Haruyama, T., Kobatake, E., Ikariyama, Y., Aizawa, M. (1995). Immunosensing with amperometric detection, using galactosidase as label and p-aminophenyl-β-galactopyranoside as substrate. Anal. Chim. Acta. 304:353–359.

23. Matsumoto, M., Tsunematsu, K., Tsuji, A., Kido, Y. (1997). Enzyme immunoassay using peroxidase as a label and a dip-strip test for monitoring residual bacitracin in chicken plasma. Anal. Chim. Acta. 346:207–213.

24. Valcarcel, M., Luque de Castro, M.D. (1994). Flow-through (bio)chemical sensors. Part V: Flow-through sensors based on integrated reaction, separation and detection. Amsterdam, pp. 259–322.

25. Puchades, R., Maquieira, A. (1996). Recent developments in flow injection immunoanalysis. Crit. Rev. Anal. Chem. 26(4):195–218.

26. Hsu, T.T. Bilitewski, U., Schmid, R.D. (1992). Development of an automatic flow-injection electrochemical analysis system for phenol and its application to the construction of an immunosensor for human IgG. Proc. Biosensors '92 Geneva, Switzerland, 385.

27. Kronkvist, K., Lovgren, U., Edholm, L.E., Johansson, G. (1993). Determination of drugs in biosamples at picomolar concentrations using competitive ELISA with electrochemical detection: applications to steroids. J. Pharm. Biomed. Anal. 11: 459–467.

28. Yu, Z., Xu, Y., Ip, M.P.C. (1994). An ultrasensitive electrochemical enzyme immunoassay for thyroid stimulating hormone in human serum. J. Pharm. Biomed. Anal. 12:787–793.

29. Ivnitski, D.M., Siditkov, R.A., Kurochkin, V.E. (1992). Flow-injection amperometric system for enzyme immunoassay. Anal. Chim. Acta 261:45–52.

30. Krishnan, R., Ghindilis, A.L., Atanasov, P., Wilkins, E. (1995). Fast amperometric immunoassay utilizing highly dispersed electrode material. Anal. Lett. 28:2459–2474.

31. Krishnan, R., Ghindilis, A.L., Atanasov, P., Wilkins, E. (1996). Development of an amperometric immunoassay based on highly dispersed immunoelectrode. Anal. Lett. 29:2615–2631.

32. Abdel-Hamid, I., Atanasov, P., Ghindilis, A., Wilkins, E. (1998). Development of a flow-through immunoassay system. Sensors Actuators B 49(3):202–210.

33. Bogdanovskaya, V.A., Fridman, V.A., Tarasevich, M.R., Scheller, F. (1994). Bioelectrocatalysis by immobilized peroxidase: the reaction mechanism and the possibility of electroanalytical detection of both inhibitors and activators of enzyme. Anal. Lett. 27:2823–2847.

34. Ghindilis, A.L., Krishnan, R., Atanasov, P., Wilkins, E. (1997). Flow-through amperometric immunosensor: fast "sandwich" scheme immunoassay. Biosensors Bioelectron. 12(5):415–423.

35. Hjelle, B., Jenison, S., Torrez-Martinez, N., Yamada, T., Molte, K., Zumwalt, R., MacInnes, K., Myers, G. (1994). A novel hantavirus associated with an outbreak of fatal respiratory disease in the southwestern United States: evolutionary relationships to known Hantavirus. J. Virology 68:592–596.

36. Krishnan, R., Ghindilis, A.L., Atanasov, P., Wilkins, E., Montoya, J., Koster, F.T. (1996). Fast amperometric immunoassay for hantavirus infection. Electroanalysis 8:1131–1134.

37. Abdel-Hamid, I., Ghindilis, A.L., Atanasov, P., Wilkins, E. (1999). Flow-through immunoassay system for determination of staphylococcal Protein A. Anal. Lett. 32: 1081–1094.

38. Helrich K. (ed). (1990). Official Methods of Analysis of the Association of Official Analytical Chemists, Chapter 17: Microbiological Methods, Vol. 2, (15th ed.), AOAC Inc., Arlington, VA, 425–497.

39. Beran, G.W., Shoeman, H.P., Anderson, K.F. (1991). Food safety: an overview of problems. Dairy Food Environ. Sci. 11:189–194.

40. Buchanan, R.L., Doly, M.P. (1997). Foodborne disease significance of *E. coli* O157:H7 and other enterohemorrhagic *E. coli*. Food Technology 51:69–76.

41. Abdel-Hamid, I., Ivnitski, D., Atanasov, P., Wilkins, E. (1999). Enzyme immunofi-ltration assay of E. coli O157:H7. Biosensors Bioelectron. 14:309–316.

42. Abdel-Hamid, I., Ivnitski, D., Atanasov, P., Wilkins, E. (1998). Highly sensitive flow-injection immunoassay system for rapid detection of bacteria. Anal. Chim. Acta, 399:99–108.

6

Optical Sensor Arrays for Medical Diagnostics

Keith J. Albert, Caroline L. Schauer, and David R. Walt
Tufts University, Medford, Massachusetts, U.S.A.

I. INTRODUCTION

Currently, fluid analysis is the fundamental tool in the diagnosis of disease. The present approach is to procure samples and transfer them to a clinical laboratory for analysis. Between the measurement and subsequent analysis lies a time lag with potential for mishandling of the samples. Consequently, there is a need for a continuous bedside instrument for blood analysis [1], especially for patients with diabetes or on kidney dialysis. In the future, clinical diagnostics may lead to more responsive monitoring systems for genetic disorders or physical/mental ailments. The development of these monitoring systems is directly dependent on emerging sensor technologies and their ability to perform in complex environments. The ultimate medical diagnostic sensor will be a universal sensor that can use a patient's breath and/or external fluids to instantly diagnose disease. Sensor technologies provide a means to create the next generation of diagnostic instruments. The need for smaller and more multiplexed sensor designs has had an impact on major technological advances in nanoelectronics [2–6], cellular analysis [7,8], electrochemistry [9–14], genomics-related detection devices [15–22], molecular recognition [23–25], immunochemistry [26,27], combinatorial drug design [28], food quality [29–31], and organic vapor detection [32–37].

Although we have not yet developed a universal sensor, our laboratory has fabricated a miniaturized sensor array platform that may be applied to nearly any optical detection scheme. Our approach employs optical imaging fibers as a platform for creating sensors for medical diagnostic assays. We attach optically based sensors to the distal tips of optical fibers and monitor fluorescence changes due to the presence of target analytes. Optical sensors have the advantage, over other sensor types, of being free from electromagnetic interferences because there are no direct electrical connections. Optical fibers can also be utilized for remote, hazardous, or in vivo sensing applications where it is difficult to place a detection system [38]. The optical fiber is used mainly to guide light to and from the sensory materials, but it also may be used for simultaneous imaging during a chemical sensing event [39–42] to support the measurement of independent variables [43].

The need for small, fast-responding detection systems is expanding and the fiber-optic platform offers a different approach to multianalyte sensing through small sensor design. Selective sensor chemistries are incorporated onto the distal face of optical fibers or onto microsphere sensors. The detection of electrolytes, glucose, pH, CO_2, O_2, penicillin, amplified DNA, unlabeled DNA, cell activity, and organic vapors have all been achieved in this laboratory by employing fiber-optic-based sensor arrays. To implement the array platform for diagnostic assays, real-time data processing and highly responsive sensors are required. Ideally, the optical sensors would perform well in complex environments without the need for periodic calibrations or extra reagents and would be fast, reversible, reliable, cost effective, sensitive, and target selective. In the future, diagnostic instrumentation might avoid potential detection problems in complex environments of changing pH, temperature, salinity and may possess smart processing capabilities to solve low target specificity, sensor drift, calibration, and interferences. The brunt of the detection would therefore be placed on the analysis rather than on developing selective sensor chemistries. This chapter is designed to review our laboratory's efforts at developing sensor technologies and detection schemes for medical diagnostic assays.

II. MATERIALS AND INSTRUMENTATION

A. Instrument Design and Signal Transduction

Every optical instrumental design incorporates a light source, supporting optics, a detector, and a data processor. The present system employs only one optical fiber or fiber bundle and therefore requires a more sophisticated instrumental design, as seen in Figure 1. We utilize a computer-controlled imaging system with an inverted fluorescence microscope, a Xe arc lamp light source, dichroic mirrors and optical filters, a CCD detector, and image processing software. Different light sources and detectors are employed, depending on the sensing application. For example, if an increase in sensitivity is desired, a high-powered monochromatic laser source and a photomultiplier tube (PMT), avalanche photodiodes, or an intensified charge-coupled device (CCD) might be employed. There are many situations where different types of optical fibers or substrates

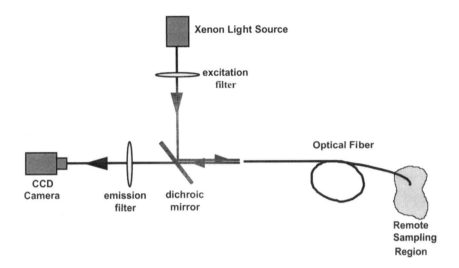

Figure 1   Optical instrumentation used for the fiber-optic array. The excitation light passes through the fiber toward the distally located sensors. Some of the emission light from the fluorescent indicators is captured back through the fiber and onto the CCD for detection. The CCD is used to monitor fluorescence intensity changes due to sensor–target interactions.

are designed, e.g., bifurcated bundles [44,45] or planar waveguides [46], but these will not be addressed. Our laboratory employs single-core fibers and optical imaging fibers for the work discussed.

An optical fiber is composed of a plastic, glass, or fused-silica core surrounded by an outer cladding with a lower refractive index, such that entering light is internally reflected at the interface of the two different materials. Light coupled into the optical fiber within the critical angle will propagate throughout the fiber because of total internal reflection and can be propagated over long distances. In all sensing applications discussed later, a multimode optical fiber or fiber bundle is employed and all sensing chemistries are attached to the distal tips of the optical fiber [39,40,42,43,47–63]. The sensory materials can consist of fluorescent indicators attached to polymers, micron-sized beads, or living cells. The fluorescence indicators absorb excitation light introduced at the proximal end of the fiber, and fluorescence light is isotropically emitted and some of the light captured back through the fiber and transmitted to the detector. In all applications discussed later, the returning longer-wavelength fluorescence light *is measured as a change in intensity at the detection wavelength.* The sensory material and/or fluorescent indicator are modulated during exposure to target, and the detector measures the returning light's change in intensity. Changes in the absorbance intensity can also be measured if the returning light is collected at the same wavelength, but these methods will not be discussed.

Optical sensors have a few inherent complications, including bleaching, leaching, or physical changes to the sensory elements. Sensor drift from photobleaching or dye leaching can be compensated through normalization steps or ratiometric fluorescence measurements. From a practical standpoint, sensors also need to withstand sterilization procedures for invasive monitoring. For example, steam can physically change sensor morphology or ultimately affect a sensor's performance. We have shown that CO_2 [63] and multianalyte [55] sensor systems were still able to monitor effectively after sterilization. These sensors provide feasibility studies for future invasive sensing applications.

B. Single-Core Optical Fibers and Their Application

Single-core optical fibers or optical bundles have been employed in our laboratory for multianalyte detection schemes. With single-core fibers, one must use one fiber for each sensor. Multianalyte arrays are made by bundling such fibers. We have shown that this platform is effective for monitoring multiple DNA sequences [54] and for detecting volatile organic vapors and vapor mixtures via pattern recognition [49,50,64].

1. DNA Detection

Oligonucleotide detection schemes, e.g., DNA microchips and arrays, are now at the forefront of sensor development because of their relevance to the scientific community's efforts at understanding the human genome. We have developed DNA sensor arrays for oligonucleotide identification. A bundle of seven single-core optical fibers was fabricated to monitor fluorescence changes due to oligonucleotide hybridization [54]. DNA targets were labeled with a fluorescent dye, and their complementary probes were immobilized onto each individual fiber tip. To test the specificity of the sensor array, human cytokine mRNA sequences were immobilized (interleukin 6, interleukin 4, human β-globin, interferon γ-1, and interleukin 2). Fluorescently labeled target solutions were assayed using the sensor array. The fiber tips were immersed in the target solution and incubated for five minutes. The sensors were then rinsed with buffer and the fluorescence was measured. The sensor array demonstrated specificity by giving a fluorescence signal only for complementary probes (Figure 2); nonspecific binding did not result in an observed fluorescence signal. Immersing the fiber in a formamide solution removed the bound target, and the sensor was regenerated for further use. To detect hybridization of DNA there are certain limitations that have

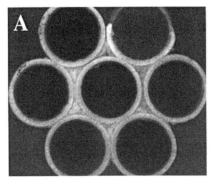 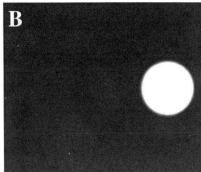

Figure 2 (A) Proximal end of a seven-single-core-fiber bundle with white light illumination. The outer diameter of the bundle is ~1 mm. For DNA detection, each fiber tip is modified with a different oligonucleotide strand. (B) When the fiber bundle is immersed in target solution, the fluorescently labeled complementary probe hybridizes to the attached oligonucleotide. The hybridization produces a measurable fluorescence signal.

to be addressed. First, high concentrations of DNA sample are needed, which are presently overcome by using polymerase chain reaction (PCR). The second limitation is DNA's slow hybridization kinetics. Our fiber-optic system requires small sample volumes and is sensitive enough to quantitatively measure small fluorescence changes. One of the disadvantages to this system is the use of labeled DNA targets; therefore a competition assay was developed using unlabeled targets with a fixed amount of labeled targets to measure hybridization in proportion to concentration. The benefits of such a system include detection of multiple DNA sequences in less than five minutes and the reversible and stable nature of the sensor.

2. Artificial Nose

Using an array platform similar to the seven single-core fiber bundle for DNA detection, we developed a 19-single-core fiber bundle "artificial nose" to detect a wide variety of volatile organic compounds [49,50]. Unlike the DNA array, the "artificial nose" sensors are *not* target selective. The sensor array is prepared containing a solvatochromic dye imbedded in a variety of differentially reactive polymers. The dye undergoes spectral shifts (intensity, wavelength) resulting from polarity changes. When an analyte vapor is presented in pulsatile fashion, each sensor produces a unique temporal fluorescence signature that is dependent on vapor diffusion through the polymer layer, polymer type, polymer swelling, vapor polarity, exposure time, and flow rate. Each unique sensor–analyte signature profile is used to train computational net-works for subsequent analysis via pattern recognition. Following an initial training step, the system can recognize 91–100% of the training set and greater than 84% of a test set of volatile organics. These and other results within our laboratory provide grounds for exploring the capacity of this system for detect-ing "breath" vapors, e.g., alcohol and ketones, which may be an indication of a physical ailment or a possible genetic disorder. Also, the incorporation of a pattern recognition sensor may be suited for medical diagnostic assays once the sensor is trained to recognize a certain target analyte, which would alleviate the need for highly selective sensory materials.

C.   Optical Imaging Fibers and Their Application

The disadvantage of employing bundled single-core fibers is that only one sens-ing element can be incorporated per optical fiber. The number and outer diame-ters of the individual sensor elements therefore limit the overall size of the sensor array. An alternative approach is to use an optical imaging fiber. Optical imaging fibers are coherent, high-density arrays of micron-scale optical fibers. Individual optical fibers are fused together in a coherent manner such that each fiber carries an isolated optical signal from one end of the fiber to the other. Thousands of individual optical fibers are drawn together and maintain an image from one end to the other (Figure 3). Optical imaging fibers can consist of 3,000–100,000 individually clad optical fibers, each with diameters of 3–10 μm. Fibers with cores as small as ~500 nm in diameter have also been employed in our laboratories [40,65]. Image resolution depends on the size of the individual fiber elements within the high-density optical imaging fiber or on the size of the detector pixels.

Optical imaging fibers are suited for multiplexing sensors and sensor arrays because many sensor elements can be incorporated onto the distal face of the same imaging fiber [40,41,43,47,48,51–53,55,59,61,62]. Thousands of separate optical pathways are used to carry signals simultaneously from multiple sensors immobilized at different locations on the fiber's tip. As discussed in more detail later, imaging fibers can incorporate one sensor or as many sensors as optical pixels, 3,000–100,000; many sensor elements with different sensing chemistries can be employed for multiple assays. Two approaches have been taken for designing sensor arrays on the distal face of these fibers: (1) the sen-sors are attached by employing a systematic photodeposition process, and (2) the sensors are randomly distributed (see sec. II.D).

Due to the coherent nature of the imaging fiber, discrete sensor spots can be attached to the distal tip in a systematic fashion by ultraviolet (UV) illumina-tion through a pinhole at the fiber's proximal end. The UV illumination initiates solution polymerization on the distal tip and polymerization occurs *only* through

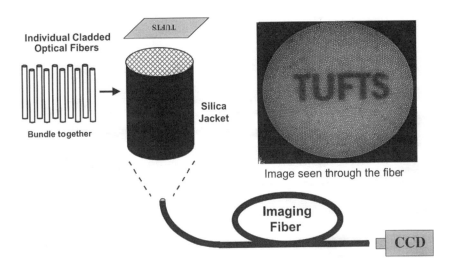

Figure 3   An optical imaging fiber. (Left) Thousands of individually clad optical fibers are drawn together in a coherent fashion such that an image is preserved through the fiber to the CCD detector. (Right) Image of *Tufts* as viewed through a modified imaging fiber. (Modified from Ref. 38.)

those regions of the fiber where the pinhole is directed. This packing arrangement allows for the design of multianalyte sensors to be deposited onto the fiber-optic tip, as seen in Figure 4. Different sensor chemistries are immobilized, and the sensor's performance is dependent on the polymerization time and solution composition of monomer and initiator. Optical imaging fibers have been employed to photopolymerize sensing regions on their distal tips to monitor pH [43,48,55,66], CO_2 [55], oxygen [55,59], penicillin [43], glucose [59], DNA [57], and organic vapors [51]. In one study, a pH sensor was deposited onto the distal end of a fiber tip [48], and in another many pH polymer spots were deposited using aryl azides [66]. The fiber tip can be highly packed with polymer spots 2.5 μm in diameter, spaced 4.5 μm apart, and 1.2 μm high [56].

Biosensors contain a biological recognition element connected to a transducer. One type of biosensor can be developed by immobilizing enzymes into polymer matrices that also contain transducer elements for monitoring enzyme-substrate products [43,58,59]. In one study, a sensor array was employed for simultaneous and continuous measurement of glucose and oxygen [59]. The glucose biosensors are synthesized from defined polymer spots, with immobilized fluorescent probes positioned onto the distal end of an imaging fiber. The first sensor type is glucose oxidase with a ruthenium dye, $Ru(Ph_2Phen)_3^{2+}$, immobilized into the polymer spot. The variations in O_2 are monitored by a second sensor

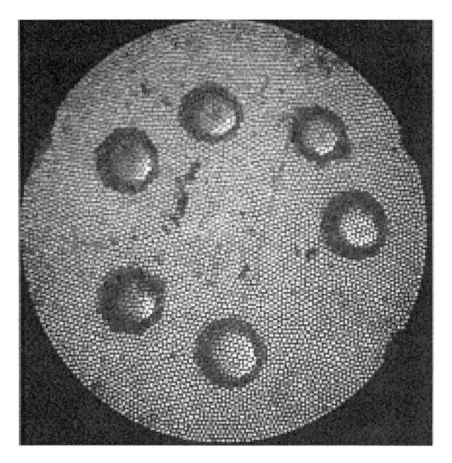

Figure 4 CCD image showing six photodeposited polymer-sensing regions when illuminated with white light. Multianalyte sensor arrays have been fabricated with similar optical imaging fibers for simultaneous measurement of multiple chemical species (see text). The outer diameter of this fiber is 350 μm.

spot, which does not have the immobilized glucose oxidase but contains only the ruthenium dye. The ruthenium dye's fluorescence in a siloxane matrix is quenched in the presence of increasing O_2. Since glucose consumption depletes the O_2 level in the polymer, fluorescence decreases in the presence of glucose. The oxygen-independent glucose fiber-optic sensor is compact and has fast response times to glucose, and this sensor provided a technique for fabricating future photodeposited biosensors.

A biosensor was developed for the analysis of penicillin based on changes in pH by using a pH-sensitive polymer containing the enzyme penicillinase [58].

This initial work with a single-analyte penicillin sensor led to the development of a dual-analyte pH-referenced penicillin sensor [43]. The sensor was made up of two distinct spot types immobilized onto the distal end of a fiber tip. One spot contained the pH-sensitive dye, fluorescein, and measured a pH change due to the environment. The other spot measured the pH change due to the presence of both penicillin and the environment. The pH/penicillin spot had immobilized penicillinase, which converts penicillin to penicilloic acid to cause a microenvironmental pH change. Four 27-μm-diameter spots of each sensor type were deposited onto the fiber tip to eliminate any slight variations in the spot synthesis. Initially, the sensor was tested in two penicillin solutions 0 and 5 mM in phosphate buffer, pH 7. The presence of penicillin is indicated by a fluorescence decrease in the pH/penicillin spot due to the enzymatic generation of penicilloic acid. The sensor was used to follow batch penicillin fermentation, which exhibited medium pH changes as the fermentation progressed. During fermentation, samples were removed and stored until the fermentation was complete. The sensor was tested against a known colorimetric method and demonstrated excellent agreement for the concentration of penicillin, independent of pH changes.

Fabrication of a multianalyte sensor for the simultaneous measurement of O_2, CO_2, and pH integrated the results from both the pH [48] and CO_2 [63] single-analyte detection schemes [55]. The sensor had six 40-μm-diameter polymer spots on the fiber tip, with two replicates of each sensor type. The two O_2 sensing spots were made up of a ruthenium dye imbedded in the siloxane polymer spot. Initially, four pH-sensitive spots, with immoblized fluorescein, were deposited onto the fiber tip. Two of these pH-sensitive regions became the pH sensors. The other two were converted to CO_2-sensing regions by saturating them with bicarbonate buffer and coating them with a gas-permeable membrane. In the presence of CO_2, the fluorescence intensity decreased due to an internal shift in pH of the CO_2-sensing spots upon generation of carbonic acid inside the membrane. The multianalyte sensor measured in the range of 0–100% for O_2, 0–10% for CO_2, and 5.5–7.5 pH. Monitoring the process of beer fermentation tested the multianalyte sensor's measurement capacity. Unfermented wort saturated with different amounts of CO_2 and O_2 was used as a calibration solution. To this solution, yeast was added, and the sensor measured O_2, CO_2, and pH. The formation of CO_2 during fermentation decreased the pH of the solution, while the yeast consumed O_2. During the fermentation, the sensor measured O_2, CO_2 and pH simultaneously.

The previously described seven-single-core-fiber DNA sensor array resulted in a bulky array, however, and with more than seven probes the bundle would become unwelding. The alternative approach was to employ an optical imaging fiber to reduce the overall size of the array. The need to site-specifically deposit many DNA-sensing sites required the photodeposition of DNA-sensitive polymer matrices [57]. The previous polymer photodeposition technologies used to fabricate enzymatic biosensors were ineffectual for fabricating DNA sensors due to the small size of the DNA probe and the weakly cross-linked polymer matrix required. The sensor was created by the site-selective photodeposition of low cross-linked amine-reactive polymers onto the fiber-optic tip and reacting the polymers with 5′ amino-terminated oligonucleotide probes until the sensor contained no more amine-reactive sites. The sensor was tested with p(dA) immobilized onto the fiber tip and the target p(dT)-FITC in solution. The sensor could be repeatedly washed and rehybridized. The lowest concentration of p(dT)-FITC detected was 1.3 nM; however, a p(dT)-biotin target with a streptavidin-FITC gave a detection limit of 0.2 nM. The decreased detection limit was due to the increase of fluorescein signal through multiple fluorescein binding sites on the streptavidin.

Two oligonucleotide probes were designed and incorporated into the polymer spots to test whether the sensor could distinguish point mutations. The H-ras-wt (wild type) and the H-ras-\Gk\D with a single base-pair mismatch were incorporated onto a fiber-optic tip to detect point mutations. A 109-base-pair PCR product was then hybridized to the array. At 28°C, the target hybridizes both immobilized sequences. At 54°C, only the perfect compliment gives a fluorescent signal. The major limitation of the photodeposited sensor arrays is the fabrication time due to the number of steps required.

D. High-Density Sensor Arrays

In the remainder of this chapter, we will discuss our laboratory's development of high-density sensor array platforms that may offer significant improvements in diagnostic-related monitoring over current methods. High-density optical sensor arrays employ the same types of optical imaging fibers discussed previously and allow thousands of individually addressable transducer elements to simultaneously monitor chemical species in a high-speed and reproducible fashion. We have also shown that these array platforms have a detection limit enhancement built into their design. Our high-density sensor arrays [40] have been employed to monitor living cells [62], detect low-level vapors [47,52], develop immunoassays [67–69], detect fluorescently labeled DNA targets in the zeptomole range [53], and unlabeled DNA targets [61] in a complex environment.

1. Optical Imaging Fiber Employed as High-Density Sensor Array Platform

The polished tip of an optical imaging fiber can be placed in acidic solution, and selective etching of the core or cladding results, depending on the fiber material's composition. The selective etching was used to show that both ordered microtip arrays [70] and micro-and nano-well arrays [65] are easily fabricated on the face of an optical imaging fiber. The array of microwells etched onto the fiber's distal face creates high-density ordered microwells, with each well being individually interrogated because it is optically "wired" to an optical fiber. Figure 5A shows an atomic force micrograph (AFM) of a portion of the etched face of an optical imaging fiber. The ordered microwells serve as the high-density array platform. Many sensing tasks have been designed with this platform by incorporating complementary-sized sensor beads such that one bead is contained in each microwell. These functionalized silica or latex beads have a defined size and incorporate a designed fluorescent probe. The fabrication of the microwell arrays has introduced a new architecture for optical sensing.

2. Randomly Ordered Addressable High-Density Optical Sensor Arrays

The thousands of fused optical fibers can each incorporate *one* sensory material to produce an enhanced, high-density sensor array capable of multianalyte sensing on the tip of a 500- to 1000-μm optical imaging fiber [40]. Assembling the high-density sensor arrays consists of two simple steps: (1) etching microwells and (2) placing an aliquot ($\sim$1 μL) of a microbead sensor suspension onto the fiber's distal face. As the solution evaporates, the microbead sensors spontaneously assemble into the etched wells (one sensor per well) and the excess beads are wiped off. Figure 5B shows the etched microwells housing sensors. Micronsized sensors with different encoding chemistries, i.e., optical bar codes, randomly position themselves in the optical fiber array (Fig. 6), and the bar codes allow the user to positionally register the different sensor elements through the use of different encoding schemes [40,52,53,61,71]. The optical bar code is a mixture of fluorescent dyes with different excitations, emissions, and intensities to independently identify each bead in an array. Such encoding enables array fabrication to be simplified, since sensors can be randomly dispersed throughout the array instead of being specifically positioned.

Due to the randomized nature of the sensor platform, new sensors, as they are developed, can be readily incorporated into the array without effort or ruining the addressable nature of the platform. The array takes minutes to fabricate, and some arrays can be stored for many months. The burden of fabricating identical sensing elements is also alleviated, because billions of microbead sensors are fabricated at one time; for example, one milliliter of a bead suspension contains $\sim 6 \times 10^9$ microspheres with identical chemistries. Sensor stocks can also be reproducibly fabricated from one batch to the next, and in some instances sensor shelf life has been shown to be at least ten months [47].

3. Detection Limit Enhancements

As mentioned earlier, fluid analysis can be one of the most important tools for diagnostic monitoring, and the volume required by some current systems is relatively high. Very small sample volumes are needed for the fiber-optic sys-

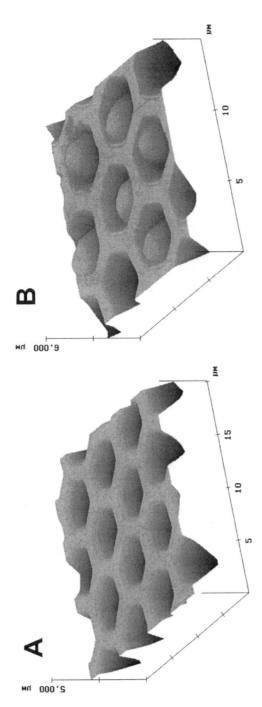

Figure 5 Atomic force micrograph (AFM) of the etched face of an optical imaging fiber before (A) and after (B) complementary-sized microspheres were randomly distributed onto the fiber tip. The randomly distributed microsensors are individually addressable because each bead sensor is optically "wired" to an optical fiber (see Fig. 6). The beads have an incorporated optical bar code so they can be positionally registered within minutes of sensor fabrication. The individual bead sensors here are 3.1-μm polymer beads. (From Ref. 60.)

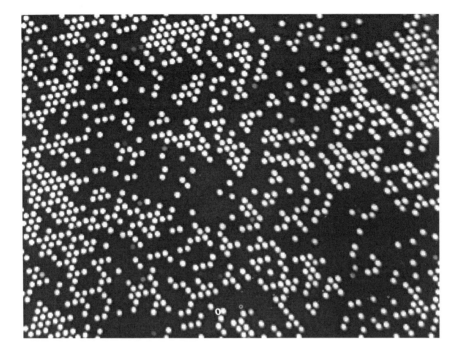

Figure 6 Fluorescence image of an optical imaging fiber with individually addressable microsensors. This CCD image was acquired with a 10× microscope objective lens, and each optical fiber core is 5 μm in outer diameter. Roughly 970 microsensors are accounted for in this portion of the ~1.2-mm-diameter optical imaging fiber.

tem, and the fluorescence-based measurement in the array platform enhances observed detection limits to an unprecedented level. The system is inherently sensitive for measuring targets in small sample volumes (<10 μL), and sensor redundancy within the array brings both detection limit enhancements and confidence in the detection. Incorporating small features to be measured and providing extremely large spatial resolution allows chemical concentrations and gradients to be measured on scales smaller than individual cells. Reduced measurement volumes also allows for highly localized target concentrations. Smaller sensors enable the interrogation of an even smaller absolute number of molecules without necessarily sacrificing sensitivity.

Sensor redundancy is another important feature for increasing the signal-to-noise ratio (S/N) of a measurement. The microsensor arrays allow one to simultaneously monitor hundreds or thousands of sensor elements during target exposure. The S/N increases by $\sqrt{n}$, where n is the number of sensors analyzed.

This signal enhancement essentially removes noise from individual sensors by averaging responses over many sensors. If each sensor within the array responds with a small signal to a low-level target, then their identical response profiles can be combined. By summing large numbers of sensors, we are able to improve the precision and speed of the measurement and thereby measure decreasing concentrations of analyte in a high-throughput fashion. Sensor redundancy and the ability to enhance detection limits through signal processing removes most false positives and false negatives and has been employed to detect low-level vapor [47,52] and zeptomole levels of fluorescently labeled DNA targets [53]. The use of these high-density sensor arrays in medical diagnostics has only begun, and their potential and other diagnostic multianalyte sensing applications is being explored.

4. Application of the High-Density Sensor Arrays for DNA Detection

The high-density bead arrays are important tools for high-speed diagnostic tests with low target concentration. These arrays have been employed for detecting ultralow levels of fluorescently labeled DNA targets [53] and also for detecting unlabeled DNA targets in a complex mixture [61]. Miniaturized high-density arrays offer powerful sensing capabilities for advanced genetic analysis and diagnosis of disease-related gene mutations or for monitoring targets known to play a role in certain diseases. The DNA biosensor array, developed in our laboratory, employs the same optical substrate geometry as discussed earlier: functionalized microsphere sensors are incorporated into the etched microwells on the face of an optical imaging fiber.

Single-stranded oligonucleotide probes are attached to optically encoded microspheres (3 μm), and multiple types of microbead sensors are then mixed together. The mixed sensor population is then randomly distributed on the etched face of an optical imaging fiber to create a randomly ordered, addressable high-density bead array. The encoded microspheres allow the sensors to be positionally registered within minutes. One such study incorporated 25 different oligonucleotide probes and was employed to detect multiple DNA sequences in parallel by monitoring hybridization of fluorescently labeled target oligonucleotides. The 25 sequences were from various disease states and disease-related genes (oncogenes, cystic fibrosis). An enhancement in fluorescence is observed when the fluorescently labeled target hybridizes to its complementary strand immobilized onto the surface of the microsphere. Hybridization occurs within seconds, and nonspecific binding does not contribute to a fluorescence signal enhancement. As briefly discussed before, these arrays employ very small volumes of sample (10 μL), and the absolute number of target molecules remains unchanged.

Therefore, the small sample volumes allow for relatively high local concentrations of target on each bead; 10 fM can be detected in less than ten minutes [53]. Employing the same array platform also enables the detection of unlabeled DNA targets in a complex environment [61]. A randomly addressable bead array was fabricated in which each microsphere was functionalized with molecular beacons. Molecular beacons are hairpin-shaped structures in which the 5' and 3' nucleic acid ends are complementary to each other, which keeps a fluorophore and quencher in proximity. As the complementary DNA target hybridizes to its complementary pair on the molecular beacon, the fluorophore and quencher are separated, resulting in an increase in fluorescence upon target hybridization. The molecular beacons employed were designed to be complementary to different wild-type and mutated genes of the cystic fibrosis transmembrane conductance regular region. This DNA biosensor was capable of making quantitative measurements with a detection limit of approximately 100 pM. There was a linear relationship between the initial rate of beacon fluorescence vs. target concentration, enabling unknown target concentrations to be determined.

III. CONCLUSIONS

Imaging fibers are excellent optical substrates for medical diagnostic assays and multianalyte sensing applications. Our laboratory's sensor technology has progressed from employing single-core optical fibers and fiber bundles to high-density microsensor arrays incorporating thousands of sensors for simultaneous measurements. These arrays have the ability to detect analytes in very small volumes, with detection limit enhancements built into their design. Other diagnostic measurements that could be employed with our optical imaging fiber arrays are monitoring processes of living cells [62] and breath analysis [49,50]. The imaging fibers can thus be employed for simultaneous measurement of multiple chemical species in an environment, or they can be employed for imaging and chemical characterizations [39,41,42,60,70,72], which is advantageous for sensing applications where visual information cannot otherwise be acquired. These imaging and sensing properties could serve as an enhanced endoscope to facilitate information gathering during surgery. Optical sensors potentially can perform well in complex environments without the need for periodic calibrations or extra reagents and are fast, reversible, reliable, cost effective, sensitive, and target selective. Sensors have to deal with complex environments, and in vivo diagnostic assays might incorporate cross-reactivity into a sensor's design so that the brunt of the analysis is left to pattern recognition and computation instead of resting on the design of highly selective and sensitive sensor materials.

ACKNOWLEDGMENTS

The authors gratefully acknowledge support from the National Institutes of Health, Office of Naval Research, Department of Energy, Defense Advanced Research Projects Agency, Environmental Protection Agency, and the National Science Foundation for the generous support of the work.

REFERENCES

1. Collins, M.E.; Meyerhoff, M.E. Anal. Chem. 62:425A–437A, 1990.
2. Hu, C. Nanotechnology 10:113–116, 1999.
3. Li, J.; Papadopoulos, C.; Xu, J.M.; Moskovits, M. Appl. Phys. Lett. 75:367–369, 1999.
4. Motesharei, K.; Ghadiri, M.R.J. Am. Chem. Soc 119:11306–11312, 1997.
5. Wong, S.S.; Joselevich, E.; Woolley, A.T.; Cheung, C.L.; Lieber, C.M. Nature 394: 52–55, 1998.
6. Downs, C.; Nugent, J.; Ajayan, P.M.; Duquette, D.J.; Santhanam, K.S. V. Adv. Mater. 11:1028–1031, 1999.
7. Clark, H.A.; Kopelman, R.; Tjalkens, R.; A., P.M. Anal. Chem. 71:4837–4843, 1999.
8. Clark, H.A.; Hoyer, M.; A., P.M.; Kopelman, R. Anal. Chem. 71:4831–4836, 1999.
9. Kukla, A L.; Kanjuk, N.I.; Starodub, N.F.; Shirshov, Y.M. Sens. Actuators B B57: 213–218, 1999.
10. Cohen, A.E.; Kunz, R.R. Sens. Actuators B B62:23–29, 2000.
11. Tercier-Waeber, M.-L.; Pei, J.; Buffle, J.; Fiaccabrino, G.C.; Koudelka-Hep, M.; Riccardi, G.; Confalonieri, F.; Sina, A.; Graziottin, F. Electroanalysis 12:27–34, 2000.
12. Hinkers, H.; Hermes, T.; Sundermeier, C.; Borchardt, M.; Dumschat, C.; Buecher, S.; Buehner, M.; Cammann, K.; Knoll, M. Sens. Actuators B B24:300–303, 1995.
13. Paeschke, M.; Wollenberger, U.; Lisec, T.; Schnakenberg, U.; Hintsche, R. Sens. Actuators B B27:394–397, 1995.
14. Tercier-Waeber, M.-L.; Buffle, J.; Confalonieri, F.; Riccardi, G.; Sina, A.; Graziottin, F.; Fiaccabrino, G C.; Koudelka-Hep, M. Meas. Sci. Technol. 10:1202–1213, 1999.
15. Ramsay, G. Nat. Biotechnol. 16:40–44, 1998.
16. Marshall, A.; Hodgson, J. Nat. Biotechnol. 16:27–31, 1998.
17. Budach, W.A.; Abel, A.P.; Alfredo, E.; Neuschaefer, D. Anal. Chem. 71:3347–3355, 1999.
18. Gerry, N P.; Witowski, N.E.; Day, J.; Hammer, R.P.; Barany, G.; Barany, F. J. Mol. Bio. 292:251–262, 1999.
19. Case-Green, S.C.; Mir, K.U.; Pritchard, C.E.; Southern, E.M. Curr. Opin. Chem. Biol. 2:404–410, 1998.
20. Fodor, S.P.A. Science 277:393, 1997.
21. Chee, M.; Yang, R.; E., H.; Berno, A.; Huang, X.C.; Stern, D.; Winkler, J.; Lockhart, D. J.; Morris, M.S.; Fodor, S.P.A. Science 274, 1996.

22. Brown, P.O.; Botstein, D. Nature Genetics 21:33–37, 1999 (supplement).
23. Teasdale, P.R.; Wallace, G.G. Analyst 118:329–334, 1993.
24. Kriz, D.; Kempe, M.; Mosbach, K. Sens. Actuators B B33:178–181, 1996.
25. Nicholls, I.A.; Andersson, L.I.; Mosbach, K.; Ekberg, B. Trends Biotechnol. 13: 47–51, 1995.
26. Winklmair, M.; Schuetz, A.J.; Weller, M.G.; Niessner, R. Fresenius' J. Anal. Chem. 363:731–737, 1999.
27. Skladal, P.; Kalab, T. Anal. Chim. Acta 316:73–78, 1995.
28. Watt, A.P.; Morrison, D.; Evans , D.C. Drug Discovery Today 5:17–24, 2000.
29. Pisanelli, A.M.; Qutob, A.A.; Travers, P.; Szyszko, S.; Persaud, K.C. Life Chem. Rep. 11:303–308, 1994.
30. Hofmann, T.; Schieberle, P.; Krummel, C.; Freiling, A.; Bock, J.; Heinert, L.; Kohl, D. Sens. Actuators B B41:81–87, 1997.
31. Mandenius, C.-F.; Ekloev, T.; Lundstroem, I. Biotechnol. Bioeng. 55:427–438, 1997.
32. Grate, J.W.; Wise, B.M.; Abraham, M.H. Anal. Chem. 71:4544–4553, 1999.
33. Abbas, M.N.; Moustafa, G.A.; Mitrovics, J.; Gopel, W. Anal. Chim. Acta 393: 67–76, 1999.
34. Park, J.; Groves, W.A.; Zellers, T. Anal. Chem. 71:3877–3886, 1999.
35. Groves, W.A.; Zellers, E.T.; Frye, G.C. Anal. Chim. Acta 371:131–143, 1998.
36. Doleman, B.J.; Sanner, R.D.; Severin, E.J.; Grubbs, R.H.; Lewis, N.S. Anal. Chem. 70:2560–2564, 1998.
37. Craven, M.A.; Gardner, J.W.; Bartlett, P.N. Trends Anal. Chem. 15:486–493, 1996.
38. Pantano, P.; Walt, D.R. Anal. Chem. 67:481A, 1995.
39. Bronk, K.S.; Michael, K.M.; Pantano, P.; Walt, D.R. Anal. Chem. 67:2750–2757, 1995.
40. Michael, K.L.; Talylor, L.C.; Shultz, S.L.; Walt, D.R. Anal. Chem. 70:1242–1248, 1998.
41. Michael, K.L.; Ferguson, J.A.; Healey, B.G.; Panova, A.A.; Pantano, P.; Walt, D.R. In: Usmani, N.A. ed. The Use of Optical-Imaging Fibers for the Fabrication of Array Sensors. Washington, DC, 1998. Vol. 690, pp 273–289.
42. Panova, A.A.; Pantano, P.; Walt, D.R. Anal. Chem. 69:1635–1641, 1997.
43. Healey, B.G.; Walt, D.R. Anal. Chem. 67:4471–4476, 1995.
44. Grojean, R.E.; Sousa, J.A. Rev. Sci. Instrum. 51:377–378, 1980.
45. Dun, N.J.; Dun, S.L.; Wu, S.Y. Neurosci. Lett. 158:51–54, 1993.
46. Skrdla, P.J.; Saavedra, S.S.; Armstrong, N.R.; Mendes, S.B.; Peyghambarian, N. Anal. Chem. 72:1947–1955, 2000.
47. Albert, K.J.; Walt, D.R. Anal. Chem. 72:1947–1955, 2000.
48. Barnard, S.M.; Walt, D.R. Nature 353:338–340, 1991.
49. White, J.; Kauer, J.S.; Dickinson, T.A.; Walt, D.R. Anal. Chem. 68:2191–2202, 1996.
50. Dickinson, T.A.; White, J.; Kauer, J.S.; Walt, D.R. Nature 382:697–700, 1996.
51. Dickinson, T.A.; White, J.; Kauer, J.S.; Walt, D.R. Anal. Chem. 69:3413–3418, 1997.
52. Dickinson, T.A.; Michael, K.M.; Kauer, J.S.; Walt, D.R. Anal. Chem. 71:2192–2198, 1999.

53. Epstein, J.R.; Lee, M.; Walt, D.R. Anal. Chem. in press (2002).
54. Ferguson, J.A.; Boles, T.C.; Adams, C.P.; Walt, D.R. Nature Biotechnol. 14:1681–1684, 1996.
55. Ferguson, J.A.; Healey, B.G.; Bronk, K.S.; Barnard, S.M.; Walt, D.R. Anal. Chimica Acta 340:123–131, 1997.
56. Healey, B.G.; Foran, S.E.; Walt, D.R. Science 269:1078–1080, 1995.
57. Healey, B.G.; Walt, D.R. Anal. Biochem. 251:270–279, 1997.
58. Kulp, T.J.; Camins, I.; Angel, S.M.; Munkholm, C.; Walt, D.R. Anal. Chem. 59: 2849–2853, 1987.
59. Li, L.; Walt, D.R. Anal. Chem. 67:3746–3752, 1995.
60. Michael, K.L.; Talylor, L.C.; Walt, D.R. Anal. Chem. 71:2766–2773, 1999.
61. Steemers, F.J.; Ferguson, J.A.; Walt, D.R. Nat. Biotech. 18:91–94, 2000.
62. Taylor, L.C.; Walt, D.R. Anal. Biochem. 278:132–142, 2000.
63. Uttamlal, M.; Walt, D.R. Biotechnology 13:597–601, 1995.
64. Johnson, S.R.; Sutter, J.M.; Engelhardt, H.L.; Jurs, P. C. Anal. Chem. 69:4641–4648, 1997.
65. Pantano, P.; Walt, D.R. Chem. Mater. 8:2832–2835, 1996.
66. Bronk, K.S.; Walt, D.R. Anal. Chem. 66:3519–3520, 1994.
67. Szurdoki, F.; Michael, K.L.; Taylor, L.C.; Schultz, S.L.; Walt, D.R. Fluorescent Immunoassays Performed on Microspheres. American Chemical Society: Boston, MA. 1998. Vol. 216, pp ANYL-034.
68. Szurdoki, F.; Michael, K.L.; Agrawal, D.; Taylor, L.C.; Schultz, S.L.; Walt, D.R. In: Chen, Y.-R., ed. Immunofluorescence Detection Methods Using Microspheres. SPIE—The International Society for Optical Engineering: Bellingham, WA. 1999, Vol. 3544, pp 52–62.
69. Szurdoki, F.; Michael, K.L.; Walt, D.R. Anal. Biochem. 291:219–228, 2001.
70. Pantano, P.; Walt, D.R. Rev. Sci. Instrum. 68:1357–1359, 1997.
71. Albert, K.J.; Gill, D.S.; Pearce, T.C.; Walt, D.R. manuscript submitted February 2002.
72. Michael, K.L.; Walt, D.R. Anal. Biochem. 273:168–178, 1999.

7
Optochemical Nanosensors for Noninvasive Cellular Analysis

Susan L. R. Barker
Veridian, Charlottesville, Virginia, U.S.A.

Heather A. Clark
University of Connecticut Health Center, Farmington, Connecticut, U.S.A.

Raoul Kopelman
University of Michigan, Ann Arbor, Michigan, U.S.A.

I. INTRODUCTION

Advances in sensor technology often involve development of new ways of detecting a particular analyte or creation of new sensing methodologies that can be applied to a variety of sensors. Here we describe an example of each of two modes of analytical sensor research, both focused on novel ways to apply fluorescence spectroscopy to the detection of cellular analytes. The first section describes developments in optical sensors for detection of cellular nitric oxide. Two biosensors and one chemical sensor have been developed that are highly selective and reversible and have fast response times. These sensors have been applied to extracellular and intracellular measurements of macrophage produced nitric oxide.

The second section describes the production of the smallest anthropogenic devices to date, spherical sensors (wireless and fiberless) with radii as small as 10 nm. This class of optochemical PEBBLE (probe encapsulated by biologically localized embedding) sensors covers a wide range of analytes (such as pH, calcium, oxygen, and potassium) with excellent spatial, temporal, and chemical resolution.

139

These PEBBLEs have been used to monitor intracellular analytes and to cause minimal perturbation when delivered and operated inside single mammalian cells, such as human neuroblastoma, mouse oocytes, or rat alveolar macrophage.

II. NITRIC OXIDE SENSORS

Investigation of the numerous biological roles of nitric oxide [1–6] creates the need for noninvasive, sensitive, and selective detection methods capable of real-time nitric oxide measurement. Previously, a number of different electrochemical and optical sensors have been developed for detection of aqueous nitric oxide [7–16]. In addition, fluorescein derivatives have been used for solution and cellular detection of nitric oxide [17]. We have developed three new nitric oxide-selective optical sensors using alternative methods for real-time detection of cellular nitric oxide.

Sensors generally incorporate molecular-recognition elements that are biomolecules, such as an enzyme, resulting in a biosensor, or a nonbiological molecule, such as an indicator dye, giving a chemical sensor. We present here two biosensors prepared with heme-containing or heme-binding biomolecules and one novel chemical sensor, based on analyte adsorption to a metal surface reported by fluorescence changes of a surface-attached dye molecule. The biosensor and chemical sensor detection schemes have been used to create ratiometric fiber-optic sensors for determination of extracellular nitric oxide. In addition, lifetime-based fiberless sensors have been applied to the measurement of intracellular nitric oxide. These sensors represent significant advances in selectivity and in real-time detection of nitric oxide.

A. Biosensor I

In the first biosensor developed [18], the chemical-recognition element is cytochrome c′, a hemoprotein known to be highly selective for nitric oxide [19–24]. The cytochrome c′ was attached to the tip of an optical fiber via colloidal gold. Proteins have been shown to retain their bioactivity [25,26] when adsorbed to colloidal gold, which has been shown to be a useful biosensor matrix [26–29]. In the original sensors [18], cytochrome c′ was labeled with a fluorescent spectator dye (Oregon Green™), and changes in the fluorescence *intensity* of the dye were observed. Oregon Green™ alone is unaffected by nitric oxide [7] but effectively reports changes in the cytochrome c′ as it binds nitric oxide [18,30]. The main drawback of this sensor was its reliance on a single fluorescence intensity.

Sensors based on measurements of a single fluorescence spectrum peak intensity are known to be problematic in most practical applications [31]. Ratiometric sensors have been one answer to the problems posed by intensity measurements [31]. Another solution has been the measurement of fluorescence lifetimes [32].

The cytochrome c' biosensors were improved [30] upon by the addition of a second fluorescent dye as a reference dye as well as by the measurement of fluorescence lifetimes. The ratiometric technique allowed the development of reliable fiber-optic sensors, which in turn have been used for measurements of extracellular macrophage nitric oxide. The fluorescence-lifetime measurements of nitric oxide were made with the dye-labeled cytochrome c', both in solution and in the cytosol of macrophages. These were the first direct as well as selective measurements of intracellular nitric oxide concentrations of macrophages in culture.

The *ratiometric* sensors were developed [30] by adding a second fluorescent component, derivatized microspheres, to the sensor tip. The 685-nm fluorescence of these spheres is not affected by micro- to millimolar levels of nitric oxide, making it an ideal reference peak. The sensor fluorescence emission spectrum is shown in Figure 1. The sensor response was determined from the ratio (R) of fluorescence intensity of the labeling dye, Oregon Green^{TM}488, to the fluorescence intensity of the reference microspheres. The sensors were calibrated (Fig. 2) over the range 0–0.7 mM nitric oxide, and the response was found to be linear ($r^2 = 0.998$) with a slope of 0.56 $\Delta R_0/R$/mM NO, where R_0 is the dye ratio at zero nitric oxide and R is the dye ratio at each nitric oxide concentration, resulting in a limit of detection of 8 µM.

The reference microspheres have excellent photostability. Therefore all effects of photobleaching on the sensor signal were due to photobleaching of

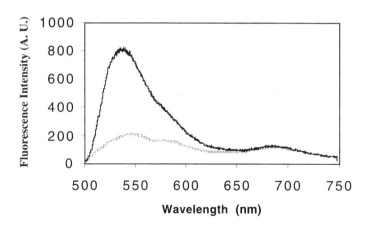

Figure 1 Emission spectrum of a fiber-optic sensor excited at 488 nm. Solid line, purged with N_2 (same as in air); dotted line, qualitatively saturated with NO. The 540-nm peak is the fluorescence emission of the dye-labeled cytochrome c', and the 685-nm peak is the fluorescence emission of the reference microspheres.

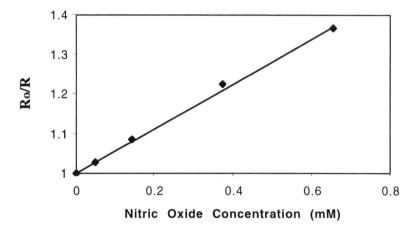

Figure 2   Response of fiber-optic ratiometric cytochrome c′ biosensors. The calibration was performed in 100 mM pH 7.4 phosphate buffer. The fluorescence ratio was R_0/R was plotted against nitric oxide concentration.

the cytochrome c′ labeling dye (Oregon Green™) and were comparable to those reported previously [18]. The ratiometric sensors have excellent reversibility, as shown in Figure 3. In addition, the sensors have fast response times to both increases and decreases in nitric oxide. The 0–90% response time was measured to be 0.25 sec (Fig. 4) but is equipment limited.

For the ratiometric cytochrome c′ sensor the response to numerous potential interferents was determined [30]. The sensors did not respond to 1M nitrate, 1 M nitrate, 1 M chloride, or 100% oxygen. The sensor is useful in the pH 6–9 range. Measurements of interference from hydrogen peroxide, peroxynitrate, and superoxide are particularly relevant to the application of this sensor to measurements of nitric oxide produced by macrophages. We found that high levels of hydrogen peroxide, superoxide, and peroxynitrite, as compared to the amounts present in the macrophage environment, had little effect on the sensors. From this data we concluded that these compounds do not significantly interfere with the measurement of macrophage-produced nitric oxide.

The fluorescence lifetime (τ) of the dye-labeled cytochrome c′ in 100 mM phosphate buffer solution was determined to be 4.0 nsec. Upon addition of nitric oxide, this lifetime became shorter. When plotted (Fig. 5) as the difference ($\tau_0 - \tau$) between the fluorescence lifetime in the absence of nitric oxide (τ_0) and the fluorescence lifetime at each nitric oxide concentration (τ), the response is linear ($r^2 = 0.996$) with a slope of 3.9 $\Delta\tau$ (nsec/mM NO) and a limit of detection of 30 µM nitric oxide.

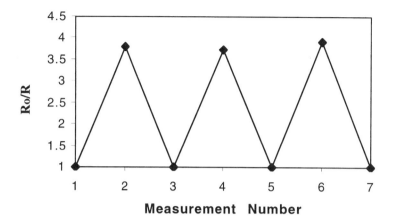

Figure 3 Reversibility of fiber-optic ratiometric cytochrome c′ biosensors. The fluorescence ratio R_0/R was plotted against measurement number. Alternating measurements were taken in 100 mM pH 7.4 phosphate buffer and 100 mM pH 7.4 phosphate buffer with arbitrary high concentrations of nitric oxide. The standard deviation of the measurements in buffer without nitric oxide is less than 1%.

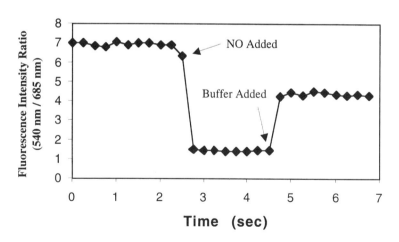

Figure 4 Response time of fiber-optic ratiometric cytochrome c′ biosensors. The ratio of fluorescence intensities (540 nm/685 nm) was plotted against time (sec). The initial points were taken in 100 mM pH 7.4 phosphate buffer, and qualitative aliquots of nitric oxide in 100 mM pH 7.4 and 100 mM pH 7.4 buffer were added sequentially.

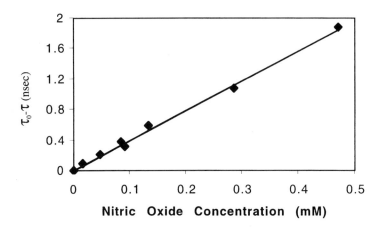

Figure 5   Lifetime response of dye-labeled cytochrome c' in 100 mM pH 7.4 phosphate buffer. The difference in the fluorescence lifetime ($\tau_0 - \tau$) was plotted against nitric oxide concentration.

B.   Biosensor II

Biosensors analogous to those prepared with dye-labeled hemoprotein cytochrome c' have been prepared [33] with the heme domain of the nitric oxide-binding protein, soluble guanylate cyclase (sGC). This protein is the only known receptor for in vivo nitric oxide [34] and has many similarities to cytochrome c', including a pentacoordinated [35] iron atom, as well as a low affinity for oxygen and a high affinity for nitric oxide [35]. Recently, the N-terminal fragment of the heme-binding $\beta 1$ subunit of sGC was prepared [36]. The heme in this fragment also contains a pentacoordinated iron atom and forms a 5-coordinate complex with nitric oxide [36]. This heme domain (HDsGC) was incorporated into fluorescent, ratiometric fiber-optic sensors that were applied to the measurement of macrophage nitric oxide production.

The HDsGC was also labeled with Oregon Green™. Thus, this sensor functions in a manner analogous to the biosensors [18,30] prepared with cytochrome c', with response governed by the characteristics of the heme domain. The HDsGC sensors have also been made ratiometric by adding fluorescent reference spheres. Again, the sensor response was determined based on the ratio (R) of fluorescence intensity of the labeling dye to the fluorescence intensity of the reference spheres. The response (Fig. 6) was measured between 0 and 0.7 mM nitric oxide and found to be linear ($r^2 = 0.994$), with a slope of 4.7 $\Delta R_0/R/$ mM NO, where R_0 is the dye ratio at zero nitric oxide and R is the dye ratio at

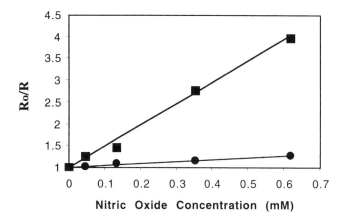

Figure 6 Response of fiber-optic ratiometric sGC peptide biosensors. The fluorescence ratio R_0/R was plotted agtainst nitric oxide concentration. Squares: Calibration in 100 mM pH 7.4 phosphate buffer. Circles: Calibration in 100 mM pH 7.4 phosphate buffer with 8 μM glutathione.

each nitric oxide concentration. This sensor's limit of detection is 1 μM nitric oxide, i.e., eight times lower than the cytochrome c′ sensor.

Again, the reference microspheres have excellent photostability; therefore, the sensor was susceptible only to photobleaching of the labeling dye, which was found to be a double exponential as a function of time. This photobleaching did not significantly affect the sensor response in buffer, for 125 measurements caused a signal decrease equivalent to only 20 μM nitric oxide. Such photo-bleaching did not have a significant effect on the application of this sensor, since only 10–20 measurements were typically made at one time. In addition, a baseline calibration point could be taken in buffer at any time.

The heme domain of soluble guanylate cyclase is still fragile. The HDsGC sensors were thus useful at room temperature for a period of only several hours, but could not be stored at room temperature overnight. However, sensors stored at 0–4°C continued to function for several days.

The HDsGC sensors again have fast response times to increasing or de-creasing nitric oxide. The response time was measured to be 0.25 sec, but again present equipment limitations prevent quantitation of faster response times. In addition, the sensors have excellent reversibility, similar to that shown for the cytochrome c′ biosensors. Changes in the sensor intensity ratio (R) were deter-mined with respect to numerous potential interferents. Again the sensors did not respond to 1M nitrate, 1 M nitrate, or 100% oxygen. However, as mentioned, the labeling-dye-fluorescence is sensitive [37] to pH below 6. Also, the sensor has a nonlinear response to pH over the pH range 6–10. In this work, pH effects were not an issue, because sensor calibrations and cellular measurements were both made in a pH 7.2 buffer.

In addition to nitric oxide, macrophages produce hydrogen peroxide, peroxynitrite, and superoxide, as already stated. Therefore, the extent of interference from these compounds was again determined. The levels of hydrogen peroxide, superoxide, and peroxynitrite tested had little effect on the sensors, though they were high compared to the amounts present in the macrophage environment. We thus predict that these compounds will not significantly interfere with the measurement of macrophage-produced nitric oxide, and cellular measurements (see later) were used to verify these results.

Glutathione has been shown to destabilize the bond between sGC and nitric oxide [38]; however, glutathione does not affect cytochrome c'. Macrophages incubated in Ringer's buffer for 3 hr produced an average of 8 μM glutathione. Therefore, the sensors were calibrated in phosphate buffer containing 8 μM glutathione, and the slope was reduced to 0.42 $\Delta R_0/R$/mM NO (Fig. 6), decreasing the sensor sensitivity by an order of magnitude.

C. Chemical Sensor

We have also developed a novel kind of molecule-specific sensor, based on analyte adsorption to a metal surface that is reported by fluorescence changes of an attached dye molecule [7]. Specifically, we have developed nitric oxide–selective sensors prepared with a difluorofluorescein derivative (Oregon Green^{TM}) on gold. In solution, this dye is optically insensitive to nitric oxide. However, the dye absorbance and fluorescence have been determined to be sensitive to nitric oxide in the presence of colloidal gold. Gold surfaces (which do not fluoresce) have been used to detect gaseous nitric oxide by measuring the reversible increase in electrical resistance of the Au film upon nitric oxide adsorption [39]. However, in the sensors described here, the fluorescence intensity of the fluorescein dye is used to report the nitric oxide adsorption on the gold. This mechanism has allowed preparation of fiber-optic dye-based nitric oxide sensors, which have been made ratiometric by the addition of reference-dye microspheres. These chemical sensors have several advantages over nitric oxide–selective biosensors, including greater stability and commercially available components.

Studies of the dye absorbance, fluorescence excitation, and fluorescence emission show *no* spectral changes between dye in aqueous solution purged with nitrogen and solution saturated with nitric oxide. However, dilute dye (0.2 mM) in a 50-nm colloidal gold solution (0.01%) did respond to nitric oxide, showing intensity decreases in the absorbance and fluorescence excitation and emission spectra upon addition of nitric oxide. A similar, although less drastic, nitric oxide–induced decrease in fluorescence emission intensity of the fluorescein derivative was also observed with the gold colloid–coated fiber sensors. The fluorescence lifetime [40] of the dye on gold was measured using sensors prepared on quartz slides. In buffer purged with nitrogen the lifetime of the dye was found to be 4.0 nsec, while in solution saturated with nitric oxide the lifetime was 3.8 nsec. Fluorescence is known to be quenched due to energy transfer when the fluorescent species is close to a metal surface [41]. However, the drastic changes in the absorbance and fluorescence excitation and emission spectra, coupled with minimal changes in the fluorescence lifetime, indicate a change in the transition dipole of the molecule rather than a quenching mechanism.

Surface-enhanced Raman spectroscopy was used to further investigate the sensor response mechanism using sensors prepared on quartz slides [42]. These results demonstrated that the addition of nitric oxide causes the fluorescein group to reorient on the gold surface. Such orientational rearrangement could result in a change in the transition dipole of the dye molecule, consistent with our earlier interpretation of the absorbance and fluorescence data.

In addition to the fluorescein derivative, fluorescent microspheres that are insensitive to at least millimolar nitric oxide levels were added to the fiber-optic chemical sensors. This allows ratiometric measurements, where the ratio (R) was calculated as the ratio of fluorescence intensity of the fluorescein dye to the fluorescence intensity of the reference spheres. The sensor response was measured in the range 0–1 mM nitric oxide as the ratio (R) of the fluorescence intensity of the fluorescein derivative to the fluorescence intensity of the reference microspheres. The response (Fig. 7) was linear ($r^2 = 0.993$) with a slope of 0.23 $\Delta R_0/R$/mM NO, where R_0 is the dye ratio at zero nitric oxide and R is the dye ratio at each nitric oxide concentration. The limit of detection is 20 μM nitric oxide. The sensors have excellent reversibility and fast response times to increasing or decreasing nitric oxide. With the present equipment, the response time (0–100%) was measured to be 0.25 sec or less. The effects of photobleaching on the sensor signal were also determined. The reference microspheres have excellent photostability. Therefore all effects of photobleaching were due to photobleaching of the fluorescein derivative, which was found to be multiexponential.

The sensor response to numerous potential interferents was determined [7]. Oxygen, nitrite, and nitrate did not interfere with the sensor, and these chemical sensors are useful at pH > 6. The responses to hydrogen peroxide, peroxynitrite, and superoxide were measured, and these chemicals were again found to have little effect on the sensors.

The creation of this nitric oxide sensor, comprising a fluorescent dye on gold, opens the door to further investigations of this new kind of combinatory sensor chemistry and the utility of other dye–metal pairs as selective sensors for other molecules or ions.

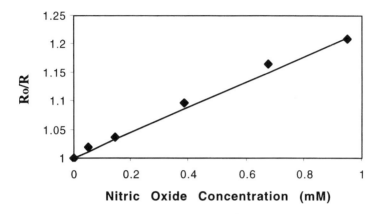

Figure 7 Response of fiber-optic ratiometric dye–based chemical sensors. The calibration was performed in 100 mM pH 7.4 phosphate buffer. The fluorescence ratio R_0/R was plotted against nitric oxide concentration.

D. Applications

Macrophages are known to produce high levels of nitric oxide [43–46] when activated with treatments such as interferon-γ (IFN-γ) and lipopolysaccharide (LPS). In separate experiments [7,30,33], the ratiometric fiber-optic biosensors and chemical sensor were all used to measure the extracellular nitric oxide released by macrophages, as shown in Table 1. The fiber-optic sensors were placed in solution approximately 0.5 cm from the macrophages. For the HDsGC biosensors, the experimental conditions were comparable to those under which the macrophage glutathione production was measured [33]. Therefore, for the HDsGC biosensor, the response slope found in the presence of 8 μM glutathione was used to calculate the macrophage nitric oxide concentrations. The unactivated cells produced about 30 μM nitric oxide, averaged for the three sensor types. Macrophages activated with both LPS and IFN-γ produced an average nitric oxide concentration of 170 μM. Activated macrophages produce superoxide and hydrogen peroxide [43–46] as well as nitric oxide. Therefore, as an alternate method of determining superoxide and hydrogen peroxide interference, cells were activated with LPS and IFN-γ, but nitric oxide production was inhibited with N^{ω}-monomethyl-L-arginine (NMMA). With the biosensors and chemical sensors, the average nitric oxide levels produced by such inhibited cells were comparable to the levels produced by the unactivated cells. Therefore, the sensors' response to compounds other than nitric oxide was found to be minimal.

Table 1 Cellular Nitric Oxide Concentrations Produced by Macrophages Exposed to Various Treatments

| Cell treatment | Extracellular NO (μM): ratiometric sensor measurements | | | Intracellular NO (μM): lifetime measurements |
	Cyt c$'$	HDsGC	Chemical	Cyt c$'$
None	≤20	50 ± 40	<20	<30
IFN-γ & LPS	210 ± 90	120 ± 50	190 ± 70	160 ± 10
IFN-γ, LPS & NMMA	≤40	30 ± 20	≤20	≤30
IFN-γ, LPS & SOD		160 ± 90		
IFN-γ, LPS, NMMA, & SOD		50 ± 20		

Extracellular measurements were made with fiber-optic, ratiometric cytochrome c$'$ biosensors, HDsGC biosensors, and Oregon Green dye–based chemical sensors. The intracellular measurements were by lifetime measurements of the dye-labeled cytochrome c$'$.

Additional experiments were performed with the HDsGC biosensors to verify this sensor's selectivity for nitric oxide [33]. Macrophages were activated with LPS and IFN-γ, but superoxide production was inhibited with SOD. Such macrophages produced high levels of nitric oxide, and cells activated with LPS and IFN-γ and inhibited by NMMA and SOD produced low levels of nitric oxide. Since the unactivated macrophages and the nitric oxide–inhibited cells produced similar low levels of nitric oxide while the activated macrophages produced larger amounts of nitric oxide in the presence or the absence of super-oxide, we concluded that the superoxide and hydrogen peroxide do not significantly affect the sensor response. For the macrophage experiments, the postexperiment cell viability was determined [7,30,33] to be at least 95%.

Intracellular nitric oxide was determined by fluorescence-lifetime measurements of macrophages scrape-loaded with dye-labeled cytochrome c$'$ (Table 1). Figure 8 shows photomicrographs of the cells with the dye-labeled cytochrome c$'$ loaded into the cytosol. In the unactivated cells, nitric oxide was undetectable. The average intracellular nitric oxide concentration of the macrophages activated with both LPS and IFN-γ was 160 ± 10 μM. Cells activated with LPS and IFN-γ and inhibited with NMMA were again used to determine the extent of interference from superoxide and hydrogen peroxide. These nitric oxide–inhibited cells produced nitric oxide levels near the sensor limit of detection, indicating that superoxide and hydrogen peroxide do not have a significant effect on the lifetime-based measurements.

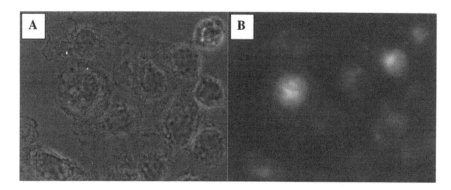

Figure 8 Brightfield (A) and fluorescence (B) images of macrophages scrape-loaded with dye-labeled cytochrome c′.

E. Conclusions

The nitric oxide sensors described here represent significant advances in the pursuit of sensitive, selective methods for real-time detection of nitric oxide. In addition, the ability to make ratiometric and/or lifetime–based measurements makes these techniques quite reliable. The cytochrome c′ biosensors [30] can be used for fiber-optic sensors as well as fiberless sensing. These sensors also offer advantages such as good stability and sensitivity, but they require use of a protein that is not commercially available. Similarly, the HDsGC is a unique peptide requiring specialized preparation. The HDsGC sensors [33] offer high sensitivity but suffer from glutathione interference and lack stability. The dye-based chemical sensors [7] are the least sensitive of the three but can be prepared from commercially available components and are very stable. A comparison of these three sensor types is shown in Table 2. The applications shown earlier demonstrate the applicability of these ratiometric and lifetime-based sensors and their utility for cellular measurements. Such direct measurements will allow experimental analysis of nitric oxide levels during cellular activities and could provide valuable additional information about cellular nitric oxide.

III. PEBBLE SENSORS

Optochemical and electrochemical sensors are playing an increasingly greater role in biological and medical science [47–50]. The common denominator of such chemical sensors is the interface that separates sample chemistry from indicator chemistry. This separation provides the matrix in which novel combi-

Table 2 Comparison of Fiber-Optic, Ratiometric Cytochrome c′ Biosensors, HDsGC Biosensors, and Oregon Green Dye–Based Chemical Sensors

	Cyt c′	HDsGC	Chemical
Limit of detection	8 μM (30 μM[a])	1 μM	20 μM
Reversibility	100%	100%	100%
Reproducibility	99%	99%	99%
Physical stability	Good	Moderate	Excellent
Response time	<250 msec	<250 msec	<250 msec

[a]Lifetime-based measurement.

nations of indicators, sensitizers, catalysts, and stabilizers can act in concert. For intracellular applications, the challenge has been to reduce the sensor's size and thereby to minimize the biological invasiveness, reduce the detection limit, and shorten the response time [51,52]. To date, the smallest sensors have been microelectrodes and submicrometer fiber-based optodes. Due to the encasing capillary or fiber-optic tip (which both have tapered shapes), both micropipettes and fibers have penetration volumes of at least many cubic micrometers, and this cone-shaped volume grows as the third power of the penetration depth. Thus, to reach into the nucleus of an 80-micrometer mouse oocyte cell with a penetration depth of about 40 μm, the fiber-tip penetration volume is typically 1000 μm³ while the cell volume is about 300,000 μm³. Such penetration may induce severe biological perturbation and seriously endanger the viability of the cell. In contrast, the volume of a 0.6-μm-diameter PEBBLE sensor is only 0.2 μm³, i.e., one ppm of the cell's volume; for a 60-nm PEBBLE this penetration volume fraction is only one ppb, a rather negligible mechanical perturbation. This point is particularly significant for smaller mammalian cells, such as the neuroblastoma discussed later. Apparently, even bacterial cells could now be investigated with PEBBLE sensors.

Historically, the PEBBLE sensors are an outgrowth of fluorescent microspheres, beads, and nanoparticles [53]. The first use of a *single* nanoparticle as sensor may have been that of Sasaki et al. [54], where a pH-sensing nanoparticle was manipulated from the bulk of a solution to the interface by means of a laser tweezer (light trap). Compared with simple fluorescent beads that contain a single kind of dye indicator, the optochemical PEBBLE sensors [55] can be more complex in their structure and function (Fig. 9). The PEBBLE composition, including the matrix, the fluorophore, and other components, is optimized for the task at hand, the same as for fiber-based optodes (e.g., ion correlation optodes [56,57]). In addition to the usual considerations (detection limit, selec-

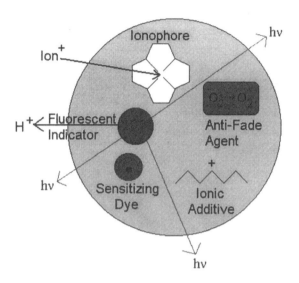

Figure 9 Schematic representation of a PEBBLE sensor containing various active ingredients within the boundaries of a biocompatible polymeric matrix.

tivity, reversibility, reproducibility, stability, etc.), PEBBLE deliverability into the cell and biocompatibility are of great importance.

PEBBLE sensors consist mainly of two types of devices: (1) single or combination indicator molecules in an acrylamide matrix, and (2) multicomponent, multifunction devices in a liquid polymer. The chemical and spectroscopic properties of PEBBLE sensors are analogous to those of fiber-optic sensors, based on the same sensor design, i.e., ionic and optically active components incorporated in a polymeric matrix. The wide array of fiber-based optodes produced to date have been, or are in the process of being, adapted to PEBBLE sensors. Some consist of an indicator dye or a pair of indicator dyes entrapped in the pores of a hydrogel. Such sensors use commercially available fluorescent ion indicators for analytes such as pH, calcium, and oxygen. For instance, a pH PEBBLE has been produced [55] with linear pH response in the range of 6.8–7.5 (slope = 0.32 for fluorescence intensity ratio plotted against pH). This PEBBLE was adapted from a pH optode described previously [58], so the matrix behavior of the indicator could be predicted. The polymer matrix provides the advantages in this type of sensor due to its biocompatibility as well as its chemically and physically controlled microenvironment.

As another example of a hydrogel-based sensor, a ratiometric calcium sensor has been developed [55] that uses two calcium-selective dyes kept in close proximity within the environment of the polymer matrix. Without the matrix, the indicators would move freely throughout the cell and undergo differential sequestration, making ratiometric measurements more difficult. Since the two dyes are used together, the sensor is considerably less prone to inaccurate measurements caused by photobleaching or position within the cell.

The more complex liquid polymer PEBBLE is minimally composed of an ionophore and a pH indicator that work synergistically [57,59,60] (Fig. 9). For example, if a potassium ion penetrates the polymer and is bound by the ionophore, a positive charge is ejected from the matrix to preserve charge neutrality. This positive charge is in the form of a hydrogen ion, which induces a change in the fluorescence spectrum (intensity) of the pH indicator. In this way a sensor can respond with high selectivity to an ion such as potassium. Thus the sensor utilizes selective ionophores developed over many years for ion-selective electrodes rather than relying on less selective fluorescent molecular probes. The same principle holds for both fiber-optic and PEBBLE sensors. However, such synergism could not be achieved with freely floating pairs of ionophore and chromoionophore molecules inside a cell.

A. Hydrogel PEBBLEs

Hydrogel PEBBLEs were fabricated in a microemulsion process [61] to produce spherical sensors ranging from 20 to 200 nm in diameter, as confirmed by transmission electron microscopy (e.g., Fig. 10). Investigations of PEBBLE suspensions were conducted in order to more carefully characterize PEBBLE number densities, morphology, and size distribution. Microscopic examination of the PEBBLEs has been complicated by their gelatinous, water-miscible properties. Transmission electron micrographs of PEBBLE suspensions dried on formvar carbon support grids demonstrate that PEBBLEs produced by the microemulsion process range in diameter from 20 nm to approximately 250 nm. Initial characterization using this technique indicates that the smaller PEBBLEs (20–50 nm in diameter) are present in the highest amounts, while the larger, 200 nm PEBBLEs are present in slightly lower amounts (Table 3). We note that the smallest PEBBLEs weigh only about 1 attogram and contain only zeptograms of active material. In other words, 1 gram of active material produces about 10^{17} such PEBBLEs, and the 200-nm PEBBLEs contain on the order of thousands of active molecules.

B. Delivery Methods

PEBBLE sensors can be used as individual probes, or in clusters of single-function (single-analyte) PEBBLEs, or in sets of multiple-function (multianalyte) PEBBLEs, or in ensembles including sets of clusters. While PEBBLE clus-

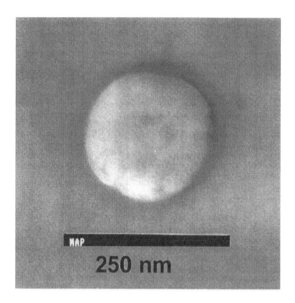

Figure 10 Transmission electron micrograph of a single 50-nm PEBBLE sensor dried on a formvar grid.

ters are appropriate for imaging single-analyte gradients and their dynamics, the sets (or "ensembles") either may give an overall multianalyte measurement or may provide simultaneous, real-time, multianalyte chemical images, describing the spatiotemporal dynamics of complex chemical reactions and events. Thus some of our studies emphasize individual PEBBLE performance, while others emphasize PEBBLE clusters or ensemble characteristics. Each of these options for utilizing PEBBLEs requires different delivery methods. One method was developed based on "biolistic" embedding into the cell via a gene gun system (BioRad, Hercules, CA). The gene gun delivers only one or two PEBBLEs to a

Table 3 Number Densities for PEBBLE Sensors in the Diameter Range of 20–200 nm

20–50 nm	50–100 nm	200–250 nm
$6.2 \times 10^{6}/\mu g$	0.9–$3.8 \times 10^{6}/\mu g$	2.0–$6.0 \times 10^{4}/\mu g$

Reported as numbers of PEBBLEs per microgram of dried PEBBLEs.

cell, making single-PEBBLE measurements possible. An alternative method is to use lyposomes to transport a large number of PEBBLEs into the cytoplasmic space, which allows the user to monitor multiple regions of a cell simultaneously. Two other delivery methods are (1) pico-injection, which allows for controlled PEBBLE delivery and therefore measurements in the cell nucleus, and (2) phagocytosis, which provides for the ability to monitor the chemistry in specialized compartments of immune-competent cells. An example of each of these methods is given shortly.

A gene gun uses a burst of helium to drive PEBBLEs into adherent cells, much like a shotgun blast. The technique injects many cells at once and delivers approximately one or two PEBBLEs to each cell that it injects. Transmission electron microscopy (TEM) images of neuroblastoma cells that have been injected with PEBBLEs using the gene gun indicate that a single PEBBLE or a pair of PEBBLEs is shot into the cytosol of the cells (Fig. 11). Both 200-nm and 20-nm PEBBLEs can be injected via this method. In order to assess the viability of cultured neural cells after pebble delivery with the gene gun, neuroblastoma cells were bombarded with PEBBLEs and immediately tested for the ability to exclude the dye Trypan Blue (as a measure of cell viability). This assay indicated that minimal cell death (1.4% and 2.6% in excess of controls) occurred with biolistic delivery of pebbles (Fig. 12).

Liposomal delivery uses commercially available lipid vesicles to transport PEBBLEs into neuroblastoma cells. The liposomes interact with the PEBBLEs and then fuse to the cell membrane, where they release the PEBBLEs into the cytoplasm. This is a very gentle method, and many PEBBLEs can be introduced

a 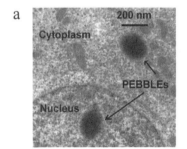   b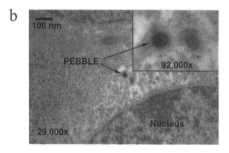

Figure 11 Transmission electron micrographs of PEBBLE sensors imbedded biolistically (via gene gun), at 900 psi, into the cytoplasm of neuroblastoma cells: (a) Two 200-nm PEBBLEs, near or inside the cell nucleus; (b) one 20-nm PEBBLE next to a 1° lysosome in the cell cytoplasm. Original magnification is indicated on the figure and the inset.

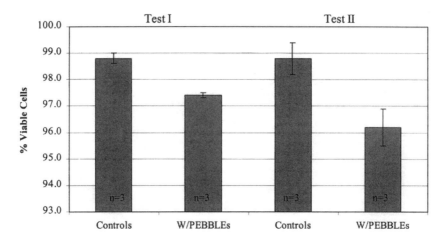

Figure 12 Trypan Blue viability assay: untreated controls and neuroblastoma cells bombarded with PEBBLEs at 900 psi.

into the cytoplasm at once. A distribution of PEBBLE sensors throughout the cytosol provides a method for monitoring ion concentrations at distinctly different locations; thus, imaging ion concentrations across the cytosol is possible (Fig. 13). Another advantage is that many cells can be injected at once, unlike some methods (such as pico-injection) where delivery takes place on a cell-by-cell basis.

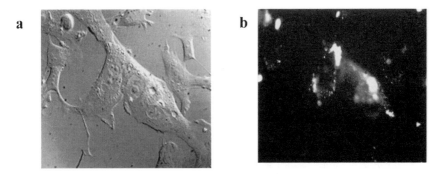

Figure 13 Calcium PEBBLEs delivered to neuroblastoma cells utilizing liposomal delivery. (a) Nomarski illumination; (b) fluorescence image with excitation at 590 nm. Note that the PEBBLEs remain in the cytoplasm of the cells and are not contained in the nucleus.

Pico-injection has been shown to be an effective method for controlled delivery of PEBBLEs, or sets of PEBBLEs, to single cells. Fine control of the injection tip allows one to insert PEBBLEs into the nucleus of a cell or the cytoplasm or both. Single areas of a dividing cell can be selectively injected (Fig. 14). In this example, a single cell of a divided mouse oocyte was injected with pH-sensitive PEBBLEs. The green fluorescence can easily be observed over the background of the cell.

Pico-injection can also be used for inserting ensembles of PEBBLEs into single cells. Figure 15a shows a mouse oocyte with a two-analyte sensor set, containing a cluster of oxygen-selective PEBBLE sensors as well as a cluster of calcium PEBBLE sensors. Using two distinct excitation wavelengths resulted in distinct fluorescence images (Figs. 15b and 15c), as well as fluorescence spectra (Fig. 15d). In this way, distinct analytes can be measured and imaged without spectral overlap. It is noted that, in contrast to fluorescent indicator dyes, here there is no physical interference between the two fluorescent indicators (no binding, quenching, or energy transfer), since each indicator is separately imbedded in its own protective PEBBLE matrix. Also, the cell can be highly loaded, due to the absence of quenching of the indicator dyes. In addition, the cell boundaries are sharply defined even after hours, due to the absence of leaching across the cell membrane.

PEBBLEs were also used to monitor calcium in phagosomes within rat alveolar macrophage. Macrophage that had phagocytosed calcium-selective PEBBLE sensors were challenged with a mitogen, Concanavalin A (Con A), inducing a slow increase in intracellular calcium, which was monitored over a

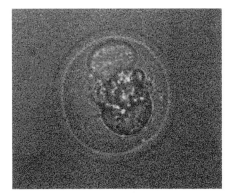

Figure 14 Mouse oocyte that has divided into two cells, with pH-sensitive PEBBLEs injected into the top cell only. The oocyte is being illuminated with 488-nm excitation, and the green PEBBLEs are fluorescing.

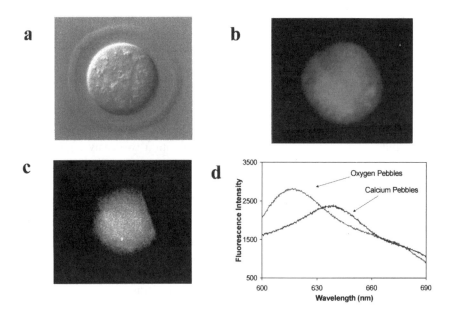

Figure 15 Mouse oocyte that has been injected with both calcium PEBBLEs and oxygen PEBBLEs. (a) Nomarski illumination; (b) fluorescence image using 488-nm illumination to excite the oxygen PEBBLEs; (c) fluorescence image using 560-nm illumination to excite the calcium PEBBLEs; (d) spectra from oxygen PEBBLEs and calcium PEBBLEs, with excitation wavelengths indicated in b and c.

period of 20 minutes (Fig. 16). PEBBLE clusters confined to the phagosome enabled correlation of ionic fluxes with specific functions of this organelle. In contrast, conventional fluorescent calcium indicators tend to monitor concentrations throughout the cell simultaneously (including the nucleus), making resolution of individual compartments difficult.

C. Physical Characteristics

Despite their small size, PEBBLE sensors were found to be highly stable, physically and photophysically. The effects of photobleaching are minimized by using ratiometric measurements and short exposure times (100 msec or less). Leaching of the indicator dyes form the PEBBLE sensor was investigated and did not present a serious problem. Oxygen PEBBLEs localized in the harsh environment of phagosomes of rat alveolar macrophages for five days did not display physical degradation or leaching of the fluorophore. This suggests that

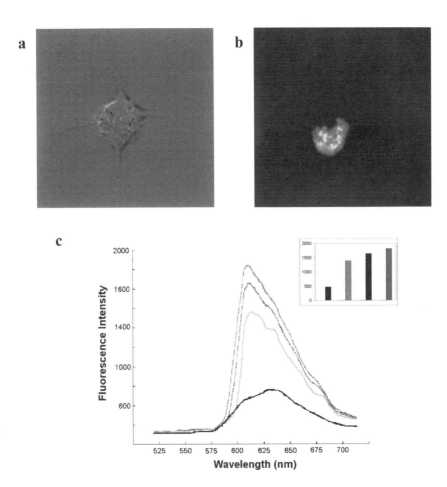

Figure 16 Rat alveolar macrophage with phagocytosed calcium-selective PEBBLE sensors (60×). (a) Nomarski illumination and (b) fluorescence illumination; (c) the increasing intracellular calcium level, monitored by calcium PEBBLEs in alveolar macrophage following stimulation with 30-μg/mL Concanavalin A (Con A). Bottom: no PEBBLEs in macrophage; second from bottom: PEBBLEs contained in phagosomes of macrophage, no stimulation; third from bottom: 10 minutes after stimulation of PEBBLE containing macrophage with Con A; top: 20 minutes after stimulation with Con A.

PEBBLEs can withstand acidic and oxidative biological conditions and remain functional. The small size is a distinct advantage when it comes to response time, since diffusion time through the matrix becomes inconsequential. When compared to the free dye, PEBBLE sensors were found to have comparable response times, suggesting that the diffusion time through the matrix was indeed minimal (less than 30 msec). On the other hand, the indicator dyes inside the PEBBLE sensor are shielded from physical and chemical perturbations by the cell environments. They are not affected by proteins [46] or heavy elements, and their calibration curves are the same for every cell type and locality.

D. Biocompatability

The small size and smooth shape of the sensor further enhances biological compatibility. The biocompatibility of PEBBLE sensors was investigated by assessing viability of cells in culture using a variety of histological and biochemical techniques (e.g., Trypan Blue exclusion, lactate dehydrogenase leakage, and energy change). The viability of cultured neuronal cells containing PEBBLE sensors was comparable to control samples or cells containing other often-used submicron particles, such as gold colloids and latex spheres.

E. Conclusion

Calculations show that fewer than 10^5 analyte ions are measured by a 200-nm PEBBLE (with 1% fluorescent molecules, by weight), putting the absolute detection limit in the zeptomole range. This low detection limit, combined with millisecond acquisition and response times as well as submicrometer spatial definition, has provided the ability to detect real-time intracellular ion fluxes. PEBBLE sensors for potassium [63], zinc [64], and oxygen [65] have been recently described and for sodium, chloride, nitrite, magnesium, and glucose are currently under development. Other PEBBLE matrices under consideration include protein- and enzyme-tagged gold colloids and sol-gel based PEBBLE sensors. Advanced optical imaging methods are expected to transform such PEBBLE-based chemical analysis ensembles into streamlined biomedical tools.

ACKNOWLEDGMENTS

We gratefully acknowledge Dr. Terry E. Meyer and Prof. Michael A. Cusanovich for providing the cytochrome c′, Yunde Zhao and Prof. Michael A. Marletta for providing the peptide derivative of sGC, and Prof. Joel A. Swanson and Albert Tsang for providing the macrophages and much assistance with the nitric oxide sensor applications. We also acknowledge extensive contributions to the PEBBLE applications and TEM characterization from Prof. Martin Philbert, Dr. Marion Hoyer, Dr. Steve Parus, and Rhonda Lightle. We acknowledge NIH grant 1 RO 1 GM50300 04A1 and DARPA grant MDA972-97-0006 for financial support, and SLRB acknowledges the Rackham Graduate School, University of Michigan, the ACS Division of Analytical Chemistry, and Merck and Co. for fellowship support.

REFERENCES

1. Nathan, C.; Xie, Q.W. Cell 78:915–918, 1994.
2. Stamler, J.S.; Singel, D.L.; Loscalzo, J. Science 258:1898–1902, 1992.
3. Moncada, S.; Palmer, R.M.J.; Higgs, E.A. Pharmacol. Rev. 43:109–142, 1991.
4. Kobzik, L.; Reid, M.B.; Bredt, D.S.; Stamler, J.S. Nature 372:546–548, 1994.
5. Bredt, D.S.; Snyder, S.H. Annu. Rev. Biochem. 63:175–195, 1994.
6. Ignarro, J.J. Annu. Rev. Pharmacol. Toxicol. 30:535–560, 1990.
7. Barker, S.L.R.; Kopelman, R. Anal. Chem. 70:4902–4906, 1998.
8. Broderick, M.P.; Taha, Z. In: 4th IBRO World Congress of Neuroscience: Kyoto, Japan, 1995.
9. Blyth, D.J.; Aylott, J.W.; Richardson, D.J.; Russell, D.A. Analyst 120:2725–2730, 1995.
10. Dave, B.C.; Dunn, B.; Valentine, J.S.; Zink, J.I. Anal. Chem. 66:1120A–1127A, 1994.
11. Friedeman, M.N.; Robinson, S.W.; Gerhart, G.A. Anal. Chem. 68:2621–2628, 1996.
12. Ichimori, K.; Ishida, H.; Fukahori, M.; Nakazawa, H.; Murakami, E. Rev.Sci. Instrum. 65:2714–2719, 1994.
13. Malinski, T.; Taha, Z. Nature 358:676–678, 1992.
14. Taha, Z. Recent Advances in Nitric Oxide Microsensing Technology. World Precision Instruments: Sarasota, FL, 1996.
15. Zhang, J.; Lever, A.B.P.; Pietro, W.J. Inorg. Chem. 33:1392–1398, 1994.
16. Zhou, X.; Arnold, M.A. Anal. Chem. 68:1748–1754, 1996.
17. Kojima, H.; Nakatsubo, N.; Kikuchi, K.; Kawahara, S.; Kirino, Y.; Nagoshi, H.; Hirata, Y.; Nagano, T. Anal. Chem. 70:2446–2453, 1998.
18. Barker, S.L.R.; Kopelman, R.; Meyer, T.E.; Cusanovich, M.A. Anal. Chem. 70: 971–976, 1998.
19. Meyer, T.E.; Kamen, M.D. In: Anfinsen, C.B.; Edsall, J.T.; Richards, F.M., eds. Advances in Protein Chemistry. Vol. 35. Academic Press: New York, 1982, pp. 105–212.
20. Ren, Z.; Meyer, T.; McRee, D. J. Mol. Biol. 234:433–445, 1993.
21. Yoshimura, T.; Suzuki, S.; Nakahara, A.; Iwasaki, H.; Masuko, M.; Matsubara, T. Biochem. 25:2436–2442, 1986.
22. Caffrey, M.; Simorre, J.-P.; Brutscher, B.; Cusanovich, M.; Marion, D. Biochem. 34:5904–5912, 1995.
23. Taniguchi, S.; Kamen, M.D. Biochim. Biophys. Acta 74:438–455, 1963.

24. Aylott, J.W.; Richardson, D.J.; Russell, D.A. Chem. Mater. 9:2261–2263, 1997.

25. Horisberger, M. Scan. Elecron. Micros. 2:9–31, 1981.

26. Crumbliss, A.L.; Perine, S.C.; Stonehuerner, J.; Tubergen, K.R.; Zhao, J.; Henkens, R.W.; O'Daly, J.P. Biotechnol. Bioeng. 40:483–490, 1992.

27. Crumbliss, A.L.; Stonehuerner, J.; Henkens, R.W.; Zhao, J.; O'Daly, J.P. Biosens. Bioelectron. 8:331–337, 1993.

28. Henkens, R.W.; Kitchell, B.S.; O'Daly, J.P.; Perine, S.C.; Stonehuerner, J.; Tubergen, K.R.; Zhao, J.; Crumbliss, A.L. J. Inorg. Chem. 43:120, 1991.

29. Clark, H.A.; Merritt, G.; Kopelman, R. SPIE Proc. 3922:138–146, 2000.

30. Barker, S.L.R.; Kopelman, R.; Meyer, T.E.; Cusanovich, M.A. Anal. Chem. 70: 971–976, 1998.

31. Lakowicz, J.R. In: Lakowicz, J.R., ed. Topics in Fluorescence Spectroscopy. Vol. 4. Plenum Press: New York, 1994, p 3.

32. Lakowicz, J.R. In: Lakowicz, J.R., ed. Topics in Fluorescence Spectroscopy. Vol. 4. Plenum Press: New York, 1994, pp 3–6, 432–445.

33. Barker, S.L.R.; Zhao, Y.; Marletta, M.A.; Kopelman, R. Anal. Chem. 71:2071–2075, 1999.

34. Waldman, S.A.; Murad, F. Pharmacol. Rev. 39:163–196, 1987.

35. Stone, J.R.; Marletta, M.A. Biochemistry 33:5636–5640, 1994.

36. Zhao, Y.; Marletta, M.A. Biochem. 36:15959–15964, 1998.

37. Haugland, R. Handbook of Fluorescent Probes and Research Chemicals. 6th ed. Molecular Probes: Eugene OR, 1996.

38. Brandish, P.E.; Buechler, W.; Marletta, M.A. Biochem. 37:16898–16907, 1998.

39. Toda, K.; Ochi, K.; Sanemasa, I. Sensors Actuators B 32:15–18, 1996.

40. Barker, S.L.R.; Clark, H.A.; Swallen, S.F.; Kopelman, R.; Tsang, A.W.; Swanson, J.A. Anal. Chem. 71:1767–1772, 1999.

41. Chance, R.R.; Prock, A.; Silbey, R. In Prigogine, I.; Rice, S.A., eds. Advances in Chemical Physics. Vol. 37. Wiley: New York, 1978, pp 1–63.

42. Barker, S. Thesis, Univ. of Michigan, 1999.

43. Xia, Y.; Zweier, J.L. Proc. Natl. Acad. Sci. USA 94:6954–6958, 1997.

44. Stuehr, D.J.; Marletta, M.A. J. Immunol. 139:518–525, 1987.

45. Marletta, M.A.; Yoon, P.S.; Iyengar, R.; Leaf, C.D.; Wishnok, J.S. Biochem. 27: 8706–8711, 1988.

46. Ding, A.; Nathan, C.F.; Stuehr, D.J. J. Immunol. 141:2407–2412, 1988.

47. Wightman, R.M.; May, L.J.; Michael, A.C. Anal. Chem. 60:769A–779A, 1988.

48. Walt, D.R.; Urban, E.R., Jr. Sea Tech. 32:47–55, 1991.

49. Neubauer, A.; et al. Biosensors Bioelectronics 11:317–325, 1996.

50. Turner, A.P.F. Anal. Chim. Acta 337:315–321, 1997.

51. Tan. W.; et al. Science 258:778–781, 1992.

52. Kopelman, R.; Dourado, S. SPIE (Int. Soc. Opt. Eng.) Proc. 2836:2–11, 1996.

53. Peterson, J.I.; et al. Anal. Chem. 52:864–869, 1980.

54. Sasaki, K.; et al. Chem. Lett. 2:141–142, 1996.

55. Clark, H.A.; Hoyer, M.A.; Parus, S.; Philbert, M.; Kopelman, R. Microchimica Acta 131:121–128, 1999.

56. Barker, S.L.R.; Shortreed, M.R.; Kopelman, R. SPIE (Int. Soc. Opt. Eng.) Proc. 2836:304–310, 1996.

57. Bakker, E.; Simon, W. Anal. Chem. 64(17):1805–1812, 1992.
58. Song, A.; Parus, S.; Kopelman, R. Anal. Chem. 69(5):863–867, 1997.
59. Bakker, E.; Willer, M.; Pretsch, E. Anal. Chim. Acta 282(2):265–271, 1993.
60. Hauser, P.C.; et al. Anal. Chem. 62(18):1919–1923, 1990.
61. Daubresse, C.; et al. J. Colloid Interface Sci. 168:222–229, 1994.
62. Clark, H.A.; Hoyer, M.; Philbert, M.; Kopelman, R. Anal. Chem. 71(21):4831–4836, 1999.
63. Brasuel, M.; Kopelman, R.; Miller, T.J.; Tjalkens, R.; Philbert, M.A. Anal. Chem. 73(10):2221–2228, 2001.
64. Sumner, J.; Aylott, E.; Monson, E.; Kopelman, R. Analyst 127:11–16, 2002.
65. Xu, H.; Aylott, J.W.; Kopelman, R.; Miller, T.; Philbert, M. Analyt. Chem. 73(17):4124–4133, 2001.

8
Ultrasensitive and Specific Optical Biosensors Inspired by Nature

Xuedong Song
Kimberly-Clark Corporation, Roswell, Georgia, U.S.A.

Basil I. Swanson
Los Alamos National Laboratory, Los Alamos, New Mexico, U.S.A.

I. INTRODUCTION

The threat of potential biological warfare (BW) and terrorists' attacks using biological agents such as pathogens and toxins have received increased attention in recent years [1]. Unlike chemical warfare agents that cause rapid symptoms, biological agents usually takes hours or even days to display any significant symptoms. This slow symptom development to BW agents makes BW attack more frightening. One scenario is that the first observation and subsequent response to symptoms developed from such an attack may be too late because of the delay. One critical step to minimize the damage for human health and environmental contamination from such an attack is a rapid detection and identification of the BW agents used so that timely mitigation measures can be taken. Since such BW attacks can theoretically take place anywhere and at any time, regular field sampling (either battlefield or environmentally important sites) and detection would be ideal to provide timely warning. This type of regular field sampling and detection for either hazardous agents in environments or toxins in humans creates an extremely high need for detection technologies. Ideal detection technologies for such a purpose must be simple, low cost, and fast as well as highly sensitive and specific. Unfortunately, current detection methods cannot meet all the requirements. For instance, although gene probe [2] and immunoassay [3] can provide very sensitive and specific detection, they are intrinsically slow and high cost and are generally not suitable for regular field applications.

The detection systems based on surface plasmon resonance spectroscopy can provide rapid detection of potential BW agents and environmental contaminants [4], but they lack the high sensitivity and specificity required in many situations. Moreover, gene probes can detect only microorganisms and not protein toxins.

Since current detection technologies cannot meet the requirements for point-of-care or fieldable detection, there is a need to develop new concepts and approaches for biosensors. In recent years, a number of groups have reported several new biosensor systems for the detection of biological agents such as pathogens and protein toxins. For example, Charych et al. [5] applied binding-induced conformation perturbation of conjugated polydiacetylene backbone to achieve a colorimetric change for detection of influenza viruses and cholera toxins. Unfortunately, this approach suffers low detection sensitivity and high nonspecific environmental perturbations, such as temperature and pH variations. One elegant biosensor design was reported by Cornell et al. [6] to couple a complicated biomimetic membrane system with an interaction-controllable ion channel for signal transduction and amplification. The key to the success of this work was the fabrication of a complex self-assembled tethered bilayer membrane where mobility of the ion channel (gramicidin) attached to antibodies in the upper leaf is used to open and close ion-channel conduction upon antibody–antigen binding. Thermotropic liquid crystals have also been successfully used to achieve signal amplification induced by a ligand–receptor binding [7]. Protein–ligand interaction causes twisted nematic liquid crystals to untwist, to amplify the reporting signal.

Motivated by the need for convenient and cheap sensors for protein toxins (e.g., botulinium, ricin, SEB, and cholera), we have developed a new biosensor capable of being implemented in a rugged, miniaturized format for field sensing and use in point-of-care detection [8,9]. Here we describe an optical biosensor system developed in our laboratory, which is, in some ways, parallel to the ion-channel-based biosensors. Instead of using electronic impedence for signal amplification, our biosensor system uses fluorescence to generate signal amplification. Although the integrated optical biosensor was initially developed specifically for detection of protein toxins [8], the technologies should have potential for applications in a wide variety of areas, such as environmental monitoring, medical diagnostics, and drug screening.

II. APPROACH

Cell signaling in nature requires different biological components to communicate and interact with each other to maintain biological functions. This communication frequently involves specific recognition and binding interactions, which subsequently induce a signal transduction and amplification [10] . The initial signal that triggers a cascade event for signal amplification is often generated through a receptor-aggregation process induced by a highly specific binding event [11]. In addition to the signal transduction, many other biological activities, such as translocation of protein toxins into cells, are initiated by specific binding of the protein toxins with the multiple receptor molecules, which results in receptor aggregation on cell membrane surfaces [12]. The consequence of such a receptor aggregation is to generate new entities with new functions, such as ion channels, or to induce a physical property change for the membrane structures, such as a polarity perturbation, pore formation, or other local environmental changes. The multivalent interactions between biological molecules and receptors usually have relatively high apparent binding affinity, a result of an aggregation-induced avidity effect. The heart of our biosensor system for detection of protein toxins is to closely mimic this receptor-aggregation-induced signal generation and amplification process on cell membrane surface.

We developed three signal transduction and amplification schemes for detection of species involved in an aggregation process or a multivalent interaction [8]. They utilize distance-dependent fluorescence self-quenching or energy transfer mechanisms or combination of both to probe the distance change between the receptors resulting from receptor aggregation on a biomimetic membrane surface. Scheme 1 illustrates how these schemes work. In the first two (Scheme 1A), fluorophore-tagged receptors are homogeneously incorporated into a membrane-mimetic architecture (e.g. phospholipid bilayers). The membrane-mimetic surface retains fluid-like phases, much like real cell membranes, which allow lateral diffusion of the tagged receptors. The surface density of the labeled receptors is low enough to avoid any significant interaction between fluorescent probes, so the fluorescent probes fluoresce independently. The receptor aggregation process induced by a multivalent binding will bring multiple labeled receptors, consequently multiple fluorescent probes, into close proximity, thereby triggering an interaction between the fluorescent probes, which results in fluorescent property changes (e.g., intensity, lifetime, and polarization). In the case using a fluorophore as a probe that can undergo distance-dependent fluorescence self-quenching, the fluorophores fluoresce independently and strongly prior to protein–receptor binding. The fluorescence intensity will decrease due to fluorescent self-quenching if the target protein can induce the receptor aggregation to bring the fluorophores into close proximity. The fluorescence decrease provides a signal generation specifically for the aggregation process. In using an energy transfer pair as probes, the fluorescence of the donor is strong and the fluorescence of the acceptor is weak before binding of the target protein, when only the donor is excited. The donor fluorescence will decrease and acceptor fluorescence will increase as a result of an energy transfer from the donor to the acceptor when the multivalent binding of the target molecule induces receptor aggregation, which also brings the donor and the acceptor into close

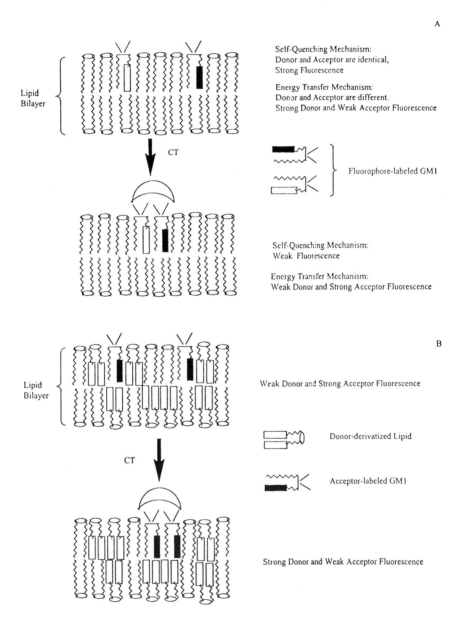

Scheme 1 See text for description.

proximity. The simultaneous double fluorescence change provides a reliable and sensitive method for the multivalent target molecules.

In the third scheme (Scheme 1B), the membrane surface formed from a mixture of natural lipids and fluorescence donor-imbedded amphiphiles provides a fluid supporting matrix and, at the same time, participates in signal transduction. The membrane surface retains the dynamic and structural properties of biomembrane, which allows lateral diffusion of the receptors covalently tagged with fluorescence acceptors. If the fluorescent donor/acceptor pairs and the surface density of the donor/acceptor in the membrane-mimetic surface are carefully chosen, the homogeneously distributed acceptors can efficiently quench most of the donor fluorescence. The system will show weak fluorescence of the donor (and strong fluorescence of the acceptor) even though only the donor is excited. Signal amplification can be realized by using a quencher or acceptor that can quench fluorescence of many donors. The binding-induced receptor aggregation results in aggregation of the fluorescent acceptor (or quencher), producing a decrease in the quenching efficiency and in an increase in the donor fluorescence (and a decrease in the acceptor fluorescence in the case of fluorescent quencher). If the fluorescence acceptor attached to the receptors can itself undergo distance-dependent fluorescence self-quenching, the acceptor fluorescence can be further reduced. The first two schemes require the relatively large surface area resulting from a low-surface-density requirement of the labeled receptors to minimize the preaggregation fluorescence self-quenching. The third scheme may prove to be more versatile for some applications, in view of the more efficient use of the surface area and the possibility of enhancing sensitivity by combining both energy transfer and self-quenching mechanisms.

In the following sections, we demonstrate these design principles using two multivalent recognition systems for direct detection of cholera toxin (CT) and avidin as well as indirect detection of the receptor molecules using both fluorimetry and flow cytometry.

III. RESULTS AND DISCUSSION

A. Detection of Cholera Toxin Using Distance-Dependent Fluorescence Self-Quenching [8a]

The pentavalent cholera toxin (CT), which specifically recognizes and binds with up to five ganglioside GM1 molecules, was chosen as a model protein toxin system for initial study. CT/GM1 recognition shares common features of many protein toxin/glycolipid interactions, such as shiga toxin/globotriosyl-ceramide [13]. In this study, lyso-GM1 is covalently tagged with a fluorescence probe through its free amino group [8d]. Such modification is expected to have minimal influence on the binding affinity and specificity of the penta-saccharide recognition moieties for CT. Although we identified several fluorophores that undergo efficient distance-dependent fluorescence self-quenching, we focus our discussions only on the results obtained from fluorescein and $B_{581/591}$-labeled GM1 (see structure from scheme 2a). Fluorescein-tagged GM1 molecules are quite water soluble in a monomeric form, while $B_{581/591}$-GM1 molecules form micelles in water. As shown in Figure 1, the monomeric F-GM1 in aqueous solution shows strong fluorescence without CT. Addition of CT in the F-GM1 solution causes significant fluorescence intensity decrease as a function of time, due to fluorescence self-quenching as a result of the formation of multivalent complexes between CT and up to five F-GM1 molecules. The extent of the intensity drop is proportional to the CT concentration prior to signal saturation. In order to test the specificity of the detection method, albumin was used for comparison. Although the presence of a low concentration of albumin (<50 times the upper detection limit of CT) was found to show little effect on fluorescence, a measurable fluorescence decrease (>3%) was indeed observed with high albumin concentration (>50 times the upper detection limit of CT concen-

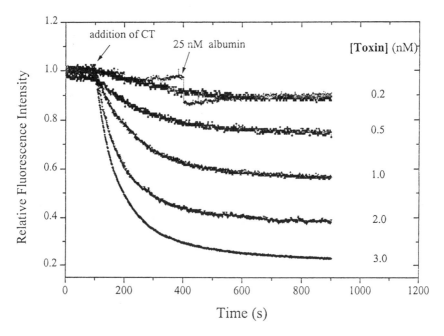

Figure 1   Fluorescence intensity at 520 nm (ex. at 480 nm) of F-GM1 (10 nM) in tris-buffer (pH = 8.0) upon addition of different concentrations of CT and albumin.

tration for a specific sample). This nonspecific response can be attributed to nonspecific binding between F-GM1 and albumin.

In addition to the fluorescence intensity drop, the fluorescence lifetime [17] and polarization of the fluorescein were found to respond to the formation of CT-/F-GM1 complexes. The Perrin equation [14] indicates that an increase in the effective volume of the fluorescent molecule and a drop of fluorescence lifetime are expected to result in an increase in fluorescence polarization. The rotational correlation time of CT/F-GM1 complexes is expected to be larger than F-GM1 itself. The formation of CT/F-GM1 complexes should result in an increase in fluorescence polarization. In contrast to the expected increase in fluorescence polarization for the CT/F-GM1 complexes, a decrease in the fluorescence polarization of F-GM1/CT complex in tris-buffer was observed. This unusual observation can be reasonably attributed to the complication caused by the self-quenching process, which dramatically changes the nature of the fluorescence.

The biosensor system can be used not only for direct detection of the multivalent target CT but also for detection of the unlabeled GM1 through a competitive binding format. A known amount of labeled GM1 and an unknown amount of unlabeled GM1 compete for the binding sites of a limited amount of multivalent CT. Depending upon the amount of unlabeled GM1, the number of the labeled and unlabeled GM1 molecules in each complex varies. As a result, the fluorescence self-quenching efficiency is proportional to the amount of the unlabeled GM1 molecules in the sample. As shown in Figure 2, the presence of the unlabeled GM1 inhibits the binding of CT to F-GM1, resulting in a smaller decrease of fluorescence due to the fact that each CT-GM1 complex has fewer fluorescein molecules.

When we tried to incorporate F-GM1 into membrane-mimetic surfaces such as POPC vesicles in aqueous solution or POPC bilayers on supporting glass microspheres, we found that F-GM1 is too water soluble to form stable membrane-mimetic architectures. In order for the labeled GM1 molecules to be anchored in a stable fashion into the membrane surfaces, which is essential for the construction of a rugged biosensor device, hydrophobic fluorophores such as $B_{581/591}$ are found to be better choices. In aqueous solution, $B_{581/591}$-GM1 molecules exist as aggregated forms, even in very low concentration (less than 10 nM), and exhibit very weak fluorescence due to self-quenching. Addition of POPC vesicles or POPC bilayers coated on glass microspheres in a $B_{581/591}$-GM1 micellar solution allows the $B_{581/591}$-GM1 micelles to break down and asymmetrically incorporate into the outer leaflet of the bilayers, where $B_{581/591}$-GM1 molecules are homogeneously distributed. This tranformation from a micellar to a membrane form boosts the fluorescence intensity about 20-fold when the surface density of $B_{581/591}$-GM1 in the POPC bilayers is low (<1%relative to phospholipid molecules). The relatively high stability of $B_{581/591}$-GM1 in the POPC bi-

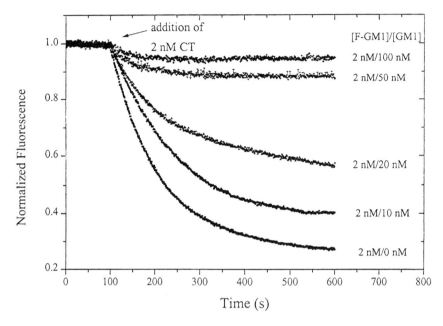

Figure 2 Relative fluorescence (em. at 520 nm and ex. at 480 nm) as a function of time for competitive binding of CT with F-GM1 and GM1 in tris-buffer (pH = 8.0).

layers coated on the glass microspheres was confirmed by little loss of $B_{581/591}$-GM1 fluorescence intensity after repeated washing steps with buffer. As shown in Figure 3, multivalent binding of CT with $B_{581/591}$-GM1 in the POPC bilayers coated on the microspheres causes a dramatic decrease in fluorescence intensity, while addition of much higher concentration of albumin causes no fluorescence change. This high specificity can be attributed to the fact that the hydrophobic $B_{581/591}$ is expected to reside in the hydrophobic interior of the POPC bilayers to shield the fluorescence probes from direct access by any interfering species. The interface provided by the POPC bilayers is critical to minimize nonspecific response. The decrease of fluorescence can be reversed by addition of an excess of nonlabeled GM1, which can compete off the labeled GM1 bounded to CT. Indeed, we have demonstrated that CT-GM1 binding on phospholipid bilayers that have been coated onto waveguide surfaces can be reversed by denaturing the cholera protein without significant loss of labeled GM1 [9]. In this scheme, only species that can induce the aggregation of the labeled GM1 can trigger the signal generation. The direct coupling of specific binding events with selective signal transduction and amplification dramatically enhances both the detection sensitivity *and* specificity.

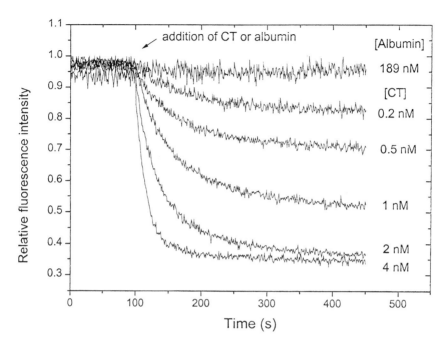

Figure 3 Fluorescence intensity (ex. at 570 and em. at 600 nm) of $B_{581/591}$-Gm1(3.2 nM) in the outer leaflet of POPC bilayers coated on glass beads (0.2 mg) as a function of time upon addition of CT or albumin. [POPC]/[$B_{581/591}$-GM1] is estimated to be 600.

The detection sensitivity and dynamic range depend on the total concentration of the labeled GM1 in the samples. Less than 0.1 nM can be reliably detected in both POPC vesicle solutions and on glass beads. High sensitivity and small dynamic range are associated with samples with a low concentration of B-GM1, while low sensitivity and large dynamic range with samples with a high concentration of B-GM1. The response time depends upon the concentration of both B-GM1 and CT in the samples as well as the surface density of labeled GM1. As expected, the samples with a higher concentration of both B-GM1 and CT give faster response.

The fluidity of the membrane surface is also found to be critical for the optimizing signal generation and response speed. This is demonstrated by the observation that the fluorescence intensity decrease for $B_{581/591}$-GM1 in the outer leaflet of fluid-like DPPC bilayers at 45°C is much larger and faster than in the crystalline DPPC bilayers at 22°C. The observation of any binding-induced fluorescence quenching for $B_{581/591}$-GM1 in the crystalline phase of DPPC vesicles at 22°C suggests that CT may quench some $B_{581/591}$-GM1 fluorescence even in the form of low-valent complexes. The crystalline phase still allows some degree of the mobility for $B_{581/591}$-GM1 in the upper leaf of the bilayer.

B. Detection of Cholera Toxin Using Distance-Dependent Resonant Energy Transfer [8b]

Many factors, such as temperature and other environmental perturbations, may influence the fluorescence intensity. As a result, using single fluorescence change as the sole signal indicator cannot absolutely exclude interference from those factors. In order to enhance the detection reliability and minimize the interference from potential environmental perturbations, we apply distance-dependent energy transfer to achieve a simultaneous double fluorescence change. We have identified several fluorescence energy transfer pairs (BODIPY dyes) to facilitate the adaptation of the system to different instruments with different excitation wavelengths. In this chapter, only results from one energy transfer pair, B_{TMR} (donor) and B_{TR} (acceptor), will be discussed. The GM1 molecules covalently labeled with B_{TMR} (B_{TMR}-GM1) and B_{TR} (B_{TR}-GM1) were incorporated into the outer leaflet of POPC bilayers either in aqueous solution or coated on microspheres. When the surface density of the labeled GM1 in POPC bilayers is low enough (<1% relative to the total concentration of POPC), strong fluorescence of B_{TMR} and weak fluorescence of B_{TR} were observed when B_{TMR}-GM1 was excited. Owing to the small Stokes shift for the BODIPY dyes, it is not possible to excite the BTMR donor exclusively, resulting in a small amount of acceptor fluorescence even at extremely low concentrations of the labeled GM1. The formation of CT complexes with up to five labeled GM1 molecules on the membrane surfaces brings both fluorescence donor and acceptor into close proximity, so energy transfer from the donor, B_{TMR}, to the acceptor, B_{TR}, occurs. As shown in Figure 4, the fluorescence of B_{TR}-GM1 increases at the expense of the fluorescence of B_{TMR}-GM1 upon addition of CT. The plot of the ratio of the acceptor/donor fluorescence intensities as a function of CT concentration gives a straight line within the upper detection limit (inset of Fig. 4). The upper detection limit is approximately one-fifth of the total labeled-receptor concentration, which is consistent with the five binding sites of each CT and almost all the receptors bind to the CT. The detection presents little temperature dependence. This is attributable to the fact that the fluorescence intensity ratios from two similar fluorophores can offset any absolute intensity change caused by temperature variation or possibly other environmental changes. Another advantage of the distance-dependent signal transduction over techniques based on changes in the index of refraction, such as surface plasmon resonance spectroscopy, is its silence to the nonspecific binding of toxin itself to the membrane surfaces.

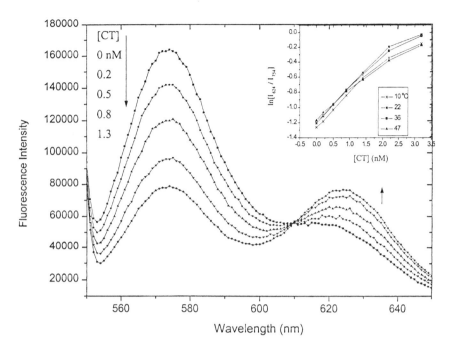

Figure 4 Fluorescence spectra (ex. at 530 nm) of BTR-GM1 and RTMR-GM1 in the outer layer of POPC bilayers on glass beads with different concentrations of CT. Sample preparation: 5-mg glass beads coated with POPC bilayers were incubated in 31 μL of BTR-GM1 (324 nM) and 28 μL of BTMR-GM1 (356 nM) aqueous solution for overnight. After they were washed three times, the beads were suspended in 1 mL tris-buffer. The sample contains 120-μL beads diluted to 240 μL. (Inset) The plot of $(R - R_0)/(R_{max} - R_0)$ versus [CT] at different temperatures. R, R_0 and $R_{,max}$ are the intensity ratio (I_{624}/I_{574}) of the two fluorescence peaks at 624 nm (acceptor) and 574 nm (donor) for the samples with CT, sample without CT, and samples with saturating CT, respectively.

The detection sensitivity and dynamic range can be adjusted by the total concentration of the labeled GM1 (see Fig. 5). A lower concentration of the labeled GM1 gives a higher sensitivity but a smaller detection range. Less than 0.05 nM of CT can be reliably detected with a response time of less than five minutes. A high concentration of albumin and other proteins, such as peanut lectin, causes no change in the fluorescence spectra.

The biosensor performance (sensitivity, specificity, and speed) is determined by many parameters, such as surface density of the labeled GM1 and the ratio of the labeled donor/acceptor. An optimal surface density from 0.2% to 1% of the labeled GM1 relative to the total lipid in the membrane surface was

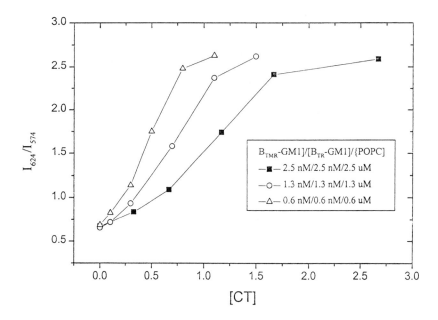

Figure 5 Fluorescence intensity ratio (I_{624} and I_{574} are fluorescence intensity at 624 nm and 574 nm, respectively) in the presence of different [CT] for B_{TMR}-GM1/B_{TR}-GM1 in the outer leaflet of POP.

found to give a large signal change for both donor and acceptor fluorescence. The samples with high density of the labeled GM1 give relatively small change due to the prebinding energy transfer, while the relatively low detection sensitivity for the samples with low density of the labeled GM1 is attributed to the affinity limitation that results in the formation of low-valence complexes. Although the system works well for samples with the ratio of [B_{TMR}-GM1]/[B_{TR}-GM1] from ⅓ to ¾, the sample with [donor-GM1]/[acceptor-GM1] = ¼ gives best results.

The system just described can be easily adapted to a variety of detection platforms, including fluorescence microscopy, microplates, flow cytometry, and miniaturized sensor arrays based on optical waveguides. Presented in Figure 6 is the cholera toxin–induced receptor aggregation as measured by resonant energy transfer using flow cytometry [10]. The sensitivity of this assay can be further improved by decreasing the microsphere concentration while holding receptor surface density constant, thus lowering the concentration of receptor without sacrificing signal.

The detection sensitivity and dynamic range can be adjusted via the total concentration of the labeled receptors. A lower concentration of the labeled

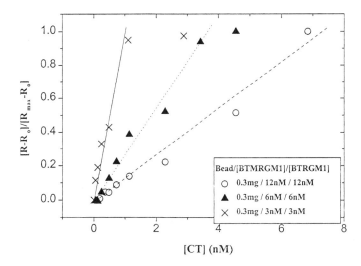

Figure 6 Receptor aggregation–induced RET measured by flow cytometry. Glass microspheres coated with a bilayer of POPC and the labeled receptors were incubated with various concentrations of CT at room temperature for 30 minutes before flow cytometry measurement. Microsphere fluorescence was excited at 514 nm with an argon ion laser, and donor and acceptor fluorescence was collected through bandpass filters and detected with photomultiplier tubes. Analog detector signals were processed with a variable-gain-ratio module to give the ratio of acceptor to donor fluorescence on a particle-by-particle basis. Data was normalized by subtracting the ratio of samples before addition of CT (R_0) and expressing the result as a fraction of the maximal ratio at saturating CT (R_{max}).

receptors gives a higher sensitivity but a smaller detection range. Less than 50 pM CT can be reliably detected in less than five minutes. The signal change starts to level off beyond the upper detection limit, due to saturation of the labeled receptor, and then drops slowly with further addition of CT. The drop in the A/D ratio of emission is reasonably attributed to the formation of low-valence complexes due to the presence of excess CT. As expected by the fact that the hydrophobic fluorophores should anchor in the interior of the membrane, a high concentration of albumin (more than 1000 times higher than the toxin upper detection limit) causes no change in the fluorescence spectra.

C. Detection of Cholera Toxin Using Both Fluorescence Self-Quenching and Energy Transfer [8c]

Although the resonant energy transfer scheme is quite sensitive, specific, and fast when using flow cytometry or fluorimetry, it may have limitations in some microsensor applications that require a high density of fluorophores in a small surface area. In this section, we describe another biosensor platform, which consists of a mixed lipid bilayer with high surface density of fluorescence donor imbedded in a synthetic lipid and low surface density of fluorescence acceptor (or nonfluorescent quencher) covalently attached to a receptor. A binding-induced receptor aggregation on such a surface triggers a change in fluorescence quenching efficiency by the acceptor, resulting in a change in fluorescence spectra of the donor or acceptor or both.

The bilayers of POPC with high percentage (20–50% relative to POPC) of pyrene-derivatized phosphatidylcholine (P-PC) or 1,2-bis-pyrene-derivatized phosphatidylcholine (BP-PC) are chosen as supporting matrix and fluorescence-donating layer (see Scheme 2B for structures). In such a bilayer, most pyrene molecules form pyrene excimers and display strong excimer fluorescence. The fluorescence of pyrene excimer overlaps significantly with absorption spectra of DABCY (nonfluorescent) and B_{FL} (strongly fluorescent), and an efficient energy transfer from the excimer to either acceptor can occur. Introduction of only 10% of DABCY-GM1 (versus P-PC) into the outer leaflet of the bilayer of POPC/ B-PC (2/1) quenches 70% fluorescence of the pyrene excimers, while more than 80% fluorescence of the excimer is quenched by only 5% DABCY-GM1 incorporated into both leaflets of the bilayers. This result suggests that efficient fluorescence quenching of the excimers by DABCY occurs not only in the same layer but also in the inner layer. It is estimated that each BADCY molecule can quench the excimer fluorescence of more than 10 pyrene molecules in the case using POPC/B-PC (2/1) bilayers, and more than 20 pyrene molecules in the case using POPC/BP-PC (2/1) bilayers. For a sample containing 10% DABCY-GM1 (versus P-PC) in the outer leaflet of the POPC/P-PC (2/1) bilayer vesicles, the DABCY-GM1 aggregation induced by CT binding results in an excimer fluorescence increase up to 45%. In contrast, the excimer fluorescence increases up to 60% with 10% DABCY-GM1 in both leaflets of the bilayers (Fig. 7). Less than 0.1 nM CT can be detected in a few minutes. The observation of only a 60% increase of the excimer fluorescence upon addition of enough CT to bind all the receptors (about one-fifth of [DABCY-GM1]) indicates that the excimer fluorescence does not fully recover, for the obvious reason that the aggregated acceptor can still quench the fluorescence of the excimers nearby.

Unlike the platform based on a nonfluorescent DABCY as the quencher, simultaneous double color change can be achieved by using a fluorescent acceptor covalently attached to GM1. When a low percentage of B_{FL}-GM1 (from 0.3% to 5% versus P-PC) is incorporated into the outer layer of POPC/P-PC (or BP-PC) (2/1) bilayers, a relatively weak fluorescence of pyrene excimer and strong fluorescence of B_{FL}-GM1 were observed, even though only pyrene is excited (at 345 nm). We attribute this to the energy transfer from the excimer to B_{FL}-GM1. In contrast, B_{FL}-GM1 in POPC vesicles with comparable surface density shows almost no fluorescence when excited at 345 nm. Cholera toxin-

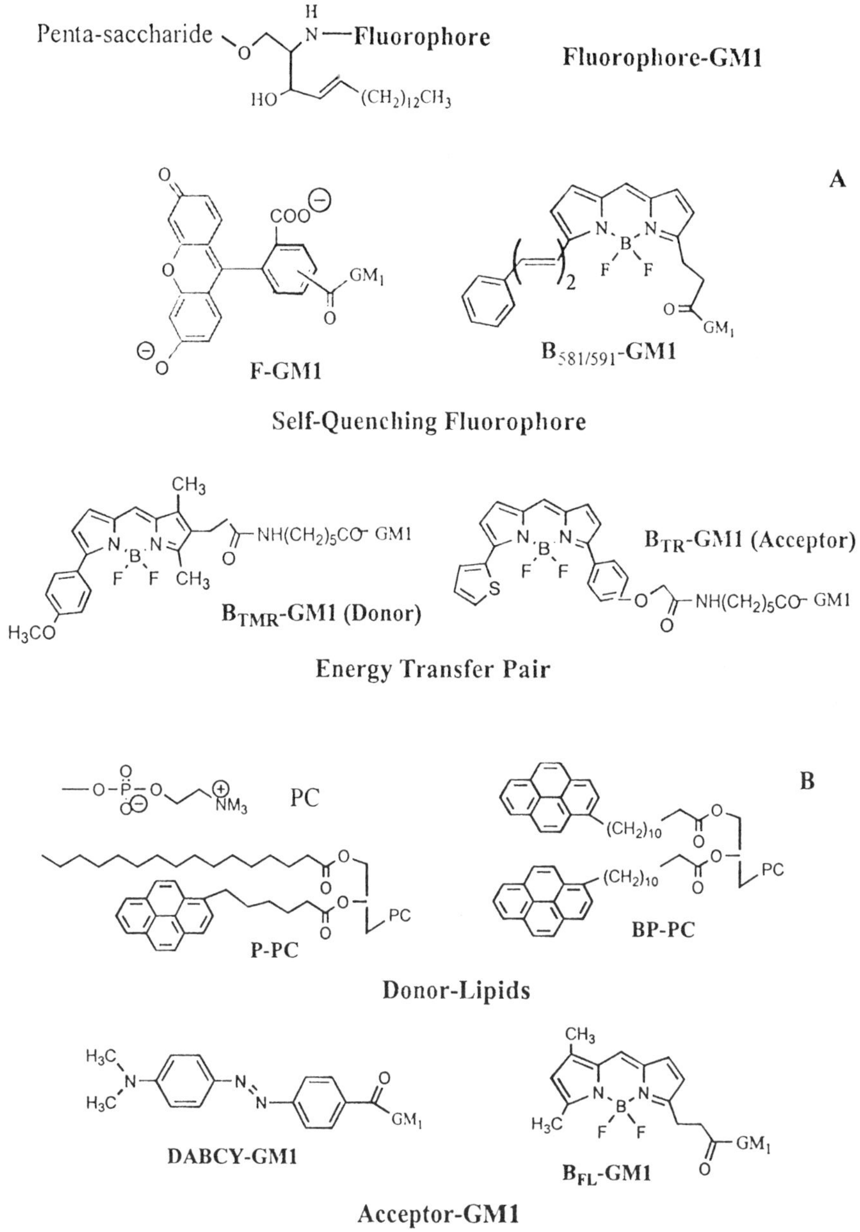

Scheme 2   Structures of molecules used in this chapter.

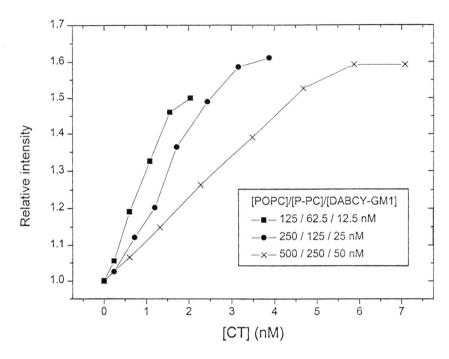

Figure 7 Relative fluorescence intensity at 482 nm (ex. at 348 nm) of pyrene excimer versus [CT] for samples with DABCY-GM1 in both sides of the bilyers formed from POPC and P-PC.

induced aggregation of B_{FL}-GM1 in the bilayers reduces the energy transfer from the pyrene excimer to B-FL and increases fluorescence self-quenching between B_{FL} molecules. The excimer fluorescence increases and the BFL-GM1 fluorescence decreases in the presence of CT (Fig. 8). The combination of both distance-dependent energy transfer and self-quenching has potential to achieve signal amplification for detection of multivalent interactions.

D. Detection of Avidin–Biotin Interaction Using Distance-Dependent Fluorescence Self-Quenching

Avidin, a protein widely used in biotechnology, has four binding sites for biotin [15]. The same approach discussed for the detection of CT and GM1 can be used for the detection of avidin and biotin. Similar to our observations for fluorescein-labeled GM1/CT system, the strong fluorescence of $B_{581/591}$-biotin in the outer leaflet of POPC vesicles or POPC bilayers on glass microspheres de-

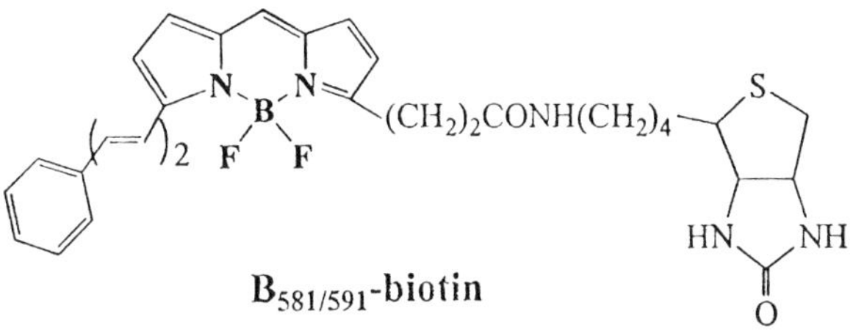

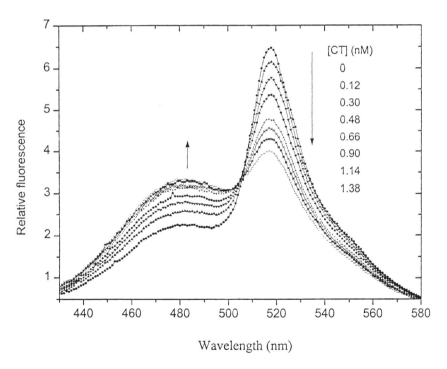

Scheme 3   Molecular structure of BODIPY$_{581/591}$-biotin.

Figure 8   Fluorescence spectra (ex. at 345 nm) of aqueous dispersions of POPC/BP-PC (250 nM/125 nM) with 6.25-nM BFL-GM1 in both leaflets upon addition of different [CT].

creases dramatically when avidin was added. Figure 9 shows the fluorescence intensity of $B_{581/591}$-biotin in the outer leaflet of POPC bilayers coated on glass microspheres as a function of time upon addition of avidin or albumin. The degree of the decrease in fluorescence intensity reflects the amount of the avidin added. The kinetic profile also depends on the amount of the added avidin. The system was tested for specificity using albumin and peanut lectin. Albumin has many hydrophobic pockets to bind with hydrophobic moieties of a molecule, and peanut lectin has four binding sites for galactoside [15]. We found that the detection system shows high selectivity against other potential interfering proteins. For example, the presence of 20 nM albumin or peanut lectin or CT causes no measurable change in fluorescence for a sample containing 3.0 nM $B_{581/591}$-biotin, while 1 nM avidin induced more than 75% decrease. For the same sample, 100 nM albumin or peanut lectin causes only a c.a. 10% drop in fluorescence. The kinetic profile of the fluorescence caused by the nonspecific binding of albumin and peanut lectin is also different from that induced by the specific binding of avidin. The fluorescence decreases gradually for avidin, while the

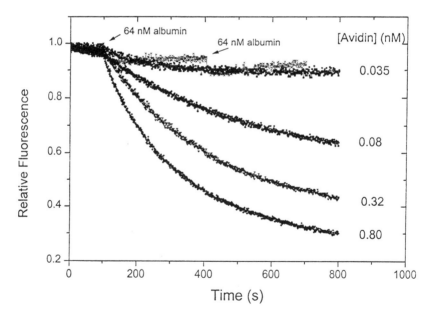

Figure 9 Relative fluorescence of $B_{581/591}$-biotin (2.4 nM) in POPC bilayers coated on 0.1-mg glass beads ([POPC]/[$B_{581/591}$-Biotin] was estimated to be 500) as a function of time upon addition of avidin or albumin. ex. at 565 nm and monitored at 592 nm at room temperature.

presence of albumin or peanut lectin causes a sudden drop in fluorescence. This difference is also observed for a CT/F-GM1 system [8a], where CT causes the fluorescence of F-GM1 to drop gradually and albumin induces a rapid drop. The nonspecific signal is apparently caused by the nonspecific binding between albumin/peanut lectin and the fluorophore. Strong evidence suggests that most free $B_{581/591}$-biotins are anchored on the surfaces of POPC bilayers, but the complex of avidin/$B_{581/591}$-biotin prefers to stay in the bulk solution. We believe that the large, water-soluble avidin drags the labeled biotin out of the bilayer surfaces as suggested by the fact that the signal saturates at ¼ biotin to avidin rather than the expected 2 if the biotin remained in the bilayer. Glass microspheres coated with POPC bilayers and $B_{581/591}$-biotin maintain most fluorescence after washing with tris-buffer. But most fluorescence was lost after complexing with avidin by washing.

It was found that either in tris-buffer or in the outer leaflet of POPC vesicles or POPC bilayers coated on glass microspheres, the concentration of avidin required to saturate the fluorescence decrease is about one-fourth of the total concentration of the labeled biotin. This is expected for each avidin with four binding sites for biotin in tris-buffer. This is not the case on surfaces, because only two binding sites on each site of avidin are available for binding on surfaces. The observation that each avidin binds four labeled biotins on the surfaces of POPC vesicles and POPC bilayers on glass microspheres can be explained by the release of avidin/biotin complexes from the surfaces to solution. The binding sites on the other side become available to the labeled biotins on the surfaces.

Figure 10 shows the fluorescence change of $B_{581/591}$-biotin in tris-buffer with different concentrations of unlabeled biotin for competitive binding upon addition of avidin. The extent of fluorescence decrease is reversely proportional to the concentration of the unlabeled biotin. This competitive assay method can reliably detect less than 0.2 nM biotin. Due to the high affinity between biotin/avidin interaction, the replacement of the labeled biotin already bound to avidin is extremely slow and takes more than four days via the unlabeled biotin. The assay should be performed by adding avidin to a sample containing a known amount of the labeled biotin and an unknown amount of free biotin. Sequentially adding the labeled biotin to avidin followed by the unlabeled biotin (the sample to be measured) is *not* a good approach.

IV. CONCLUSIONS

Ultrasensitive and specific biosensors for the detection and identification of species (e.g., multivalent proteins and their receptors) involved in a multivalent interaction have been developed. The integrated optical biosensor mimics nature

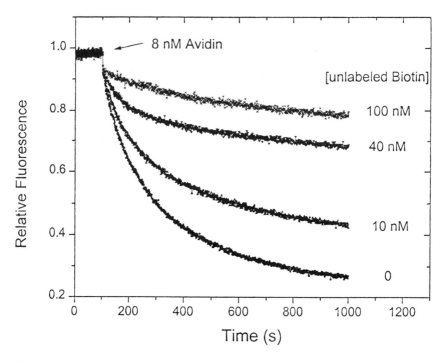

Figure 10 Fluorescence (em. at 590 nm, ex. at 570 nm) of $B_{581/591}$-Biotin (10 nM) in tris-buffer with different concentrations of norbiotinamine hydrochloride (unlabeled biotin) upon addition of 8 nM avidin.

in three important ways. First, phospholipid bilayers with optically tagged receptor molecules are attached directly to optical transducers and used to mimic the cell membrane surface. Second, biomolecular recognition is coupled directly to signal transduction and amplification, because they are in many cell-signaling processes in nature, by using the protein–receptor binding to trigger proximity-based fluorescence self-quenching and resonant energy transfer. Thirdly, as in cell signaling in nature, our sensor scheme relies on receptor aggregation to trigger signal transduction. The use of receptor aggregation to trigger transduction optimizes specificity and also results in higher effective binding affinities (the avidity effect) relative to a single receptor–protein binding event. In the case of cholera toxin and avidin, two multivalent proteins, protein–receptor recognition brings multiple optically tagged molecules into close proximity, thereby triggering the fluorescence signal. Using fluid bilayers coated onto glass beads, sensitivities of <10 pM (picomolar) and <50 pM have been achieved for CT and avidin, respectively. This sensitivity compares favorably with lab-based immunoassay, such as the enzyme-linked immunosorbant assay (ELISA) method. In contrast to ELISA, the integrated optical biosensor is fast (minutes), simple (one step, with no added reagents), insensitive to temperature variation, and robust owing to the stability of the recognition molecules and membranes.

Although originally developed for the detection of multivalent protein toxins, this approach can be adapted to the detection of any antigen involved in a multivalent interaction. Many protein toxins, unlike shiga and cholera, which bind multiple glycolipids, recognize a single glycolipid and one or more other receptors that decorate the target cell surface (e.g., botulinum toxoids also recognize a transmembrane protein). In this case, two different receptors must be used to trigger proximity-based fluorescence changes upon protein binding. More generally, two or more recognition molecules that recognize different epitopes of the same antigen could be used in this sensor scheme. The availability of huge libraries of antibodies and the rapid development of recombinant approaches to recognition molecules (e.g., RNA aptamers) make this sensor approach attractive for the detection of virtually any signature protein. We are currently exploring the use of a wide range of recognition molecules and the adaptation of this approach to other protein toxins and signature proteins for diagnosis of infectious disease. The potential adaptability of this approach to a rugged miniaturized sensor array format and the higher sensitivities (relative to lab-based immunoassays) afforded by the avidity effect also made this approach attractive for the early diagnosis of infection, where it is critical to identify signature proteins early after infection or exposure. In general, the method has potential applications for environmental sensing, low-cost medical diagnostics, and high-throughput drug screening.

ACKNOWLEDGMENTS

This work was supported by the Chemical and Biological Nonproliferation Program (NN-20) of the Department of Energy and the Laboratory Directed and Development Fund of Los Alamos National Laboratory. The authors thank Drs. John Nolan, David G. Whitten and Andrew Shreve for access of their instruments and helpful discussions.

REFERENCES

1. (a) J.D. Simon. JAMA 278:428 (1997); (b) G.W. Christopher, T.J. Cieslak, J.A. Palvin, E.M. Eitzen Jr. JAMA 278:412 (1997); (c) R. Danzig, P.B. Barkowsky JAMA 278:431 (1997).

2. (a) E. Kress-Rogers, ed. Handbook of Biosensors and Electronic Noses (CRC Press, Boca Raton, FL, 1997; (b) P. Wood. In: C.P. Price and D.J. Newman, eds. Principles and Practice of Immunoassay. Stockton Press, New York, 1991; (c) J.R. Astles W.G. Miller. Anal. Chem. 66:167 (1994); (d) S.P.A. Fodor, J.L. Read, M.C. Pirrung, L. Stryer, A.T. Lu, D. Solas. Science 251:767 (1991).

3. (a) R. Elghanian, J.J. Storhoff, R.C. Mucic, R.L. Letsinger, C.A. Mirkin. Science 277:1078 (1997); (b) B.D. Hames, S.J. Higgins, eds. Gene Probes. IRL Press, New York, 1995; (c) J. Wang, E. Palecek, P.E. Nielsen, G. Rivas, X.H. Cai, H. Shiraishi, N. Dontha, D.B. Luo, P.A.M. Farias, J. Am. Chem. Soc. 118:7667 (1996).

4. G.M. Kuziemko, M.R. Stroh, R.Stevens. Biochemistry 35:6375. (1996).

5. (a) D.H. Charych, J.O. Nagy, W. Spevak, M.D. Bednarski. Science 261:585 (1993); (b) W. Spevak, J.O. Nagy, D.H. Charych. Adv. Mater. 7:85 (1995).

6. B.A. Cornell, V.L.B. Braach-Maksvytis, L.G. King, P.D.J. Osman, B. Raguse, L. Wieczorek, R.J. Pace. Nature 387:580 (1997).

7. V.K. Gupta, , J.J. Skaife, T.B. Dubrovsky, N.L. Abbott. Science 279:2077 (1998).

8. (a) X. Song, J. Nolan, B. I. Swanson. J. Am. Chem. Soc. 120:11514 (1998); (b) X. Song, J. Nolan, B. I. Swanson. J. Am. Chem. Soc. 120:4873 (1998); (c) X. Song, B.I. Swanson. Langmuir 15:4710 (1999); (d) X. Song, B. I. Swanson. Anal. chem. 71:2097 (1999).

9. D. N. Kelly, X. Song, D. Frayer, S. B. Mendes, N. Peyghambarian, B. I. Swanson, K. Grace. Optical Letters 24:1723 (1999).

10. (a) G. M. Shepherd, , M.S. Singerand, C.A. Greer. Neuroscientist 262:2 (1996); (b) A. Berghard, L.B. Buck. J. Neurosci. 16:909 (1996); (c) J. G. Hildebrand. Annu. Rev. Neurosci. 20:595 (1997).

11. V. Kent, S. Mao, C. Wofsy, B. Goldstein, S. Ross, H. Metzger. Prod. Natl. Acad. Sci. U.S.A. 91:3087 (1994); M. Daeron. Ann. Review Immuno. 15:203 (1997); K. Sagawa, W. Swaim, J. Zhang, E. Unsworth, R. Siraganian. J. Biol. Chem. 272: 13412 (1997).

12. (a) P. Cuatrecasas. Biochemistry 12:3547 (1973); (b) P. Cuatrecasas. Biochemistry 12:3558 (1973); (c) P.H. Fisherman, J. Moss, J.C. Osborne. Biochemistry 17:711 (1978); (d) J. Staerk, H.J. Ronneberger, T. Wiegandt, W. Ziegler. Eur. J. Biochem. 48:103 (1974); (e) L. Eidels, R.L. Proia, D.A. Hart. Microbio. Rev. 47:596 (1983); (f) M. Noda, SC. Tsai, R. Adamik, J. Moss, M. Vaughan. Biochim. Biophys. Acta 1034:195 (1990).

13. H. Ling, A. Boodhoo, B. Hazes, M.D. Cummings, G.D. Armstrong, J.L. Brunton, R.J. Read. Biochemistry 37:1777 (1998).

14. F. Perrin. J. Phys. Radium 7:390 (1926)

15. (a) N.M. Green. Adv. Protein Chem. 2:985 (1975); (b) M. Wilchek, E.A. Bayer. Anal. Biochem. 171:1 (1988); (c) E.A. Bayer, M. Wilchek. Trends Biochem. Sci. 3:N257 (1978); (d) O. Livnah, E.A. Bayer, M. Wilchek, J.L. Sussman. Proc. Natl. Acad. Sci. USA 9:5076 (1993); (e) L. Pugliese, A. Coda, M. Malcoati, M. Bolognesi. J. Mol. Biol. 231:698 (1993).

16. T.M. Bayer, M. Bloom. Biophys. J. 58:357 (1990).

17. A. Shreve, personal communication.

9

Evanescent-Wave Biosensors

Brent A. Burdick
Sandia National Laboratories
Albuquerque, New Mexico, U.S.A.

I. INTRODUCTION

There is a need in health care for quick, reliable, and cost-effective in vitro diagnostic testing platforms. For example, in the critical situation of emergency room chest pain diagnostics, rapidly available information saves resources and lives. This becomes even more medically significant when multiple patients present with symptoms simultaneously. Currently, the availability in most hospitals of quick-assessment technology sensitive to subnanomolar concentrations is rather limited. Furthermore, although experimental devices have recently been demonstrated by Ligler et al. [1], there does not exist at this time any market-ready version of such technology for use in remote applications (i.e., battlefield and/or rural medicine, point-of-incident trauma care, etc.). Other applications that could benefit from affordable, portable, and sensitive (subnanomolar) immunoassay technology include: (1) the detection of biological and chemical warfare agents, (2) pollution monitoring, (3) life science research,

(4) agricultural/food testing, (5) veterinary medicine, and (6) drug screening. Alternatively, rapid and sensitive assays for nucleic acids in biological samples in the burgeoning molecular diagnostics area are contemplated.

A direct answer to the broad need for economical yet sensitive in vitro diagnostic instrumentation is one capable of measuring subnanomolar concentrations of analyte (directly in whole-blood samples) in less than five minutes without the need for separation and/or wash steps. As such, it would be well suited for inclusion in lightweight, inexpensive devices for conducting sophisticated laboratory-quality testing in point-of-care sites, such as the patient's bedside, emergency rooms, outpatient laboratories, physicians offices, and intensive care units.

Our approach to developing the appropriate biosensor platform to meet these needs uses evanescent-wave illumination coupled with total internal reflectance fluorimetry (TIRF, Fig. 1) to sensitively and simultaneously detect multiple analytes. By incorporating evanescent-wave illumination with off-axis collection of excited fluorescence, our approach offers a high-contrast detection and quantification of dilute concentrations of analyte. As an example, Plowman et al. have demonstrated femtomolar sensitivity using a sophisticated laboratory evanescent planar waveguide device [2] .

Figure 2 is a schematic representation of one assay format using this approach. A planar waveguide provides a solid surface for immobilization of recognition molecules and acts as the transmission means for optical excitation. Light injected into the waveguide is trapped by total internal reflection, with an accompanying evanescent component that penetrates exponentially into the sensing region for a distance of $\sim$100–200 nm, greater than the thickness of a protein layer resident on the waveguide surface. This evanescent behavior gives the biosensor selectivity to surface-bound protein binding events over similar protein binding in bulk solution. By employing a planar waveguide geometry with a large, flat surface area, it is also possible to configure the biosensor for multiple analyte analysis. We have chosen to name this the Evanescent Planar Waveguide (EPW^{TM}) Platform.

The EPW^{TM} Platform involves depositing on the waveguide surface "capture" antibodies specific to the analyte or antigen to be detected (Fig. 2). These capture antibodies become immobilized on the waveguide through simple adsorption to the surface (or specific chemical attachment, if desired). The capture antibody surface is exposed to the analyte sample introduced, resulting in a

Total Internal Reflection (TIR)

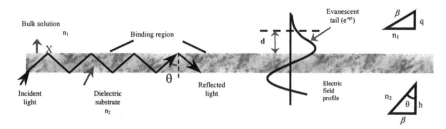

Figure 1   The evanescent field (of depth d) is set up through total internal reflection of incident light within the waveguide or index of refraction n_2 ($n_2 > n$, for bulk solution).

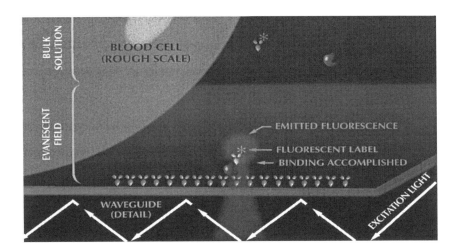

Figure 2 Schematic representation of the sensing configuration for evanescent wave-guide (EPW™) immunoassay. When an analyte molecule binds to an immobilized capture antibody, a fluorescently labeled reporter antibody can then also bind and is pulled within the evanescent zone of the waveguided light, thus exciting fluorescent emission. Note that, since fluorescence is excited only in a shallow region less than ~200 nm from the surface, interference from sources such as blood cellls and unbound reporter antibodies is virtually eliminated.

certain number of antigen molecules binding according to concentration. This binding is detected and quantified by fluorescent-molecule-labeled "reporter" antibodies, with ternary complex (sandwich) formation. The reporter antibodies in the complex are optically excited by the evanescent field at the waveguide surface. In practice, the solution of labeled reporter antibodies can be mixed with the analyte solution prior to exposure to the sensor surface, providing the labeled antibody does not compete with the same binding sites as the immobilized capture antibody. Selecting antibodies that are specific to widely spaced binding sites on the analyte of interest avoids this interference. Monoclonal antibodies are of preference in this regard. Nonspecific binding is removed by "passivation" of areas on the waveguide surface that remain uncoated with capture antibody through treatment with agents such as albinum and carbohydrate.

It is important to note that, in the EPW™ detection scheme, no separation or wash steps are required. Only those fluorophores located within the evanescent field (not the bulk solution) are excited and fluoresce, resulting in a high contrast ratio between bound reporter species and all other interfering materials (e.g., unbound reporter species, blood cells). This feature helps to dramatically simplify the principles of operation of the EPW^{TM} Platform. The other important feature is that of real-time, kinetic measurements as the standard of operation, as opposed to endpoint measurements.

There have been a number of planar waveguide fluoroimmunosensors demonstrated to date: a thick-film-waveguide sensor based on a device pioneered at the University of Utah forming the basis of the EPW^{TM} approach [3–8], a planar device developed at Naval Research Laboratory [1,9], and other thin-film waveguide fluorosensors [2,10,11]. Ives et al. have proposed that the higher evanescent intensity and reflection density of thin-film ($\sim$1 μm thick) wave-guides with 500–1000 reflections per centimeter should enhance the sensitivity of evanescently based immunosensors [12]. In general, one can increase the reflection density at the waveguide surface either by making the waveguide thinner or by increasing the waveguide refractive index. However, these steps will improve the detection limit of a fluorosensor only if the thin-film wave-guide exhibits low propagation losses and low values of self- (native) fluores-cence. These constraints have to date required sophisticated methods for fabri-cating thin-film waveguide sensors. Thus, while thin-film waveguide biosensors have proven to be very powerful tools for basic studies of TIRF methods, they have been essentially laboratory instruments and have not been compact or inex-pensive enough for eventual commercial development and/or field deployment in decentralized testing settings.

A semiautomated, benchtop instrument (the Lifelite^{TM} analyzer) employs the EPW^{TM} injection-molded polystyrene waveguide and integrated optics in a disposable cartridge unit. The EPW^{TM}/Lifelite^{TM} system is the only planar wave-guide fluorescence immuno/molecular diagnostic assay device known to utilize a plastic integrated lens waveguide as the sensor element. Other approaches commonly employ an optically polished fused-silica substrate as the waveguide [1]. In anticipation of the predicted demand (tens of millions per year), the use of costly materials and labor-intensive procedures to produce components such as a fused-silica waveguides would represent a major limitation to large-scale acceptance and use. The EPW^{TM} approach utilizes inexpensive fabrication and materials for all disposable components of the system, including the critical integrated optical element itself, the waveguide.

II. EPW^{TM}/LIFELITE^{TM} BIOSENSOR CONFIGURATION AND OPERATION

A. EPW^{TM} and Disposable Cartridge Unit

The EPW^{TM} (Fig. 3) consists of a a monolithic, injected-molded ($\sim$2.5 cm $\times$ 2.5 cm) polystyrene unit consisting of a cylindrical incoupling lens, a planar reac-tion plate, and an outcoupling element. The incoupling lens accurately and effi-

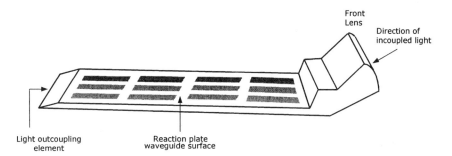

Front
Lens
Direction of
incoupled light

Light outcoupling
element

Reaction plate
waveguide surface

Figure 3   First-generation EPW™ with integrated lens, the reaction plate detection area segmented into 12 discrete zones, and outcoupling element.

ciently couples the incident laser beam (from a 635-nm, 20-mW laser diode) at an optimum angle of 20° from normal into the waveguide. This promotes the coupling of higher-order modes, resulting in increased electric field intensity at the waveguide surface [5]. The cylindrical lens configuration also allows greater tolerance for positioning with respect to excitation sources. The reaction plate can currently be segmented into up to 12 separate regions with sensing zones of ~0.25-cm^2 area. This allows for different combinations/permutations of on-board controls and calibrators mixed with actual unknown detection zones. The EPW™ is currently 500 μm in thickness and is produced as a high-quality optical element through state-of-the-art plastic injection molding processes.

The EPW™ is combined with a proprietary fluidics module to yield a disposable cartridge unit, designed to be readily manufactured on a high-volume commercial scale (Fig. 4). The cartridge unit consists of commercial-grade ABS plastic and contains a sample well, with gasket for the addition of up to 800 μL of fluid sample, and a movable sample cover to close in order to contain and isolate the sample following introduction into the cartridge sample well.

The EPW™ is positioned within the cartridge body to provide introduction of the sample to the bottom, inverted face of the waveguide containing active capture agent. A schematic of the flow of fluid through the specialized compartments of cartridge unit and, eventually, onto the waveguide surface is presented in Figure 5. The cartridge unit also contains mixing reservoirs or chambers to allow the introduction of ancillary reagents (in dry form) necessary for the assay(s) being performed. Proprietary active fluidics allow for mixing of dry reagents with sample fluid within the cartridge. Fluorescent emission from specific binding on the waveguide surface is collected by a lens assembly, transmitted through a bandpass filter (to reject scattered laser light), and imaged onto a CCD array.

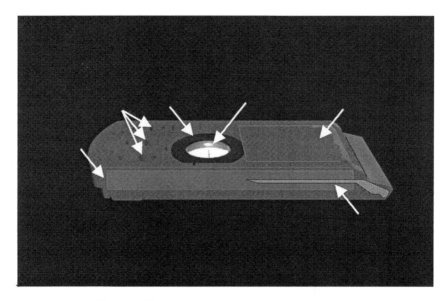

Figure 4   EPW^{TM} Lifelite^{TM} Cartridge.

B.   EPW^{TM}/LIFELITE^{TM} Analyzer

The Lifelite^{TM} Analyzer, which incorporates all the required excitation/emission optics, heating control, and fluidics interface with the cartridge unit is pictured in Fig. 6. The unit also contains microprocessor control units and user interface. The Celux^{TM} unit itself is compact (approximately $12'' \times 10'' \times 11''$), portable (on

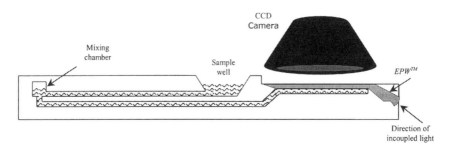

Figure 5   Cross section of Lifelite^{TM} cartridge showing the fluid motion, mixing chambers, and positioning of the EPW^{TM} within the cartridge element.

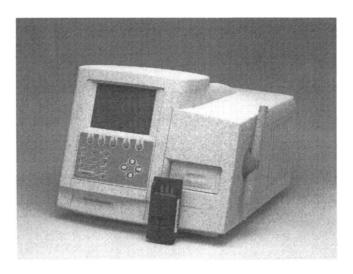

Figure 6 EPW™ Lifelite™ Prototype Analyzer.

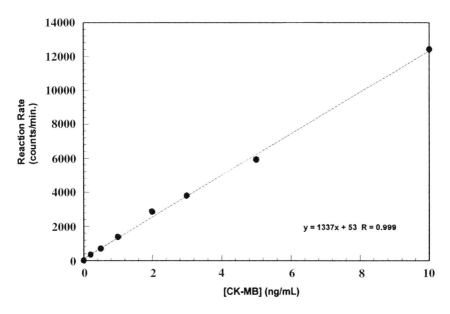

Figure 7 CKMB *EPW*™ immunoassay showing linearity and abbreviated dynamic range.

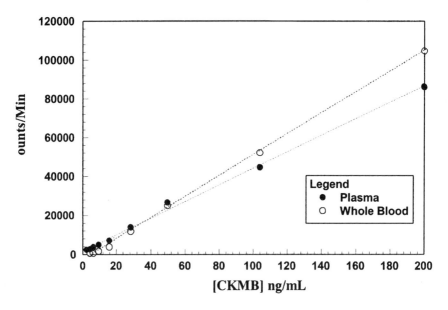

Figure 8   CKMB sandwich immunoassay: whole-blood vs. plasma standard curves.

the order of 20-lb weight), and equipped with a CRT display/keyboard and printer. The cartridge is inserted into the retractable drawer (right-hand portion of the unit) after being scanned by the barcode reader for identification processing. Results are available typically in five minutes following insertion of the cartridge.

III.   RESULTS AND DISCUSSION

A.   System Performance with EPW™/Lifelite™ Prototype Unit—Immunoassays

Originally, validation of the cartridge unit and Lifelite™ Analyzer was undertaken with the use of protein analytes with relevant diagnostic importance, e.g., the MB isoenzyme form of creatine kinase (CK), which has served as a "gold standard" in monitoring episodes of acute myocardial infarction (AMI). Whole-blood samples (800 µL) containing varying amounts of CKMB were applied to the waveguide surface containing active anti-CKMB capture antibodies and tracer (or labeled) antibody with Cy5 dye attached as the reporter fluorophore. A 635-nm laser diode served as the excitation source, and emitted fluorescence

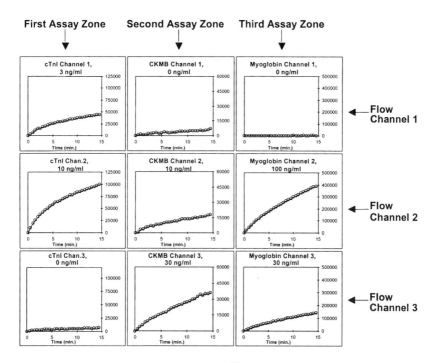

Figure 9 Multizone detection on the EPW™ showing detection of three different protein analytes in blood at three separate concentrations for each analyte (cTnI: 0, 3, 10 ng/mL, CKMB: 0, 10, 30 ng/mL; myoglobin: 0, 30, 100 ng/mL.

was collected on a CCD camera fitted with a Nikon 55mm/f2.8 lens. Results are displayed (Fig. 7) as a dose–response curve showing linearity over a range of analyte concentration and a low threshold detection (≤0.3 ng/mL). This is representative of performance for a wide range of proteins assayed, with good correlation to reference assays/devices commercially available (data not shown).

To compare the response performance of CKMB in plasma vs. a whole-blood matrix, dose–response curves were generated in both sample matrices and compared directly (Fig. 8). There was little difference in response, particularly within the more clinically relevant regions of the dose–response curve (0–60 ng/mL CKMB) as registered in whole-blood vs. plasma samples. As a further confirmation of insensitivity to matrix composition, detection thresholds for CKMB were measured in partially lysed whole blood (15mg/dL free hemoglobin) all the way up to totally lysed blood (~15,000 mg/dL free hemoglobin) with negligible change in detection thresholds (data not shown).

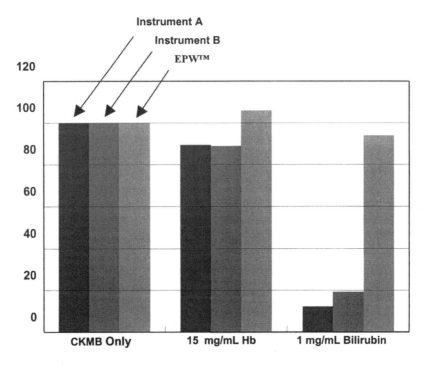

Figure 10 Investigation of comparative interferences of *EPW*™ CKMB assay widely accepted commercial immunoassay platform for CKMB (Instruments A and B).

Because the EPW™ Platform is designed for the simultaneous measurement of multiple analytes on a single (disposable) waveguide, waveguides were prepared that possessed three separate capture zones for three different protein analytes (CKMB, cTnI = cardiac troponin I, myoglobin). These waveguides were then subjected to different combinations of concentrations of the three analytes and fluorescence measurements recorded with time (up to 15 minutes, Fig. 9). This demonstration adequately resolved the issue of feasibility for multiple analyte measurement on a single waveguide surface with a minimum of optical (or immunochemical) cross-talk or intereference.

As another, independent assessment of the tolerance of the EPW™ Platform to potential interfering substances in human biological specimens (i.e., blood), a comparison of the magnitude of interference (suppression) of response with the addition of two common interfering substances (hemoglobin, bilirubin) in the CKMB immunoassay was performed (Fig. 10). Here the EPW™ performance was compared to two widely accepted commercial in vitro diagnostic

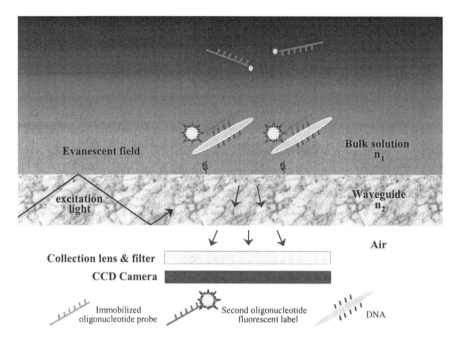

Figure 11 EPW^{TM} nucleic acid (DNA/RNA) sandwich assay schematic.

immunoassay platforms (Instruments A and B). Results indicate a marked suppression of response for Hb and bilirubin, in particular, for both Instruments A and B, whereas the EPW^{TM} response was virtually unchanged. This verifies that, through the use of evanescent-wave principles, biological or chemical sources of optical interference can in essence be totally removed from the operation.

B. Other EPW^{TM}/Lifelite^{TM} Formats—Nucleic Acid Assays

The EPW^{TM} Platform allows for the direct substitution of capture oligonucleotides for capture antibodies in order to fashion EPW^{TM} based assays designed for DNA or RNA probe-based diagnostic techniques. For example (Fig. 11), DNA or RNA sandwich assays on the EPW^{TM} surface consist of an oligonucleotide capture probe (or probes) on the surface of the waveguide in combination with a second tracer oligonucleotide with reporter tag (dye). In a fashion strictly analogous to the sandwich immunoassay (Fig. 2), the DNA/RNA analyte of interest (plasmid, genomic DNA, ribosomal RNA, PCR amplicon, etc.) is "sandwiched" between the capture and tracer probe and fluorescence measured correlated with the quantity of DNA/RNA analyte introduced.

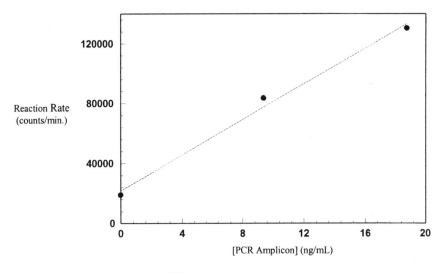

Figure 12 PCR amplicon *EPW*™ binding assay. Biotin and dye-labeled PCR primers were used to create the (~200-bp) PCR amplicon, followed by capture and detection on an avidin-coated EPW™ surface.

Table 1 Detection Limit*a* Using the EPW™ Diagnostic Platform

Analyte	Molecular weight	Detection Limit	
		ng/mL	Molar
Digoxin	781	1	1.3 nM
Oligopeptide	1,200	2	1.7 nM
Oligonucleotide	12,000	0.5	40 pM
Myoglobin	16,900	2	0.1 nM
Interleukin-4	20,500	0.042	2 pM
Troponin-I	23,500	0.2	8.5 pM
Ovalbumin	45,000	1	22 pM
Chorionic gonadotropin	50,000	0.7	10 pM
Serum albumin	66,000	20	0.3 nM
Ricin	70,000	0.25	3.6 pM
Creatine kinase MB	80,000	0.3	4 pM
Immunoglobulin G	150,000	50	0.3 nM
MS-2 (virus)	0.2 microns	10^6 pfu/mL	N/A
B. globigii	1–2 microns	10^5 cfu/mL	N/A
E. herbicola	0.5 × 3 microns	5×10^5 cfu/mL	N/A

*a*Limited assay development with some analytes.

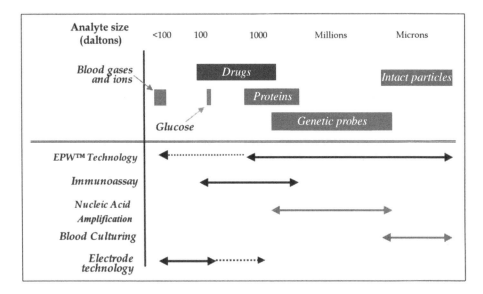

Figure 13   In vitro diagnostic spectrum showing ranges accessed by particular testing methodologies.

As a demonstration of this approach, the quantitative measurement of a ~200-bp PCR amplicon (after 20 cycles of PCR) was undertaken with appropriate complementary oligo capture and tracer probes (complementary to non-overlapping internal regions on the PCR amplicon). Results (Fig. 12) revealed linear dose–response in the range of low ng/mL concentration of PCR amplicon analyte.

IV.   CONCLUSIONS AND FUTURE DIRECTIONS

The evanescent waveguide–based biosensor approach (EPW^{TM}) detailed in this chapter has been shown to provide rapid, sensitive quantification of a number of important clinical analytes in whole blood directly, with little of no interference from common interfering substances. Table 1 presents a compilation of the detection limits on the EPW^{TM} Platform (five-minute total assay time) for a number of analytes, spanning a wide range of molecular weight (or size). Results indicate sensitivities as low as low pM levels in five minutes. The use of thinner waveguide formats using the same principles described here should lead to even greater sensitivity achievement, perhaps by as much as three orders of magnitude (femtomolar sensitivity has been shown) [2].

Future modifications and improvement will include an expansion of the assay menu (Table 1) to include not only proteins, DNA/RNA species, intact microbiological particles, and low-molecular-weight drugs, but common clinical chemistry analytes (metabolites, electrolytes, blood gases) as well (Fig. 13). This will involve novel chemistries currently under development coupled to waveguide surfaces to generate response curves on both the current EPW^{TM} (Fig. 3) and future-generation thin-film waveguides.

REFERENCES

1. F. S. Ligler, D. W. Conrad, J. P. Golden, M. J. Feldstein, B. D. Maccraith, S. D. Balderson, J. Czarnaski, C. A. Rowe. Array biosensor for multianalyte sensing. In: P. L. Gourley, ed. Micro- and Nanofabricated Structures and Devices for Biomedical Environmental Applications, Soc. Photo-Opt. Instru. Eng., Bellingham, WA 1998, pp. 50–55.
2. T. E. Plowman, W.. Reichart, C. R. Peters, H.-K. Wang, D. A. Christensen, J. N. Herron. Femtomolar sensitivity using a channel-etched thin-film-waveguide fluoroimmunosensor. Biosens Bioelectron 11:149 (1996).
3. D. A. Christensen, S. Dyer, D. Fowers, J. N. Herron. Analysis of excitation and collection geometries for planar waveguide immunosensors. In: F. P. Milanovich, ed. Fiber-Optic Sensors in Medical Diagnostics. Soc. Photo-Opt. Instru. Eng., Bellingham, WA, 1993, pp. 2–9.
4. J. N. Herron, K. D. Caldwell, D. A. Christensen, S. Dyer, V. Hlady, P. Huang, V. Janatova, H.-K. Wang, A.-P. Wei. Fluorescent immunosensors using planar waveguides. In: J. R. Lakowicz, R. B. Thompson, eds. Advances in Fluorescence Sensing Technology. Soc. Photo-Opt. Instru. Eng., Bellingham, WA, 1993, pp. 28–39.
5. D. A. Christensen, J. N. Herron. Optical immunoassay systems based upon evanescent wave interactions. In: G. E. Cohn, S. A. Soper, C. H. W. Chen, eds. Ultrasensitive Biochemical Diagnostics. Soc. Photo-Opt. Instru. Eng., Bellingham, WA, 1996, pp. 58–67.
6. J. N. Herron, D. A. Christensen, K. D. Caldwell, V. Janatova, S.-C. Huang, H.-K. Wang. Waveguide immunosensor with coating chemistry providing enhanced sensitivity. US Patent 5,512,492, April 30, 1996, University of Utah Research Foundation, Assignee.
7. J. N. Herron, D. A. Christensen, H.-K. Wang, K. D. Caldwell, V. Janatova, S.-C. Huang. Apparatus and methods for multianalyte homogeneous fluoroimmunoassays. US Patent 5,677,196, October 14, 1997, University of Utah Research Foundation, Assignee.
8. J. N. Herron, H.-K. Wang, A. H. Terry, J. D. Durtschi, L. Tan, M. E. Astill, R. S. Smith, D. A. Chirstensen. Rapid clinical diagnostics assays using injection-molded

planar waveguides. In: Systems and Technologies for Clinical Diagnostics and Drug Discovery. Soc. Photo-Opt. Instru. Eng., Bellingham, WA, 1998, pp. 54–64.

9. R. R. Wadkins, J. P. Golden, F. S. Ligler. Patterned planar array immunosensor for multianalyte detection. J Biomedical Optics 2:74 (1997).

10. A. N. Sloper, J. K. Deacon, M. T. Flannigan. A planar indium phosphate mono-mode-waveguide evanescent-field immunosensor.' Sens Actuators B1:589 (1990).

11. Y. Shou, P. J. R. Laybourn, J. V. Magill, R. M. de la Rue. An evanescent fluores-cense biosensor using ion-exchanged buried waveguides and the enhancement of peak fluorescence. Biosens Bioelectron 6:595 (1991).

12. J. T. Ives, W. M. Reichert, J. N. Lin, V. Hlady, D. Reinecke, P. A. Suci, R. A. van Wagenen, K. Newby, J. N. Herron, P. Dryden, J. D. Andrade. Total internal reflec-tion fluorescence surface sensors. In: A. N. Chester, S. Martellucci, A. M. Verga Scheggi, eds. Optical Fiber Sensors. Kluwer Academic, Hingham, MA, 1987, pp. 391–397.

10

Glow-Discharge-Treated Quartz Crystal Microbalance as Immunosensor

Selma Mutlu, M. Hadi Zareie, Erhan Pişkin, and Mehmet Mutlu
Hacettepe University, Ankara, Turkey

I. INTRODUCTION

Recently, considerable attention has been focused on the development of piezo-electric sensors for the diagnostic determination of biological analytes (e.g., enzymes, hormones, antibodies/antigens), which are based on the change of resonance frequency of piezoelectric crystal with the change of mass loaded on the crystal [1–5]. A specific binding between antibody and antigen has been exploited in piezoelectric immunosensors constructed by immobilizing antibody to the crystal surface, which then interacts very selectively with the antigen requiring detection in the medium [6–13]. The sensing layer of the immunosensor is prepared by immobilizing antibody molecules on the surface of the piezoelectric crystal by physical or chemical means.

In this study, we modified the piezoelectric crystal surface by means of a glow-discharge treatment by using ethylenediamine plasma, in order to chemically immobilize antibody molecules to the surface. Antisyphilis antibody was used as a model antibody to detect the antigen (i.e., cardiolipin) in an aqueous medium. Frequency shifts were detected, and changes of the crystal surfaces after each modification step were also followed via a novel technique, i.e., scanning tunneling microscopy.

II. Experiment

A quartz crystal microbalance (QCM) system was designed and constructed [14]. As shown schematically in Figure 1, the QCM measuring system consists of an AT-cut 10-MHz quartz crystal of an 8.7- × 0.17-mm wafer that was placed between 4.7-mm silver electrodes and mounted in a ceramic holder with a plug (Mizu, Germany). Five volts DC is applied to the oscillator circuit to "drive" the crystal, and the frequency is followed with a Phillips frequency counter (Model: PM 6672, The Netherlands). The system is enclosed in a case that is maintained in a chamber at a constant temperature of 25° ± 0.1°C during measurements to reduce frequency fluctuations due to drafts and dust. In air, this QCM system gives less than a 1-Hz drift after the initial stabilization period of about few minutes.

Mass changes of the piezoelectric crystals after each treatment (see later) were determined by the measured frequency shifts using the Saurerbey equation [15]:

$$\Delta f = (-2.3 \times 10^6) f^2 \, \Delta m / A \tag{1}$$

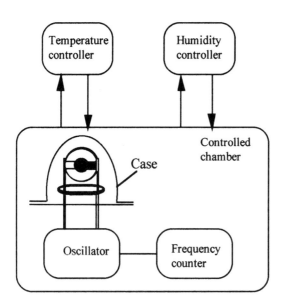

Figure 1   Schematic drawing of QCM system.

where Δf is the change in frequency (Hz), f is the resonance frequency of the original piezoelectric crystal (MHz) (10 MHz in our case), Δm is the mass increase, and A is the area coated (cm^2) (0.594 cm^2 in our case).

In order to immobilize the antibody to the piezoelectric crystal surface, a glow-discharge treatment method was applied. The glow-discharge apparatus is schematically shown in Figure 2. The reactor was a Pyrex® glass tube with a diameter of 5.6 cm and a length of 52 cm. Two copper electrodes 7×17 cm were placed externally on the reactor. One electrode was connected to a radio-frequency generator with frequency of 13.6 MHz (Tasarim Ltd., Model T-RF-1200, Turkey) through a matching network unit (Tasarim Ltd., Model T-RF-1100, Turkey), while the other electrode was grounded. The monomer tank was connected to the reactor through a flow meter (Gilmont, F-1200, Size 2, USA) and a needle valve (Brooks, Model 1355, CA).

Ethylenediamine (EDA, Sigma, UK) was used as a monomer to create amine-and/or amino-like active groups on the quartz crystal surface for covalent binding of the antibody molecules. In a typical glow-discharge treatment procedure, quartz crystal was placed on the sample holder located between the electrodes and the reactor cap was sealed. Nitrogen and oxygen gases in the reactor were swept out with an argon stream prior to the glow discharge. The reactor was evacuated to 10^{-3}–10^{-4}4 mbar. The monomer, EDA, was allowed to flow

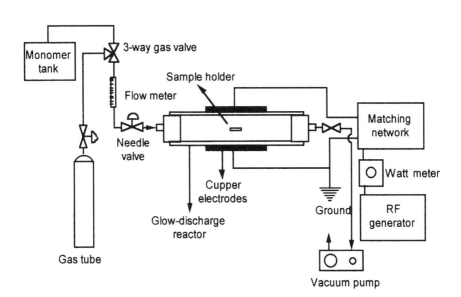

Figure 2 Schematic drawing of glow-discharge system.

through the reactor at a rate of 15 mL/min. The quartz crystals were exposed to the EDA plasma for 30 min at a glow-discharge power of 5 W. Surface-modified crystals were immediately transferred to the antibody medium for covalent binding of antibody.

For antibody immobilization, 0.2 mL of antisyphilis antibody solution (Porton, Cambridge, UK) was diluted with 5 mL of buffered saline and immediately used for antibody binding. The glow-discharge-treated crystals were incubated with this diluted antibody solution for 2 h at 25°C at a pH of 7.4. The system was agitated on a rotary shaker (Köttermann Laboratories, Germany) during incubation. After incubation, the crystals were washed with a phosphate buffer solution (pH 7.4) for 30 min in an agitated beaker, and dried in air (temperature 30°C and relative humidity 30%); the resonance frequency of the crystals was then measured until the frequency of the crystal remained constant.

The antigen test solution (VDRL, Omega, UK) was prepared via the procedure described by the manufacturer. Briefly, 0.5 mL of VDRL antigen was added (dropwise) to 0.4 mL saline over a 6-sec period while rotating the bottle on a flat surface. Rotation was continued for a further 10 sec, and then 4.1 mL of buffered saline was added. This freshly prepared VDRL antigen test solution was kept at 2–8°C until use and was consumed within 24 h. Four mL of VDRL antigen solution was added to 1 mL of 1% NaCl solution, mixed vigorously, and allowed to stand for at least 5 min prior to use. The crystals with bound antibody were immersed in the antigen test solution for 10 min of incubation time. The crystals were subsequently rinsed with buffered saline and dried in air, and then the frequency of the crystals was measured.

Changes of the surfaces of the piezoelectric crystals at the different steps just given were also followed by means of a scanning tunneling microscope (STM). The STM was constructed in our laboratory and used in a wide variety of applications [16–18]. Mechanically, it consists of two main modules: a scanner and a coarse positioner. These modules can be separated to perform distinct measurements, performance tests, and experiments. Even different modules for coarse positioning can be installed on the scanner module. The scanner part is constructed with a PZT tube (EBL #3 PZT-5H, Staveley Sensors Inc. CT) glued to an aluminum body. The electrical connections of the PZT are made through a special connector. The tip holder is also glued to the interior of the PZT tube but isolated electrically. The rough approach unit is a magnetically driven slider that is fastened to the scanner by two screws, and the whole system is mounted on a vibration isolation stage. Electrical connections to the system are made through a printed circuit board placed near the vibration-isolation stage. Very thin wires are used between the STM and this board to reduce the vibrational coupling between them.

The STM was operated in air at atmospheric pressure with a tip-to-substrate bias of 0.5–1 V (sample positive) and tunneling currents of 10–20 pA.

Etched tips of Pt/Ir (80:20) wires (0.5 mm in diameter, Digital Instruments, Santa Barbara, CA) were used in constant-current mode.

III. Results and Discussion

Over the past decade there has been rapid exploration and commercialization of plasma technology to improve the surface properties of materials without changing their bulk properties [19–23]. In these technologies, two major types of discharges are considered, i.e., high-frequency discharge (low-temperature plasma) and low frequency discharge (corona discharge). In both cases, glow-discharge treatments produce either deposition or etching on the substrate surface. Glow-discharge treatments conducted especially in an inert gas atmosphere usually cause etching of the surface, while other plasmas (e.g., organic vapors) deposit a film on the substrate surface. In both cases, the newly formed surface is dependent not on the substrate properties but on the glow-discharge conditions and the type of atmosphere (plasma) used. Note that, as stated in the literature, several hydrophilic (polar) groups (e.g., —NH, —CN, —N:N, —C=O, —COOH, —C—OH, —CHO) are formed on the substrate surface during glow-discharge treatment, depending on the monomer or gas phase used, and also through postplasma reactions.

In this study, in order to chemically immobilize antibody molecules on the piezoelectric crystal, we first treated one surface of the crystal with a low-temperature plasma by using ethylenediamine as a reactive monomer in a glow-discharge reactor system to deposit a polymeric film carrying amine-and/or amino-like active groups. By using our earlier experience to get a thin polymer film on the surface, we applied the glow discharge at the following conditions [14,24–25]: discharge power 5 W; plasma exposure time 30 min; and monomer flow rate 15 mL/min. The resonance frequencies of at least five crystals treated at these glow-discharge conditions were measured in the QCM system described in the Sec. II. The mean (± the standard deviations) of the frequency shifts was 566 ± 96 Hz after the glow-discharge treatment. Frequency shifts caused by the glow-discharge treatment and the other surface treatments applied to the crystals are given in Table 1.

The mass depositions, which were calculated from the Sauerbrey expression [Eq. (1)] corresponding the frequency shifts are shown in Table 2. The mass change was about 1.48 µg (for one crystal) after the glow-discharge treatment.

In order to confirm deposition during the glow-discharge treatment, we observed the crystal surfaces before and after the treatment via a novel technique, i.e., scanning tunneling microscopy. Following our earlier experience [16–18], we operated the STM in air at atmospheric pressure with a tip-to-

Table 1   Frequency Shifts of Different Quartz Crystal Surfaces

Material	Average frequency f (Hz)	Differential frequency ^2f (Hz)
QC	10,004,778	—
QC + amine	10,004,212	566 ± 96
QC + amine + antibody	10,001,220	$2,994 \pm 83 \ (3558)^a$
QC + amine + antibody + antigen	9,998,916	$2,306 \pm 334 \ (5862)^a$

Experimental data given as an average of data from five crystals.
[a]Differential frequencies according to the original frequency of the quartz crystal.

substrate bias of 0.5–1 V (sample positive) and tunneling currents of 10–20 pA in constant-current mode. Figures 3A and 3B give representative STM images of the untreated and glow-discharge-treated piezoelectric crystal surface, respectively, in which surface modification is clearly seen.

In this study, an antigen–antibody couple in the test kit for diagnosis of syphilis, an infection caused by *Treponema pallidum*, was selected as an example to develop the piezoelectric immunosensors. After the glow-discharge treatment, the surface-modified crystals were immediately immersed in the prepared antibody solution. In order to achieve a stable antibody immobilization, incubation was conducted for 2 h at 25°C at a pH of 7.4, following our earlier experience [14,25].

As expected, frequency shifts have been observed due to antibody immobilization on the crystal surface that caused the mass deposition. After the immobilization, measured frequencies of the crystals were comparable with the original crystal frequencies. The mean ($\pm$ the standard deviations) of the fre-

Table 2   Mass Changes of Different Quartz Crystal Surfaces

Material	Average frequency f (Hz)	Mass change ^2m (μg)
QC	10,004,778	0
QC + amine	10,004,212	1.483
QC + amine + antibody	10,001,220	$7.871 \ (9.354)^a$
QC + amine + antibody + antigen	9,998,916	$6.062 \ (15.416)^a$

Experimental data given as an average of data from five crystals.
[a]Mass changes according to the original mass of the quartz crystal.

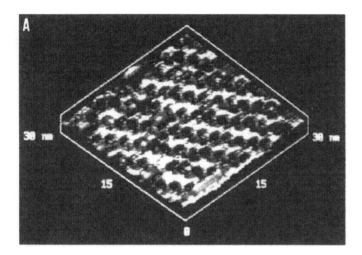

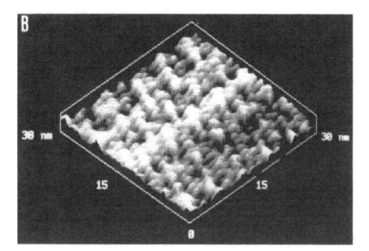

Figure 3 STM images of piezoelectric crystal surfaces: (A) untreated. (B) Glow-discharge treated. The scan area for both images is 30×30 nm. Tunnelling current 20 pA; bias voltage 500 mV. The images were taken in constant-current mode.

quency shifts obtained for at least five crystals treated in the same way at the same conditions was 2994 ± 83 Hz, which corresponds to an increase in mass of about 7.87 μg (for one crystal) after antibody immobilization calculated via Eq. (1). Note that with repeated washing of the antibody-immobilized crystals, no significant frequency shifts were observed after washing. Therefore, we concluded that strongly covalent binding of the antibodies on the crystal surfaces was achieved.

Figure 4 gives two representative images of antibody-immobilized piezo-electric surfaces. These confirm immobilization of the Y-shaped antibody molecules on the crystal surface.

In order to follow interactions of antibody-immobilized quartz crystals with antigens in aqueous solutions, the antibody-immobilized crystals were incubated in the aqueous solutions of antigen (i.e., cardiolipin) in a shaker for 10 min. After the incubation period, the crystals were dried in air and resonance frequencies were measured. The mean frequency shift (and standard deviation from five parallel experiments) after the antibody–antigen interactions was 2306 $\pm$ 34 Hz, which corresponds to an increase in mass of about 6.06 μg (for one crystal) after antibody–antigen interaction calculated via Eq. (1). Note once again that these frequency shifts indicate that mass deposition occurred on the crystal as a result of coupling of antigen and antibody.

The STM images given in Figure 5 exemplify antibody–antigen interactions on the piezoelectric surfaces. These representative images are considered here, besides the frequency shift of crystal, another indication of antibody-antigen interaction on the piezoelectric crystal surfaces.

IV. CONCLUSION

A model piezoelectric immunosensor was investigated in this study. Piezoelectric crystal surfaces were first modified by a glow-discharge treatment by using ethylenediamine plasma, in order to chemically immobilize antibody molecules to the surface. Anti-Syphilis antibody was used as a model antibody to detect the antigen (i.e., cardiolipin) in an aqueous medium. Frequency shifts were detected by using an home-made QCM system. We were also able to calculate the amount of material that deposited on the crystal surface at each step by using the Sauerbrey expression. Changes of the crystal surfaces after each modification step was successfully followed by a novel technique, i.e., scanning tunneling microscopy. From these results we concluded that the piezoelectric immunosensor developed by the methodology presented in this paper, may successful be utilized in the measurement of antigens in aqueous medium with high sensitivity and selectivity.

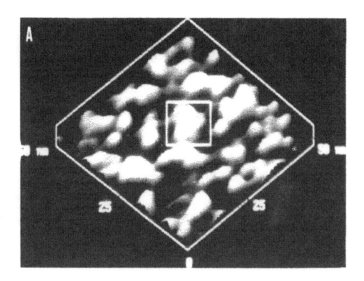

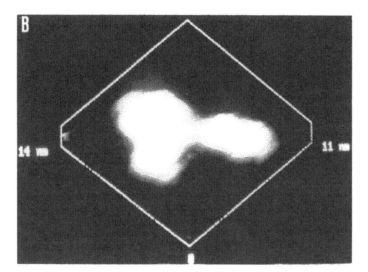

Figure 4 STM images of antibody molecules on piezoelectric crystal surfaces: (A) Representative STM image of antibody with a scan area of 50 × 50 nm. (B) An enlarged image of antibody in the box shown in image A with a scan area of 11 × 14 nm. Tunneling current 10 pA; bias voltage 500 mV. The images were taken in constant-current mode.

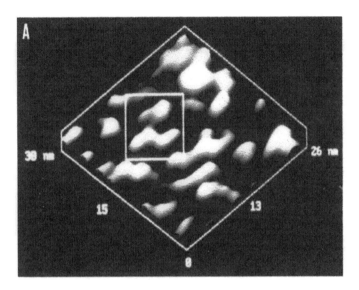

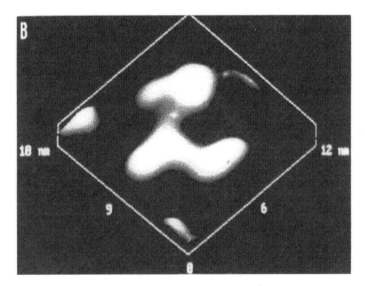

Figure 5 STM images of antibody–antigen molecules on piezoelectric crystal surfaces: (A) Representative STM image of antibody–antigen molecules with a scan area of 26×30 nm. (B) An enlarged image of antibody in the box shown in image A with a scan area of 12×18 nm. Tunneling current 10 pA; bias voltage 1 V. The images were taken in constant-current mode.

ACKNOWLEDGMENTS

This research is partly supported by Turkish Scientific and Technical Council (TÜBITAK) research project. Project No: TBAG 1534.

REFERENCES

1. Ngeh-Ngwainbi, J.; Suleiman, A.A.; Guilbault, G.G. Biosensors Bioelectron. 5:13, 1990.
2. Hughes, R.C.; Ricco, A.J.; Butler, M.A.; Martin, S.J. Science 254:74,1991.
3. Muramatsu, H.; Dicks, J.M.; Tamiya, E.; Karube, I. Anal. Chem. 59:2760, 1987.
4. Masson, M.; Yun, K.; Haruyama, T.; Kobatake, E.; Aizawa, M. Anal. Chem. 67: 2212, 1990.
5. Nabauer, A.; Berger, P.; Ruge, I.; Muller E.; Woias, P.; Kosslinger, C.; Drobe, H. Sensors Actuators B1:508, 1990.
6. Shons, A.; Dorman F.; Nawarian, J. J. Biomed Mater. Res. 6:565, 1972.
7. Roederer J.E.; Bastiaans, G.J. Anal. Chem. 55:2333, 1983.
8. Muramatsu, H.; Kajiwara, K.; Tamiya, E.; Karube, I. Anal. Chim. Acta 118:257, 1986.
9. Thompson, M.; Arthur C.L.; Dhaliwal, G.K. Anal. Chem. 58:1206, 1986.
10. Sochaczewski, E.P.; Luong, J.H.T.; Guilbault, G.G. Enzyme Microb. Technol. 12: 173, 1990.
11. Davis K.A.; Leary, T.R. Anal. Chem. 61:1227, 1989.
12. Geddes, N.J.; Paschinger, E.M.; Furlog, D.N.; Ebara, Y.; Okahata, Y.; Than, K.A.; Edgar, J.A. Sensors Actuators, B17:125, 1994.
13. Minunni, M.; Skladal, P.; Mascini, M.A. Analytical Lett. 27(8):1475, 1994.
14. Özgüven, A., M.Sc. thesis, Hacettepe University, Ankara, Turkey, 1996.
15. Sauerbrey, G. Z. Phys. 155:206, 1959.
16. Zareie, M.H. Ph.D. dissertation, Hacettepe University, Ankara, Turkey, 1995.
17. Zareie, M.H.; Erdem, G. Öner, R.; Öner, C.; Öğüş, A.; Pişkin, E. Int. J. Biol. Macromol. 19:69, 1996.
18. Zareie, M.H.; Pişkin, A.K.; Verimli, R.; Kansu, E.; Pişkin, E. Nanobiol. 1:1, 1996.
19. Hollahan J.K.; Bell, A.T., eds. Techniques and Applications of Plasma Chemistry. Wiley, New York, 1974.
20. Clark, D.T.; Feast, W.J., eds. Application of Plasmas to the Synthesis and Surface of Polymers. Wiley, New York, 1978.
21. Yasuda H.; Gazicki, M. Biomat. 3:68, 1982.
22. Yasuda, H., ed. Plasma Polymerization. Academic Press, Orlando, FL, 1985.
23. Mutlu, M.; Mutlu, S.; Alp, B.; Boyaci, I.H.; Pişkin, E., In: d'Agustino, R., ed. Plasma Processing of Polymers. Kluwer Academic, Dordrecht, Netherlands, 1997.
24. Pişkin, E. J. Biomat. Sci. Polym. Ed. 4:45, 1992.
25. Mutlu, S.; Saber, R.; Koçum, C.; Pişkin, E. Analytical Lett. 32(2):317, 1999.

11
Diagnostic Polymer Reagents Carrying DNA

Mizuo Maeda, Takeshi Mori, Daisuke Umeno, and Yoshiki Katayama
Kyushu University, Fukuoka, Japan

I. INTRODUCTION

Recent striking developments in molecular biology have demonstrated that small mutations of certain genes are the definite origin of many heritable disorders and cancers. These findings have highlighted the importance of gene mutation assays in the field of medical diagnosis. For the detection of change in the DNA base sequence, various methods have been proposed. The methods may be classified into two categories. One relies on a sequence-specific enzymatic reaction, the other relies on an oligonucleotide probe. Enzyme-based methods may be more convenient and reliable in some cases, whereas the methods based on nucleic acid hybridization should be more general and widely applicable. Most of the latter methods take advantage of immobilized single-stranded DNA (ssDNA).

On the other hand, double-stranded DNA (dsDNA) provides potent affinity functions for the sensing and purification of DNA-binding proteins and DNA-binding drugs. In fact, a variety of dsDNA-comprising materials, such as sepharose beads, synthetic polymer resins, polyacrylamide (AAm) gels, and silica gels, have been developed and successfully utilized.

In addition, when one pays attention to the structural properties of the DNA molecule, one notices that DNA itself can provide a variety of functions that are never attained by the synthetic materials or chemicals. For instance, dsDNA is interesting as a building block with a highly regulated one-dimensional structure. The size of the DNA strand can be precisely regulated at will by digestion using restriction endonucleases, elongation using polymerases, and ligation using DNA ligases, ranging from the oligomer to the gigantic chromosome of centimeter scale. All these factors allow us to imagine the possible use of DNA strands as molecular wires or as building blocks enabling various nanoscale architectures that are monodisperse, processable, and even amplifiable. Molecules bearing dsDNA should provide a tool for constructing a new class of materials having novel structures and functions. However, only a very limited number of studies with this point of view have been reported. This is partly because there is no proper method for the chemical modification of dsDNA that is suitable for the utilization of its structural features.

We have been developing the simple and highly useful strategies for conjugation between DNA and vinyl polymers, which are known to have a wide variety of features and functions. We synthesized poly(N-isopropylacrylamide) (NIPAAm) carrying dsDNA [1]. This water-soluble conjugate was found to form precipitate at temperatures over $31°C$ and was easily collected by centrifugation. In this process, DNA-binding molecules and macromolecules present in the system accompany the conjugate in becoming separated from the solution. Thus the conjugate is useful for separating DNA-binding proteins. We also prepared a polyAAm hydrogel that immobilized a large amount of dsDNA [2]. The gel was found to adsorb DNA-binding drugs effectively, so it should be useful for preconcentration and determination of such drugs as well as of some other mutagens and carcinogens.

On the other hand, a conjugate between ssDNA and polyNIPAAm is useful for gene diagnosis, since it forms precipitates, being accompanied with its complementary ssDNA in a sample solution [3]. A soluble conjugate between ssDNA and polyAAm was also prepared. This conjugate was successfully applied for gene mutation assay using capillary electrophoresis [4]. In this chapter, we describe some examples of our DNA conjugates.

II. dsDNA–VINYL POLYMER CONJUGATE

A. Conjugation Methods

In order to develop a widely useful conjugation method, DNA-selective modification reagents are needed. As an easy approach to incorporate dsDNA into the vinyl polymer, we adopted DNA-binding vinyl monomers 1, 2, and 3 [5–7]. Our strategy is to immobilize these monomers on DNA and to make the DNA "polymerizable": The result is the "DNA macromonomer," which displays multiple polymerizable groups. Radical copolymerization of the "DNA macromonomer" and vinyl monomers, such as acrylamide and N-isopropylacrylamide, results in the polymer's grafting onto the DNA (Fig. 1).

We studied the effect of these monomers on the melting temperature (Tm) of dsDNA. We found that 1 showed the largest contribution to the increase of Tm, probably due to the strongest binding among the three (1, +13.8; 2, +4.9;

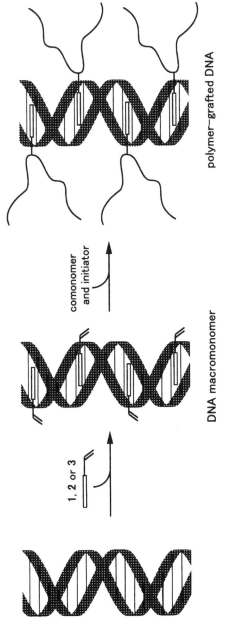

Figure 1 Conjugation of vinyl polymers with dsDNA using DNA-binding monomers (1–3) and DNA binding polymers (4).

Figure 1 Continued.

3, +10.0). However, 1 could be detached from the DNA via the addition of NaCl and/or ethidium bromide [6] or upon gel electrophoresis [8]. On the other hand, psoralen-containing monomers (2 and 3) eventually cross-linked dsDNA covalently after the UV irradiation and showed no sign of dissociation. For the preparation of stable conjugates, monomers 2 and 3 would be preferable. Monomer 3 binds more strongly than 2 because it contains two cationic charges on its spacer, while 2 has only one.

Copolymerization of vinyl monomers and DNA macromonomers can be monitored via gel electrophoresis: We observed retarded migration of the DNA, which is due to the fattening of the DNA caused by the polymer grafting. The extent of the polymer introduction turned out to be dependent on the number of monomers immobilized on the DNA before the copolymerization.

However, this approach contains several fundamental problems for the construction of the graft copolymer between DNA and vinyl polymers.

1. There would remain a considerable number of vinyl groups that had been photochemically immobilized on DNA strands but failed to participate in the subsequent polymerization reaction. This fact prevents us from preparing well-defined polymer-grafted DNA.
2. Polymer chain is introduced via random copolymerization between DNA macromonomer and vinyl monomer in a bulk. There would be a considerable distribution in the architecture of the graft chains as well as in their molecular weight. This is also undesirable for preparing the conjugates' well-characterized and well-defined structure.
3. The DNA-macromonomer itself may act as cross-linking agent because multiple vinyl groups are introduced on a DNA strand. Copolymerization might result in the formation of an intermolecular or intramolecular network. This is not preferred for the preparation of the soluble conjugate.

As an alternative method, we recently developed a much easier method for grafting the polymer onto dsDNA [1]. We have synthesized a semitelechelic oligomer of NIPAAm (4, $n = 50$) having a psoralen moiety on its end. This polymer was prepared via the coupling between an amino derivative of psoralen and an activated carboxyl end group on the oligomer of NIPAAm. The conjugation process is very simple: 4 is added to DNA, followed by UV irradiation.

B. Temperature-Sensitive DNA Conjugate

PolyNIPAAm is known as a temperature-responsive polymer that precipitates by heating to over 31°C. The conjugates between DNA and polyNIPAAm prepared in the aforementioned procedures were all found to be temperature responsive. In addition, upon heating, these polymers turned out to capture, coprecipitate with, and separate the DNA-binding molecules from the aqueous solution. This system was applied to the separation of DNA-binding dyes [9], DNA fragments [10], and DNA-binding proteins [1] in successful ways (Fig. 2).

C. Protein Imprinting at Polymer Modification

We have observed that the dense introduction of polymers almost entirely shuts out the access of DNA-binding proteins to the trunk DNA of the conjugate. In this situation, DNA is practically "coated" by the polymer. We have developed the protein-imprinting or -masking technique to modify the binding selectivity of DNA as the host molecule [11]. A brief protocol is as follows. Site-specific DNA-binding protein was added to DNA to form a complex. Then polymer 4 was added and the mixture irradiated with UV light. The protein protects its binding site from polymer modification, and the resulting conjugate has the "uncoated" site that retains the binding affinity. Other parts were coated to be "inaccessible" domains. This strategy allows us to enhance the binding selectivity of a certain DNA, and we can obtain materials with the desired affinity to a certain molecule even if its binding site is unknown.

III. ssDNA VINYL POLYMER CONJUGATES

A. Preparation of Reagents Carrying ssDNA

The DNA conjugates just described are all those with dsDNA. We also prepared conjugates between ssDNA and vinyl polymers. Polymers carrying ssDNA were easily prepared via radical copolymerization of vinyl monomer with vinyl derivative of oligonucleotide [3,4].

The vinyl derivative of oligonucleotides (5) was synthesized by the coupling of 5'-aminohexyl-(dT)$_{12}$ with methacryloyloxy succinimide. 5 (0.13 mM) and AAm (450 mM) were copolymerized in water at 25°C for 2 h using ammonium persulfate (2.9 mM) and N,N,N',N'-tetramethylethylenediamine (5.8 mM) as a redox initiator couple under nitrogen atmosphere to give a polyAAm–DNA conjugate (6) with the structure illustrated in Figure 3. The conversions of 5 and AAm were determined by HPLC to be 73% and 66 %, respectively, indicating that the amount of (dT)$_{12}$ incorporated in the resulting copolymer is 0.03 mol% as the ratio of 5 to AAm unit. Free-zone capillary electrophoresis of the resulting DNA-carrying polymer (6) indicated that 6 behaved similarly to neutral (nonionic) polyAAm in terms of migration rate. In other words, 5 does not migrate substantially by electrophoresis if the electro-osmotic flow is fully suppressed.

Thus the conjugate was substantially referred to as affinity stationary phase in capillary electrophoresis, since its electrophoretic mobility was largely

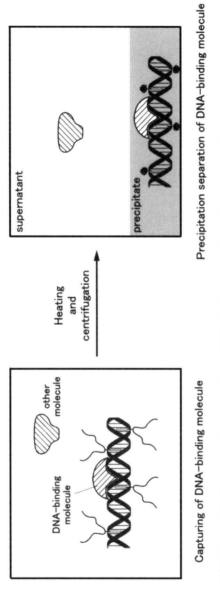

Figure 2 Affinity precipitation separation of DNA-binding molecules and macromolecules.

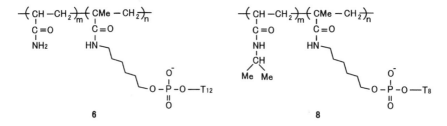

Figure 3 Chemical structures of ssDNA–vinyl polymer conjugates.

reduced due to the anchoring effect by nonionic polymer chains. The oligonucle-otide-immobilized capillary was successfully applied to the separation of c-K-ras and its one-point mismatched mutant (oncogene) as described later.

B. Affinity Capillary Electrophoresis

Affinity capillary electrophoresis is a useful method for the separation of sub-stances that participate in specific interactions. DNA analysis has been an im-portant subject of affinity capillary electrophoresis. An introduction of affinity mode into the separation mode of DNAs in capillary electrophoresis would make possible their sequence-dependent separations, whereas conventional cap-illary gel electrophoresis allows only the chain length-based separation by mo-lecular-sieving mode. In the design of affinity capillary electrophoresis, the af-finity ligand should be a ssDNA complementary to the target sequence. However, the ssDNA has to be immobilized in a capillary; otherwise, the analytes, the affinity ligand, and their complexes would migrate with the same mobility.

Recently, Baba et al. accomplished affinity capillary electrophoresis using poly(9-vinyladenine), which was immobilized into polyacrylamide gel as an af-finity ligand, to separate some DNA sequence isomers containing A and T bases [12]. We previously reported an affinity capillary electrophoresis, in which oli-gonucleotide was immobilized onto capillary inner surface, as a more versatile system for the DNA sequence-dependent separation [13].

On the other hand, polyAAm carrying oligonucleotide can serve as a pseudo-immobilized affinity ligand for more successful and sophisticated sepa-ration of DNAs based on their sequences. A capillary filled with the DNA–vinyl polymer conjugate would be promising for gene analysis recognizing the DNA base sequence.

The capillary was precoated with linear polyAAm. The resulting capillary was filled with 6 by introducing the polymerization mixture in 25-cm lengths from the cathodic end, and the rest of the capillary was filled with 3.4% poly-

AAm. Electrophoresis of sample oligonucleotides was performed using this capillary in the presence of MgCl2 with various concentrations in 5 mM tris-borate buffer (pH 7.4). Sample solution was introduced into the capillary at the cathodic side by positive pressure.

Figure 4 shows electropherograms on the separation of two oligonucleotides that have the same chain length. In the experiments, oligonucleotides examined were $(dA)_{12}$, $(dA)_6(dT)(dA)_5$, and $(dA)_8(dT)(dA)_3$. $(dA)_{12}$ is the perfect match sequence to the affinity ligand $(dT)_{12}$, while $(dA)_6(dT)(dA)_5$ and $(dA)_8(dT)$ $(dA)_3$ have one mismatched base but the mismatch position is different in each. We added Mg^{2+} in order to enhance the ligand–analyte interaction, since Mg^{2+} is known to stabilize the double-stranded form of DNA due to the reduction of an electrostatic repulsion between the two DNA strands. In Mg^{2+}-free buffer, two components could not be separated on either polyAAm-or 6-loaded capillaries. However, an increase in the concentration of Mg^{2+} ion improved the separation of the two peaks effectively. The peaks became completely separated when concentrations of Mg^{2+} were 75 µM for $(dA)_{12}$ and $(dA)_6(dT)(dA)_5$, as shown in Fig. 4(a), and 1mM for $(dA)_6(dT)(dA)_5$ and $(dA)_8(dT)(dA)_3$ in Figure 4(b). On

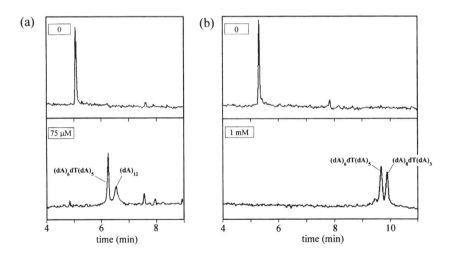

Figure 4 Effect of Mg^{2+} concentration on the separation of $(dA)_{12}$ and $(dA)_6(dT)(dA)_5$ (a) and of $(dA)_6(dT)(dA)_5$ and $(dA)_8(dT)(dA)_3$ (b) in the presence of the $(dT)12$-carrying polyAAm (**6**). Mg^{2+} concentrations were 0 and 75µM for (a) and 0 and 1mM for (b). A mixture of two oligonucleotides was introduced into the affinity capillary (effective length 38 cm) with positive pressure, and was charged at 15 kV in the presence or absence of Mg^{2+} at 25°C using 5 mM tris-borate (pH 7.4) as working solution.

the other hand, electropherograms using the capillary filled with polyAAm showed only a single peak for both cases, even though Mg^{2+} was added.

In Figure 4(b), $(dA)_8(dT)(dA)_3$, which has a longer consecutive sequence of dA, showed a larger retardation than did $(dA)_6(dT)(dA)_5$. This means that the degree of peak retardation has a good correlation with the stability of the duplex between each analyte and the affinity ligand. Thus the affinity capillary electrophoresis using oligonucleotide as affinity ligand worked successfully. Mg^{2+} concentration was found to be a convenient factor to control the strength of interaction between sample DNA and the pseudo-immobilized ligand.

In order to evaluate the potential of this affinity capillary electrophoresis for gene mutation assay, we applied this system to an analysis of K-ras sequence and its one base mutant on the codon 12 that is one of the major origins of cancer. Figure 5 shows electropherograms of the mixture of both sequences. In this experiment, polyAAm carrying an antisense sequence of c-K-ras codon 11–12 (i.e., 5'-ACCAGC-3') was employed as a pseudo-immobilized ligand. The normal c-K-ras codon 10–13 (5'-GGAGCTGGTGGC-3'), which is the

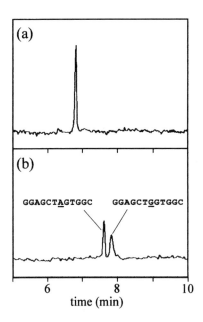

Figure 5 Separation of c-K-ras codon 10–13 (5'-GGAGCTGGTGGC-3') and its single base mutant (5'-GGAGCTAGTGGC-3') using a conventional polyAAm gel capillary (a) and that filled with (5'-ACCAGC-3')-carrying polyAAm (b). Mg^{2+} concentration was 150 µM. Other experimental conditions were the same as those in Figure 4.

complementary partner of the affinity ligand, was successfully separated from its single base mutant (5'-GGAGCTAGTGGC-3') in the presence of Mg^{2+} at a concentration of 150 μM using the affinity capillary [Fig. 5(b)], whereas an ordinary polyAAm gel capillary could not separate those isomers at all in the same conditions [Fig.5(a)]. The novel approach of the affinity capillary electrophoresis using oligonucleotide and Mg^{2+} can offer a powerful tool for gene analysis.

C. Affinity Precipitation

We also prepared a conjugate between ssDNA and thermoresponsive polyNIPAAm. The conjugate was demonstrated to distinguish its target (complementary) sequence from mismatch DNAs and to separate it from aqueous solution when heated. This conjugate hybridizes with the target sequence in homogeneous solution, and precipitates with the target with the slight change in solution temperature.

Vinyl derivative of $(dT)_8$ (7) was synthesized by the coupling of 5'-amino-terminated $(dT)_8$ with methacryloyloxysuccinimide. 7 (75 μM) and NIPAAm (150 mM) was copolymerized at 20°C using ammonium persulfate and N,N,N',N'-tetramethylethylenediamine as a redox initiator couple in nitrogen atmosphere to give polyNIPAAm-$(dT)_8$ conjugate (8) with a structure illustrated in Figure 3. Conversions of 7 and NIPAAm were determined to be 71% and 75%, respectively, indicating that the amount of $(dT)_8$ incorporated in the resulting copolymer is almost the same as the feed ratio of 1 to NIPAAm (0.05 mol%) at the polymerization step.

The resultant conjugate between polyNIPAAm and $(dT)_8$ was applied to the one-pot separation of its complementary sequence $(dA)_8$. The conjugate (0.45 w/v%; 20 μM of $(dT)_8$ in strand) was mixed with the target DNA (($dT)_8$; 10μM in strand). Then 1 w/v% of polyNIPAAm was added to the mixture because we found that a certain concentration (>1 w/v%) of homopolymer was required for the reproducible precipitation of polyNIPAAm-$(dT)_8$ conjugate. The concentration of NaCl and $MgCl_2$ was adjusted to be 1.5 M and 0.1 M, respectively.

As a result, 84% of $(dA)_8$ in the system was concentrated into the precipitate fraction in the presence of conjugate. On the other hand, only a small amount of $(dA)_8$ (ca. 6%) was distributed to the precipitate when the separation experiment was performed in the absence of the conjugate. The precipitation % of $(dT)_8$ did not depend on the presence of the conjugate, being a small value of ca. 5%.

The applicability of this separation system was further examined for the mixture of $(dA)_8$ and its one-point mutant $(dA)_3 dT(dA)_4$ (10 μM each). As a result, $84.0 \pm 1.4\%$ ($n = 3$) of $(dA)_8$ was concentrated into the precipitate by the procedure, while $91.7 \pm 0.8\%$ ($n = 3$) of $(dA)_3 \, dT(dA)_4$ remained in the supernatant. This result clearly indicates that the polyNIPAAm–$(dT)_8$ conjugate distinguished $(dA)_8$ from $(dA)_3 \, dT(dA)_4$ and isolated the complementary DNA selectively from the aqueous solution. In fact, 99% of the precipitated $(dA)8$ was recovered when the precipitate was resuspended in deionized water and centrifuged at 40%.

IV. CONCLUSION

A viable and widely applicable conjugation method for DNA is very important for developing new materials with unique functions. The methods described here would contribute to various fields of life science where molecular recognition events of DNA are dealt with.

REFERENCES

1. D. Umeno, M. Kawasaki, M. Maeda. Bioconjugate Chem. 9:719–724 (1998).
2. D. Umeno, T. Kano, M. Maeda. Anal. Chim. Acta 365:101–108 (1998).
3. D. Umeno, T. Mori, M. Maeda. Chem. Commun. 1433–1434 (1998).
4. Y. Ozaki, T. Ihara, Y. Katayama, M. Maeda. Nucleic Acids Symp. Ser. 37:235–236 (1997).
5. M. Maeda, D. Nishimura, D. Umeno, M. Takagi. Bioconjugate Chem. 5:527–531 (1994).
6. M. Maeda, A. Hirai, M. Takagi. Reactive Polym. 15:103–109 (1991).
7. M. Maeda, D. Umeno, C. Nishimura, M. Takagi. ACS Symp. Ser. 627:197–208 (1996).
8. K. Minagawa, Y Matsuzawa, K. Yoshikawa, Y. Masubuchi, M. Matsumoto, M. Doi, C. Nishimura, M. Maeda. Nucleic Acids Res. 21:37–40 (1993).
9. D. Umeno, M. Maeda. Anal. Sci. 13:553–556 (1997).
10. D. Umeno, M. Maeda. Chem. Lett. 381–382 (1999).
11. D. Umeno, M. Maeda. Supramol. Sci. 5:427–431 (1998).
12. Y. Baba, M. Tsuhako, T. Sawa, M. Akashi, E. Yashima. Anal. Chem. 64:1920–1924 (1992).
13. Y. Ozaki, Y. Katayama, T. Ihara, M. Maeda. Anal. Sci. 15:389–392 (1999).

12
Electrochemical Gene Sensors

Toshihiro Ihara
Kumamoto University, Kumamoto, Japan

Masamichi Nakayama, Koji Nakano, and Mizuo Maeda
Kyushu University, Fukuoka, Japan

I. INTRODUCTION

Recent progress in molecular biology has revealed that some disorders correlate directly with gene expression, so we may link some diseases to their responsible specific genes. For medical application, the benefit of such knowledge is immeasurable; for example, specific gene detection permits gene therapy and diagnosis for several hereditary, infectious, and neoplastic diseases (Baba, 1996; Epplen et al., 1995).

The most commonly used assay for certain disease-responsible genes takes advantage of hybridization of a probe DNA that is usually a complementary oligodeoxynucleotide (ODN) with radioactive label such as ^{32}P (Keller and Manak, 1989). Radioactive isotopes are widely used as labels because of their high detection sensitivity. Due to their hazardous nature and short shelf life, several alternative nonradioactive labeling methods (e.g., colorimetric detection conjugated with signal amplification using enzymatic reaction) have also been developed (Benotmane et al., 1997). Most of these methods, however, involve the fixation of DNA sample on a membrane and the following hybridization with a probe. Both procedures are time consuming and tedious. Therefore, a novel method that is quick and convenient and does not rely on radioisotopes is eagerly hoped for (Elghanian et al., 1997; Ihara et al., 1998; Nelson et al., 1996).

Electrochemical technique is potentially sensitive and versatile. DNA is, however, redoxinactive under ordinary conditions. Therefore, a method of labeling DNA for electrochemical detection needs to be developed (Takenaka et al., 1990; Takenaka et al., 1997). We have already proposed methods for the electrochemical detection of DNA by using ferrocene-modified ODN as a probe, in which femtomolar detection of the target was attainable on HPLC equipped with an electrochemical detector (Takenaka et al., 1994).

In this chapter, we have developed a gene sensor for detecting specific gene. ODN-modified Au electrode and ferrocene-ODN conjugate (Scheme 1) were used as the sensor tip and the probe, respectively (Ihara et al., 1997). Schematic illustration of the principle of the gene sensor is shown in Figure 1. Single-stranded ODN, which is complementary to the target, is immobilized onto the gold electrode. This electrode was used as a sensor tip. The sequence of the probe used here is also complementary to another site on the target. Therefore, sandwich-type ternary complex should form on the electrode surface when the target is present. The number of the ferrocene units concentrated on the sensor tip should be proportional to that of the target in the sample solution. On the other hand, if the added DNA is not the target or has a point mutation, such complex does not effectively form on the tip. Thus, one should be able to differentiate the target from the mutant by monitoring the magnitude of the current.

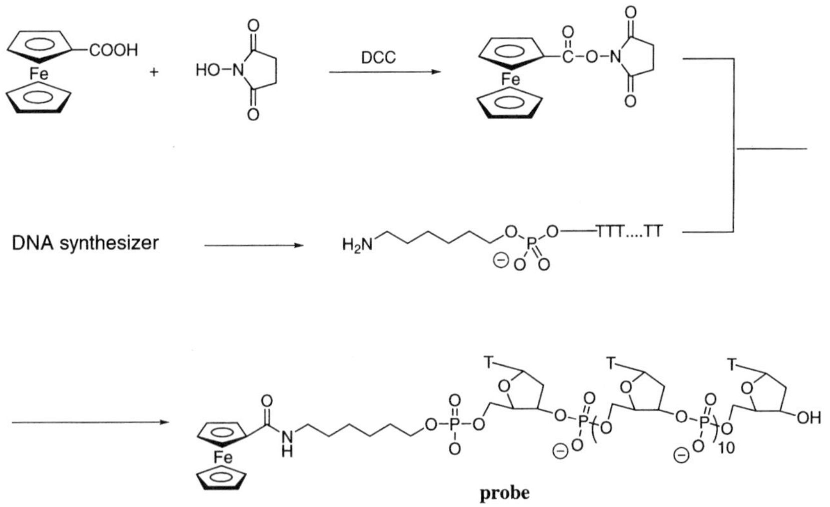

Scheme 1   Synthesis and structure of the probe.

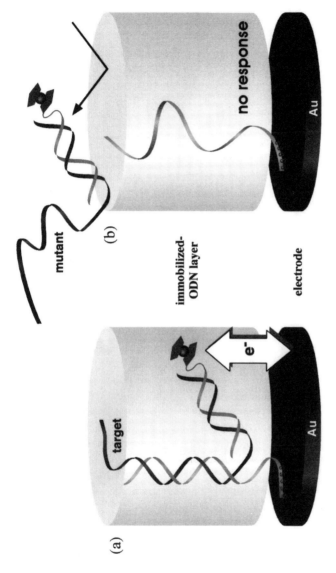

Figure 1 Schematic illustration of the electrochemical gene-sensing system based on the formation of complementary sandwich-type complex. (a) Target DNA combines the ferrocenyl ODN (probe) with the immobilized-ODN on the electrode. The oxidation current due to the concentrated ferrocenyl units should reflect the concentration of the target. (b) Ferrocenyl units are not concentrated onto the electrode in the presence of nontarget DNA.

II. MATERIALS AND METHODS

A. Materials

All dimethoxytrityl nucleoside phosphoramidites, Beaucage's reagent, and support resins for automated DNA synthesis were purchased from Glen Research Co. or Beckman Co. All other reagents used in this study were of the highest grade commercially available and used without further purification. Electrodes used for electrochemical study were purchased from BAS Co.

B. Preparation of ODNs

ODNs used in this study were prepared on a fully automated DNA synthesizer (Beckman, Oligo 1000). Synthesized oligodeoxynucleotides are as indicated here:

> probe: Fc-TTTTTTTTTTTT
> e16S: TsTsTsTsTsTCTCATACATG
> e16:   TTTTTCTCATACATG
> t19:   CATGTATAAAAAAAAAAAA
> m19:   CATCTATAAAAAAAAAAAA

"s" stands for phosphorothioester bond

A standard dimethoxytrityl nucleoside phosphoramidite coupling method was used on a 1.0 μmol CPG support column. For the synthesis of e16S, Beaucage's reagent was used to sulphurate successive 5-phosphate bonds from the 5'-end of the ODN; sulphurating was accomplished by the reagent on the oxidation steps in usual ODN synthesis (Iyer et al., 1990). Liberation from the resin and the following purification and deprotection were carried out according to the procedure descried previously (Ihara et al., 1996). All isolated ODNs were confirmed for their homogeneity by RP-HPLC analysis and were stored at −20°C after evaporation. The concentration of single-stranded ODNs was calculated using molar extinction coefficients at 260 nm derived from a nearest-neighbor model (Cantor et al., 1970).

C. Preparation of Ferrocenyl ODNs

The synthesis and purification were carried out according to the method previously reported (Scheme) (Ihara et al., 1996; Takenaka et al., 1994).

D. Hybridization

Aqueous solution [containing 100 mM KCl, 5 mM Tris-HCl (pH 8.0)] of equimolar mixture of probe and t19, and that of probe and m19 (50μM each) were kept at 90°C for 10 min. Then the solutions were allowed to cool gradually for annealing and stored at 5°C as a stock sample solution (Sambrook et al., 1989).

E. ODN Modification onto Au Electrode

A well-polished Au electrode (1.6 φ disk) was used for the sensor tip. Ten microliters of 50 μM aqueous solution (containing 100 mM KCl) of e16S was cast onto the electrode. After evaporation, the electrode was washed thoroughly with 100 mM KCl solution. Then this electrode was used as a sensor tip. Anchoring of the ODN onto the electrode was confirmed by cyclic voltammetry.

F. Differential Pulse Voltammetry

For detecting the target, the sensor tip was immersed in 30 μL of stock sample solution at 5°C for 24 h. Then the tip was rinsed with 100 mM KCl solution at 5°C for washing away the nonspecific binding. Differential pulse voltammetry (DPV) was carried out using a BAS CV-50-W voltammetry analyzer with a conventional design of a three-electrode system. The water jacket of the cell was maintained at 5°C throughout the measurement. The sensor tip, a Pt plate, and a standard Ag/AgCl (saturated KCl) electrode were used as working, counter, and reference electrode, respectively. The measurements were carried out in 100 mM KCl solution under the following conditions: pulse amplitude, 50 mV; pulse width, 50 msec; pulse period, 200 msec; rate, 25 mV sec^{-1}; temperature, 5°C.

G. Cyclic Voltammetry

1. Characterization of the Sensor Tip

To confirm the ODN modification, cyclic voltammetric measurements (CVs) with the electrode were carried out before and after the procedure of ODN modification in the presence of 10 mM ferrocyanide/ferricyanide redox couple as the marker ions (Katayama et al., 1998; Maeda et al., 1992).

2. Quantification of the Probe on the Sensor Tip

After the formation of ternary complexes on the sensor tip, the number of ferrocene units was estimated from the peak area of CV according to the procedure previously reported (Bard and Faulkner, 1980).

Both measurements were carried out in 100 mM KCl solution using the same three-electrode system as used for DPV measurements, under the following conditions: scan rate, 25 mV sec^{-1}; temperature, 25°C (characterization of the sensor tip) and 5°C (quantification of the probe).

III. RESULTS

A. Electrode Modification

In this study, phosphorothioate bonds were used as anchors to the Au electrode. Although the thiol group can be introduced onto the terminus of ODN using amidite reagent, that has thiol, this reagent is very expensive. On the other hand, phosphorothioate bonds are easily introduced into the synthetic DNA by use of Beaucage's reagent in the oxidation step of ODN synthesis (Iyer et al., 1990). Successive 5-phosphorothioates were introduced, because the affinity of a phosphorothioate group to Au may be weaker than that of a thiol (Fidanza et al., 1992; Fidanza and McLaughlin, 1989).

Cyclic voltammograms of ferrocyanide/ferricyanide redox coupled with the ODN-modified electrode (sensor tip) and an unmodified one are indicated in Figure 2. While the electrode treated by e16, which does not have any sulphur

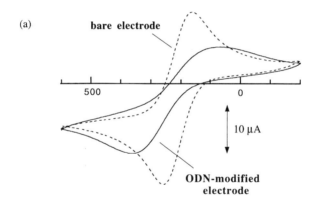

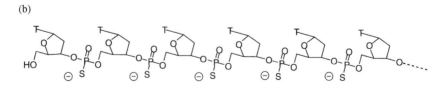

Figure 2 Cyclic voltammograms of the bare (_ _ _ _) and the ODN-modified (_____) Au electrodes at 25°C (a) and the structure of phosphorothioated ODN (5′-terminus of e16S) (b). The measurements were carried out in aqueous solution containing 100 mM KCl and 5 mM $K_4[Fe(CN)_6]$ and $K_3[Fe(CN)_6]$. CE: Pt plate, RE: Ag/AgCl, scan rate: 25 mV/sec.

atoms, gave the same voltammogram as the bare electrode, the peak current obtained by e16S-modified electrode was significantly suppressed. This indicated that the redox couple was excluded from the electrode surface due to the electrostatic repulsion between the anionic redox couple and the ODN polyanion anchoring on the electrode. The heat treatment of the e16S-modified electrode at 80°C for 30 min in water did not make any difference in the voltammogram. It is likely that the multipod anchoring by phosphorothioates should encourage a stable immobilization of DNA on Au electrode. This newly developed method would be widely useful for fixation of synthetic DNA onto electrode.

B. Gene Detection

Figure 3 shows the differential pulse voltammograms for t19 and m19. A significant anodic peak due to the oxidation of ferrocene moiety was observed for t19. it seemed that the expected ternary complex (Fig. 1) formed on the electrode surface. On the other hand, only a slight peak was observed for an m19,

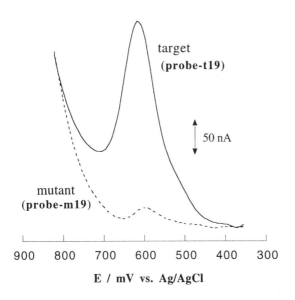

Figure 3 Differential pulse voltammograms of the tip treated by probe-t19 (target) (_____) and that treated by probe-m19 (mutant) (_ _ _ _). The ODN electrode was sensitive only for the target, t19. The measurements were carried out in 100 mM KCl solution at 5°C. CE: Pt plate; RE: Ag/AgCl; pulse period: 200 msec; scan rate: 25 mV sec^{-1}; pulse amplitude: 50 mV; pulse width: 50 msec.

mismatch 19-mer. By using our gene-sensing system, one can easily discern only one base substitution among 19 bases as a significant difference in magnitude of anodic current.

In the previous study, the redox current of the probe in homogeneous solution was observed at about 400 mV vs. Ag/AgCl reference electrode (Ihara et al., 1996). On the other hand, the redox potential observed on the sensor was about 600 mV. The potential was shifted to the positive side for as much as about 200 mV. Similar behavior was reported by R. L. Letsinger et al. for the electrode modified with ferrocene-mononucleotide conjugate (Mucic et al., 1996). Oxidation of ferrocene to ferrocenium cation requires the concomitant invasion of the counter anion into the DNA layer. This invasion seems to be difficult, due to highly dense anionic charges on the surface of the sensor tip. This effect should destabilize the oxidized state, so the redox potential is appreciably increased.

Slight current observed in the mismatch sample may be diminished by the optimization of the measurement conditions, such as the immersing period, temperature, salt concentration, and/or coexisting nonspecific binding blocker. The optimized conditions should lead to higher sensitivity. In fact, we have carried out a preliminary study on the detection limit of the gene sensor. In this

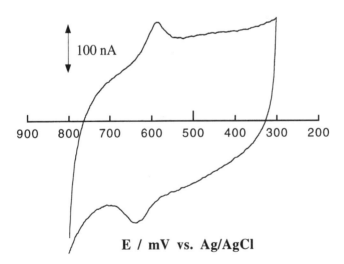

Figure 4 Cyclic voltammogram of the tip treated by probe-t19 (target). The measurements were carried out in 100 mM KCl solution at 5°C. Electrode surface coverage was calculated from the peak area. CE: Pt plate; RE: Ag/AgCl; scan rate: 25 mV sec^{-1}.

experiment, the anodic peak current observed here did not substantially decrease by diminishing the amount of the target to as little as 10^{-15} mol. This detection sensitivity seems to be sufficient for practical uses.

C.   Characterization of the Sensor Tip

Figure 4 shows a cyclic voltammogram of the sensor that was treated with probe-t19. From the peak area of this voltammogram, the density of ferrocene units concentrated on the electrode surface was estimated according to the

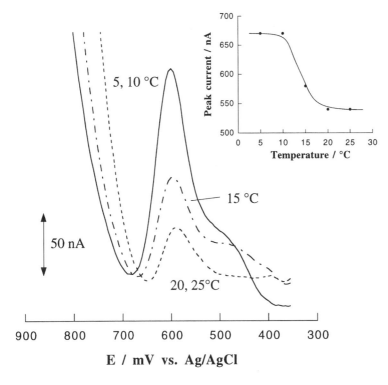

Figure 5   Temperature dependence of DPV of the tip treated by probe-t19 (target). All measurements were carried out 10 min after reaching the temperatures in 100 mM KCl solution. _____: 5, 10°C; — · —: 15°C; _ _ _ _: 20, 25°C; CE: Pt plate; RE: Ag/AgCl; pulse period: 200 msec; scan rate: 25 mV sec^{-1}; pulse amplitude: 50 mV; pulse width: 50 msec. *Inset*: Peak currents obtained by the DPVs were plotted against the measurement temperature.

method previously reported (Bard and Faulkner, 1980). It was revealed that 23–55 pmol of ferrocene exist per 1 cm^2 of the electrode surface. The coverage was almost the same as that reported by Kelley et al. (Kelley and Barton, 1997) It means that the area occupied by one ferrocene unit is the circle whose diameter is 20–30 Å. Since the diameter of the DNA helix is about 20 Å, ODNs seem densely packed. This provides the extreme anionic charge density on the electrode surface to give unusual shift of the redox potential observed here. However, one should take the roughness of electrode into consideration: Real density might be somewhat lower.

The effect of temperature on the anodic current of the voltammogram was studied. The results are shown in Figure 5. The peak for the target sample did not change at all by rinsing the electrode with aqueous KCl solution at 5 and 10°C. However, similar treatment at 20°C diminished the peak current appreciably. On the other hand, the slight current observed for m19 scarcely decreased by the same treatment (data not shown). These results indicate that the binding of the target was temperature sensitive. Such a property is the peculiar feature of DNA hybridization. That is, the observed interaction taking place on the electrode should be precise molecular recognition based on the Watson–Crick base-pairing, as expected.

For practical gene diagnosis, durability and reproducibility as the sensor are important properties. Figure 6 shows the possibility for repeated use of the sensor tip. Anodic response observed for the target was diminished appreciably by washing with aqueous KCl at 25°C. And rehybridization at 5°C completely restored the anodic peak of the voltammogram. This behavior clearly indicated the potential for repeated use of the tip as a practical sensor.

Comparing Figures 3, 5, and 6, the discrepancy is apparent in the magnitude of the response between the tips. This should be due to the difference in the gold surface conditions of the electrodes used as the basis of the sensor tips. A subtle irregularity in the procedure for immobilizing ODN may also account for it partly. This inequality in the performance between the tips remains to be eliminated.

Figure 6 The study for repeated use as the gene sensor. The sensor tip, which was treated by probe-t19 at 5°C (a) was washed with 100 mM KCl solution at 25°C (b) and rehybridized with probe-t19 at 5°C (c); DPV measurements were carried out at each step. CE: Pt plate; RE: Ag/AgCl; pulse period: 200 msec; scan rate: 25 mV sec^{-1}; pulse amplitude: 50 mV; pulse width: 50 msec.

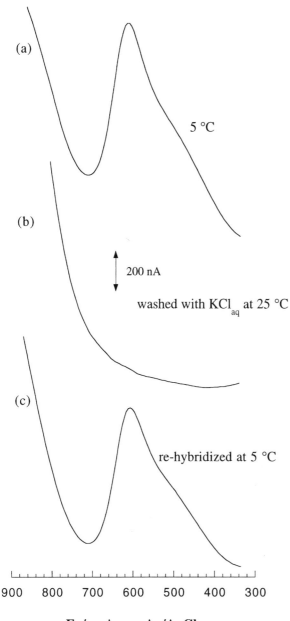

(a)

5 °C

(b)

200 nA

washed with KCl$_{aq}$ at 25 °C

(c)

re-hybridized at 5 °C

900   800   700   600   500   400   300

E / mA vs. Ag/AgCl

IV. DISCUSSION

So far, several gene sensors have been proposed by other groups (Hashimoto et al., 1994; Hashimoto et al., 1998; Kolakowski et al., 1996; Millan et al., 1994). The principle of these sensors is common, being summarized as follows: Single-stranded ODN that is complementary to the target is immobilized onto the electrode. If the single-stranded target is added to the solution where the electrode is immersed, double-stranded complex forms on the electrode surface. Then coexisting redox-active probes such as daunomycin and cobalt-polypiridine complex are concentrated onto the double-stranded DNA on the electrode surface. The electric current due to the probes should be relevant to the amount of the target. Although this method has generality, the detection limit should depend on the probe's preference for double-stranded DNA against single-stranded DNA. However, in general, the selectivity of probes is not so high. Binding of the probe to immobilized single-stranded ODN on the electrode causes background current, resulting in the limitation of the sensitive response to the target. That is, the probes have an intrinsic and unavoidable limit, depending on the preference.

On the other hand, the strategy described here is totally different from conventional gene sensors. The electrochemical response in our sensor is based on the hybridization between ODNs, which is highly specific and used in most of the usual methods for gene analysis. Therefore, the techniques of DNA hybridization have attained full growth; many tips and much know-how are available for improving the sensitivity. These assets from the study of probe hybridization should help us to brush up the system and to apply this sensor to practical samples that contain many contaminants.

When applying the sensor to gene diagnosis, we have to consider some points relating to practical demands. First is the versatility of our sensor toward the target. There is a possibility that the geometry or direction of the probe in the ternary complex may change the distance between the ferrocene unit and the electrode surface. The distance should affect the response in electric current. Thus one may worry that the length of the target would change the distance; a longer target makes the distance longer. However, the sequence targeted by the gene sensor is usually already known, at least for the wild type. Therefore, one can design the sequences of the probe and the immobilized ODN to be complementary to the adjacent sites in the target in order to bring the ferrocene unit near the electrode surface. In addition, we have shown in the previous study that the redox properties of the probe depend only slightly on the neighboring extra sequence with which the ferrocene moiety of the probe could be in contact (Ihara et al., 1996). Therefore, we can tune the sensing system, whose response does not depend on the length and the sequence of the target. Notwithstanding, the steric effect of the long target might remain even in our system. Steric hindrance may prevent the concentration of the target to some extent. As a result, the number of ferrocene units on the electrode should be decreased. Pretreatment of the sample by a certain exonuclease would suppress such an effect.

Another point is the time required for the measurement. We are now in the preliminary stage of studying the gene sensor. The measurement conditions described here are not optimized yet. We immersed the sensor tip in the sample solution for 24 hours to make doubly sure, although such a long period should not be required for attaining equilibrium, because the formation of double-stranded complex of DNA is quick. We can therefore shorten the measurement time according to the demands on practical use.

V. CONCLUSIONS

Electrochemical gene sensor has been developed using our ferrocene–ODN conjugate and anchoring the ODN on a gold electrode. The sensor allowed us to discriminate point mutation. We believe that the present gene-sensing method, which is quick and convenient and provides high detection sensitivity, is applicable to practical gene diagnosis.

ACKNOWLEDGMENTS

This work was partially supported by a Grant-in-Aid for Encouragement of Young Scientists (No. 08750941) and by a Grant-in-Aid for Scientific Research (B) (No. 09555266) from The Ministry of Education, Science, Sports, and Culture of Japan. The authors are also grateful to the Sagawa Foundation for Promotion of Frontier Science (T.I.) and to Terumo Life Science Foundation (M.M.).

REFERENCES

Baba, Y. (1996). Analysis of disease-causing genes DNA-based drugs by capillary electrophoresis. Towards DNA diagnosis and gene therapy for human diseases. J. Chromatography B: Biomed. Appli. 687:271.

Bard, A. J., Faulkner, L. R. (1980). Electrochemical methods: fundamentals and applications. Wiley, New York.

Benotmane, A. M., Hoylaerts, M. F., Collen, D., Belayew, A. (1997). Nonisotopic quantitative analysis of protein-DNA interactions at equilibrium. Anal. Biochem. 250: 181.

Cantor, C. R., Warshaw, M. M., Shapiro, H. (1970). Oligonucleotide interaction III.

Circular dichroism studies of the conformation of deoxyoligonucleotides. Biopolymers 9:1059.

Elghanian, R., Storhoff, J. J., Mucic, R. C., Letsinger, R. L., Mirkin, C. A. (1997). Selective colorimetric detection of polynucleotides based on the distance-dependent optical properties of gold nanospheres. Science 277:1078.

Epplen, J. T., Buitkamp, J., Epplen, C., Maueler, W., Riess, O. (1995). Indirect DNA/ gene diagnosis via electrophoresis—an obsolete principle? Electrophoresis 16:683.

Fidanza, J. A., McLaughlin, L. W. (1989). Introduction of reporter groups at specific sites in DNA containing phosphorothioate diesters. J. Am. Chem. Soc. 111:9117.

Fidanza, J. A., Ozaki, H., McLaughlin, L. W. (1992). Site-specific labeling of DNA sequence containing phosphorothioate diesters. J. Am. Chem. Soc. 114:5509.

Hashimoto, K., Ito, K., Ishimori, Y. (1994). Sequence-specific gene detection with a gold electrode modified with DNA probes and an electrochemically active dye. Anal. Chem. 66:3830.

Hashimoto, K., Ito, K., Ishimori, Y. (1998). Microfabricated disposable DNA sensor for detection of hepatitis B virus DNA. Sensors Actuators B, Chemical. 46:220.

Ihara, T., Maruo, Y., Takenaka, S., Takagi, M. (1996). Ferrocene-oligonucleotide conjugates for electrochemical probing of DNA. Nucleic Acids Res. 24:4273.

Ihara, T., Nakayama, M., Murata, M., Nakano, K., Maeda, M. (1997). Gene sensor using ferrocenyl oligonucleotide. J. Chem. Soc. Chem. Commun. 1609.

Ihara, T., Takata, J., Takagi, M. (1998). Novel method of detecting mismatch on DNA by using photo-induced electron transfer through DNA. Anal. Chim. Acta 365:49.

Iyer, R. P., Egan, W., Regan, J. B., Beaucage, S. L. (1990). 3H-1,2-Benzodithiol-3-one 1,1-dioxide as an improved sulfurizing reagent in the solid-phase synthesis of oligodeoxyribonucleoside phosphorothioates. J. Am. Chem. Soc. 112:1253.

Katayama, Y., Nakayama, M., Irie, H., Nakano, K., Maeda, M. (1998). Bioaffinity sensor to anti-DNA antibodies using DNA modified Au electrode. Chem. Lett. 1181.

Keller, G. H., Manak, M. M. (1989). DNA Probes. Stockton Press, New York.

Kelley, S. O., Barton, J. K. (1997). Electrochemistry of Methylene Blue bound to a DNA-modified electrode. Bioconjugate Chem. 8:31.

Kolakowski, B., Battaglini, F., Lee, Y. S., Klironomos, G., Mikkelsen, S. R. (1996). Comparison of an intercalating dye and an intercalant-enzyme conjugate for DNA detection in a microtiter-based assay. Anal. Chem. 68:1197.

Maeda, M., Mitsuhashi, Y., Nakano, K., Takagi, M. (1992). DNA-immobilized gold electrode for DNA-binding drug sensor. Anal. Sci. 8:83.

Millan, K. M., Saraullo, A., Mikkelsen, S. R. (1994). Voltammetric DNA biosensor for cystic fibrosis based on a modified carbon paste electrode. Anal. Chem. 66: 2943.

Mucic, R. C., Herrlein, M. K., Mirkin, C. A., Letsinger, R. L. (1996). Synthesis and characterization of DNA with ferrocenyl groups attached to their 5′-termini: electrochemical characterization of a redox-active nucleotide monomer, J. Chem. Soc., Chem. Commun. 555.

Nelson, N. C., Bencheikh, A., Matsuda, E., Becker, M. M. (1996). Simultaneous detection of multiple nucleic acid targets in a homogeneous format. Biochemistry 35: 8429.

Sambrook, J., Fritsch, E. F., Maniatis, T. (1989). Molecular Cloning: A Laboratory Manual. 2nd ed. Cold Spring Harbor Laboratory Press, New York.

Takenaka, S., Ihara, T., Takagi, M. (1990). Bis-9-acridinyl derivative containing a viologen linker chain: electrochemically active intercalator for reversible labelling of DNA. J. Chem. Soc. Chem. Commun. 1485.

Takenaka, S., Uto, Y., Kondo, H., Ihara, T., Takagi, M. (1994). Electrochemically active DNA probe: detection of target DNA sequence at femto mole level by high-performance liquid chromatography with electrochemical detection. Anal. Biochem. 218:436.

Takenaka, S., Sato, H., Ihara, T., Takagi, M. (1997). Synthesis and DNA binding properties of Bis-9-acridinyl derivatives containing mono-, di-, and tetra-viologen units as a connector of bis-intercalators. J. Heterocyclic Chem. 34:123.

13
Sensing of Second Messengers Using Oligopeptides

Yoshiki Katayama, Yuya Ohuchi, and Mizuo Maeda
Kyushu University, Fukuoka, Japan

Hideyoshi Higashi
Mitsubishi Kagaku Institute for Life Sciences, Tokyo, Japan

Yoshihisa Kudo
Tokyo University of Pharmacy and Life Science, Tokyo, Japan

I. INTRODUCTION

Living cells accept a wide variety of stimuli and can respond to them accurately via complex functions. Extracellular stimuli generally bind to their receptors on cellular membrane as chemical messenger molecules. Then other molecules, so-called *second messengers*, are introduced into intracellular space in many ways for processing information. These second messengers are recognized as key molecules that carry information in intracellular signal transduction systems. To understand how cellular information is processed, we need to see how much the second messengers are involved in living cells under various conditions. Among such second messengers, the calcium ion would be the most well understood one, because many methods [1–4], e.g., fluorescent probe [5–7], for monitoring its concentration and distribution have been developed. However, for many other organic second messengers, such as cyclic AMP (cAMP), cyclic GMP (cGMP), inositol-1,4,5-trisphosphate (IP3), cyclic ADP ribose, and alachidonic acid, convenient sensing techniques have not been established due to the difficulty of designing artificial ligands for the recognition of those second messengers. Thus, we need a novel concept to design selective ligands for such organic messengers.

In this chapter, we discuss a possible novel strategy for the design of synthetic ligands, which bind selectively to certain second messengers, and for constructing a sensing system for such messengers using cAMP as a target.

II. CONVENTIONAL METHODS FOR MONITORING CYCLIC AMP CONCENTRATION

Cyclic AMP (Fig. 1) is one of the most important second messengers in cellular signal transduction. Many hormones, cytokines, or neurotransmitters promote the cellular production of cAMP with the binding to their membrane receptors. The molecule regulates the wide variety of cellular functions, such as gene transcription [8], secretion [9], neuronal plasticity [10], and cellular proliferation [11], differentiation [12], and death [13], through an activation of cAMP-dependent protein kinase (protein kinase A) (Fig. 2). Disorders of cAMP production are also strongly related to many diseases [10]. Thus, the monitoring of cAMP concentration is really meaningful not only for the understanding of information processing in cells, but also for clinical applications or the validation of drugs in the pharmacological industry. In spite of such a strong need for the convenient sensing of cAMP, the most commonly used, and maybe the only practically used, technique for the cAMP assay is classical immunoassay using anti-cAMP antibody [14,15]. This methods can determine cAMP with high sensitivity (pmol level). However, this has not satisfied the potential but ardent needs in the fields just described, because the overall procedures are laborious and time consuming. Much more rapidity and ease is needed to satisfy the demands in the many fields using cAMP assay.

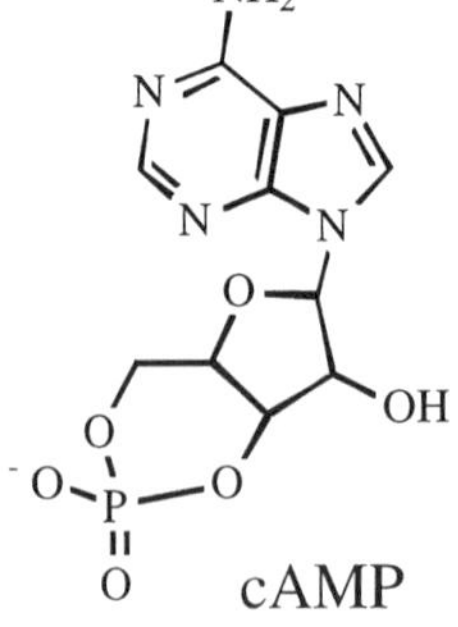

Figure 1 Structure of cyclic AMP (cAMP).

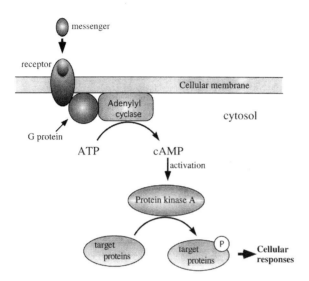

Figure 2 Cellular signal cascade participating cAMP. Binding of extracellular messengers to their receptors causes activation of adenylyl cyclase that locates just beneath the cellular membrane. Then, cyclic AMP (cAMP) is produced by the activated adenylyl cyclase from ATP. Generated cAMP binds to protein kinase A (cAMP dependent protein kinase) to activate.

Sensing systems using antibody, typically an ELISA, cannot avoid the steps separating the antibodies bound to the target from those unbound (B-F separation), because the signal that is labeled on the antibody intrinsically does not change with binding to the target molecules. This makes the system time consuming, because the method involves many washing steps. In this sense, other ligands recognizing cAMP will be needed for the development of an improved system of cAMP sensing. Probably the next easier way would be the use of biomolecules, which bind cAMP selectively, other than antibody. Tsien et al. used intracellular target protein of cAMP, protein kinase A, as another "recognizer" to design a more convenient monitoring of cAMP [16]. As shown in Figure 3, protein kinase A comprises two subunits, the regulatory (R) subunit and the catalytic (C) subunit. The kinase activity is in the C subunit. On the other hands, the R subunit acts as an inhibitor of the C subunit. cAMP binds to the two distinct sites on the R subunit. This leads to a global conformational change of the R subunit in which it dissociates from the C subunit, producing catalytic activity. Tsien et al. labeled each subunit with different fluorophores, for example, fluorescein and rhodamine. The system, which was named FICRhR, could be used as an intracellular fluorescent probe for cAMP, since

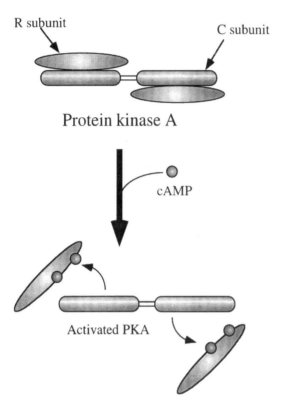

Figure 3 Activation mechanism of protein kinase A by cAMP. Protein kinase A comprises a regulatory subunit (R subunit) and a catalytic subunit (C subunit).

cAMP canceled the fluorescent energy transfer between the two labeled fluorophores due to the dissociation of both subunits [16]. FICRhR is potentially useful for cAMP sensing [17]. However, the reagent has to be injected into living cells with a micromanipulator because of the lack of membrane permeability of the reagent. The reagent also has some risk of fluctuating the orchestrated signal cascades in the cell, because it is physiologically active protein kinase A itself, which is the intracellular target of cAMP. For these reasons, FICRhR has still not fully satisfied the requirement in many research fields.

Kudo et al. used synthetic oligopeptide for the monitoring of protein kinase A activity [18]. The peptide was designed using an amino acid sequence of domain II, which is an autophosphorylation site of the R subunit of protein kinase A. This site is phosphorylated by protein kinase A highly selectively at the serine side chain. In the design of the probe substrate, three amino acids from the carboxy-terminus of the essential region of domain II were changed from CAE to AAC. Then the sulfhydryl group at the cystein residue of the C-terminus was labeled with fluorescent acrylodane. The resulting fluorescent substrate for protein kinase A, DLDVPIPGRFDRRVSVAAC-Acrylodane was called AR2 [18]. The wavelengths of maximum emission and excitation of AR2 were 520 and 360 nm, respectively. When the reagent was mixed with buffer solution containing ATP, cAMP, and protein kinase A, the fluorescence intensity at 520 nm decreased gradually with phosphorylation by the enzyme. The good correlation between the degree of phosphorylation and the fluorescence decline was confirmed by HPLC analysis. Thus, AR2 can monitor PKA activity, which reflects cAMP concentration indirectly, in buffer solution. However, this peptide could not permeate through cell membrane in many cell lines. To overcome this disadvantage, another part of the amino acid sequence of AR2, GRF, exchanged with the more hydrophobic AKA, and DACM (diethylaminocoumalin maleimide) was labeled instead of acrylodan. This reagent, DR2, penetrated spontaneously into the cell very well by simply incubating the reagent solution with cell sample, such as a primary culture of hyppocampal cells [18]. DR2 also decreased the fluorescent intensity at 520 nm with protein kinase A activation, if it was excited at 400 nm. This probe could monitor PKA activation in real time in cultured neuronal cells, which were pretreated with FK506 to inhibit calcinurin, a neuron-specific phosphatase. The strategy of using such fluorescent substrates is epoch-making in the point of imaging or continuous sensing of intracellular kinase activation. However, for cAMP sensing, the technique is indirect. A good ligand that recognizes cAMP directly with high selectivity is still needed for the development of an ideal method of cAMP sensing.

III. DESIGN OF AN OLIGOPEPTIDE RECOGNIZING CYCLIC AMP

We devised a novel approach to designing artificial ligands for organic messengers that have complicated chemical structures. We were at first planning to learn from a cellular system, since living cells use such messengers efficiently. Actually, living cells possess specific proteins for each messenger. Such proteins recognize every messenger selectively. Proteins generally recognize their target molecules with multiple subsites that are made from certain-length amino acid sequences. If there is a relatively long subsite that recognizes a major part of the guest molecule in a protein, the amino acid sequence of the subsite could be used as a candidate for the host molecule of the target molecule when it is cut out from the protein.

Via this strategy, we investigated amino acid sequences of cAMP-binding proteins and noticed a certain region that comprised a 16-amino-acid sequence in cAMP-dependent protein kinases [19]. Actually, the region had been demonstrated to bind to ribose and phosphate ester in cAMP molecule in an X-ray diffraction study [20]. This sequence in the protein originally forms a random structure and shifts to a loose helix with the binding to cAMP. The amino acid sequence in this region was also highly conserved among various subtypes of cAMP-binding protein kinases. Then the consensus amino acid sequence, FGEI ALVYNTPRAATV, was designed by comparing it with those first ordered structures in the region. Then cystein was introduced into the amino terminus as an anchor group to immobilize onto a gold surface. The peptide (RAA peptide) was easily synthesized on Fmoc chemistry using automatic peptide synthesizer, and purified with HPLC using reverse-phase C18 column [19].

IV. ELECTROCHEMICAL APPLICATION OF CYCLIC AMP–BINDING OLIGOPEPTIDE

As a first trial, we used the designed 17mer peptide to make the cAMP biosensor. Thus the peptide was immobilized onto the gold electrode surface via chemisorption using sulfhydryl group on cystein residue at the N-terminus. The modification of the electrode was accomplished by simple incubation of the electrode with the buffer solution (pH 7.4) containing the peptide (10 μM) at 5°C overnight [19]. For the electrochemical sensing of cAMP, a device is needed, because cAMP is not redox active. We decided to adopt the ion channeling mechanism strategy reported by Sugawara et al. [21]. The basic concept of cAMP sensing using the peptide-modified electrode is shown in Figure 4. Ferrocyanate/ferricyanate redox couple was added into the sample solution as a redox marker anion. In this system, cyclic voltammetry gives a reversible redox current according to the anionic marker ion. However, if monoanionic cAMP is recognized by the immobilized peptide, anionic charges would accumulate on the electrode surface, to suppress the electrochemical reaction of anionic redox marker. (Note that the net charge of the peptide should be zero at neutral pH.) Thus, cAMP should be able to be monitored with the depression of redox current in cyclic voltammetry. In fact, the redox current of the marker ion on the peptide-modified electrode responded to cAMP. Figure 5 shows cyclic voltammograms of ferrocyanide/ferricyanide anion using the peptide-modified electrode in the presence or absence of cAMP. One mM of cAMP dramatically suppressed the redox current of the anionic marker ion. Then the cAMP concentration dependence of the redox current was investigated. This current suppression was beautifully concentration dependent on added cAMP (Fig. 6). This demonstrated that the current depressions observed in Figures 5 and 6 were certainly caused by the presence of cAMP on the electrode surface. Using this system, cAMP could be determined by the decrease of redox peak current value with

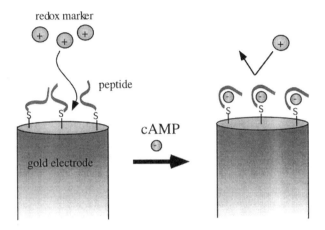

Figure 4 Basic concept of cAMP detection using an ion channeling mechanism. When monoanionic cAMP is captured by immobilized peptide (net charge is zero), the electrochemical reaction of anionic redox marker would be suppressed due to the electrostatic repulsion.

the detection limit of 1 μM. These results indicated that the effect of cAMP on the redox current is related to the interaction of cAMP and the electrode surface. However, in spite of such a clear response, it is still obscure whether the cAMP is interacting with something on the electrode other than the immobilized peptide. Thus, we synthesized a scrambled 17mer peptide, CFGAARLTVYPALN TEV, which has same amino acid composition but a different sequence, and immobilized it onto the gold electrode for an experiment similar to that in Figure 5. The redox current of the marker anion using the electrode, which was modified with the scrambled peptide, was not affected by the addition of 1mM cAMP. This clearly indicates that the response of cAMP to the redox current, which was shown in the experiments using the protein kinase A sequence peptide (RAA peptide) modified electrode, is actually due to the interaction of the designed peptide and the cAMP molecule.

For the next stage, a guest selectivity of the peptide was examined. Since there are many kinds of molecules whose chemical structure resembles cAMP in living cells, we estimated the electrochemical responses to the redox currents for many structural analogs of cAMP, such as cGMP, cCMP, cUMP, ATP, AMP, GTP, and GMP, (Fig. 7) using the electrode. These results demonstrated that the designed synthetic oligopeptide recognized cAMP with extremely high selectivity. Figure 7(a) shows the relation between the diminution of anodic peak current and cyclic nucleotide concentration. Any cyclic nucleotide, except

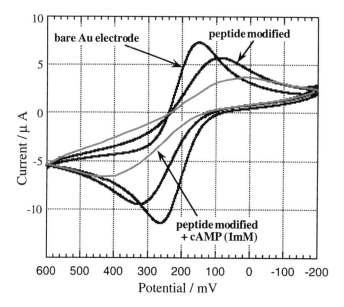

Figure 5 Cyclic voltammograms of ferrocyanide/ferricyanide redox couple (5 mM) with the Au electrode modified with the RAA peptide in the presence or absence of cAMP at 25°C. Scan rate, 25 mV·s⁻¹; [K₄[Fe(CN)₆]] = [K₃[Fe(CN)₆]] = 5 mM; [KCl] = 50 mM.

cAMP, practically did not suppress the redox current of anionic marker, indicating that the modified peptide did not recognize any cyclic nucleotides other than cAMP. These results are surprising because X-ray diffraction study showed that the corresponding amino acid sequence of the 17mer oligopeptide interacted with the cyclic phosphate diester and ribose ring of cAMP molecule in the protein kinase A [20]. On the other hand, nucleotides containing adenine base, ATP, or AMP showed slight responses, although no guanine nucleotides gave any response in the electrode system. It is not clear whether this response is caused by a molecular recognition of the peptide sequence or by other properties of the adenine moiety, such as polarity and hydrophobicity, which may affect the solubility of guest molecules in the peptide layer.

V. MOLECULAR BASIS OF THE CYCLIC AMP RECOGNITION WITH THE 17MER OLIGOPEPTIDE

The electrode modified with the 17mer peptide responded to cAMP with good selectivity. High selectivity to cAMP against other cyclic nucleotides is espe-

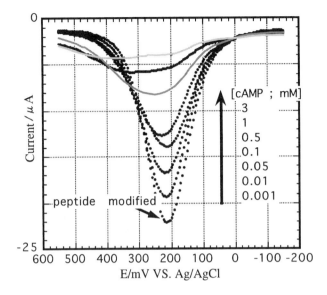

Figure 6 Differential pulse voltammograms of ferrocyanide/ferricyanide redox couple (10 mM) with the 17mer peptide-modified electrode in the presence of various concentrations of cyclic AMP at 25°C. Scan rate, 25 mV·s^{-1}; [K$_4$[Fe(CN)$_6$]] = [K$_3$[Fe(CN)$_6$]] = 5 mM; [KCl] = 50 mM.

cially noticeable, because cyclic GMP (cGMP), which has a very similar chemical structure to cAMP, is another important intracellular second messenger. cAMP should be distinguished from cGMP in any practical analysis. We investigated on a molecular basis how the relatively short peptide distinguished cAMP from cGMP with such high selectivity. In this regard, it would be worth seeing the mechanism of cAMP identification vs. cGMP in protein kinase A. Shabb and Corbin reported on this point in detail [22]. Although cAMP and cGMP are very similar molecules, their chemical properties are considerably different. In cGMP, an extra NH$_2$ group on the guanin ring can produce intramolecular hydrogen bonding with cyclic phosphodiester anion, in contrast to cAMP [Fig. 8(a)]. This interaction should depress intermolecular interaction between the anionic phosphate ester of cGMP and the arginine residue in the binding protein. In protein kinase A, the charge interaction between anionic cAMP and positive arginine residue in the cAMP-binding sequence actually plays an important role in cAMP recognition. Thus another trick is needed to establish the recognition of cGMP by the protein. Protein kinase G is the protein that binds to cGMP selectively. The first structure of the protein has rather high homology with

(a)

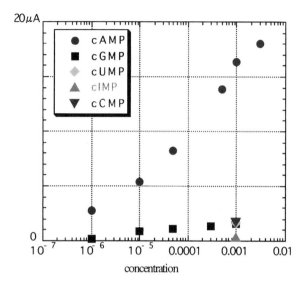

(b)

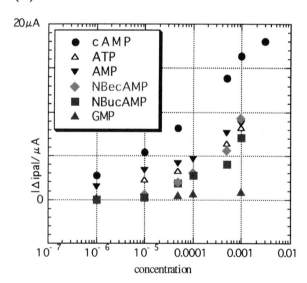

Figure 7   Changes in the anodic peak current (ipa) of ferrocyanide/ferricyanide redox couple on the differential pulse voltammetry using the Au electrode modified with the RAA peptide in the presence of various cyclic nucleotides (a) and various adenine or guanine nucleotides (b). Experimental conditions are the same as those in Figure 6.

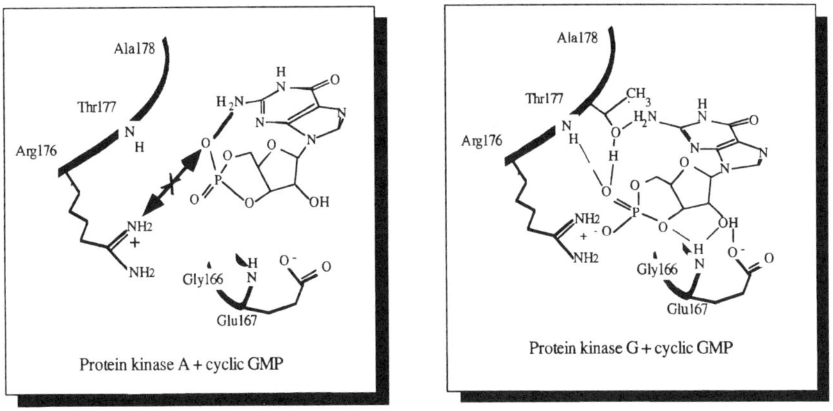

Figure 8 Chemical structures of cAMP and cGMP (a) and predicted protein-cyclic GMP contact for protein kinase A [left side of (b)] and protein kinase G [right side of (b)]. (From Ref. 24.)

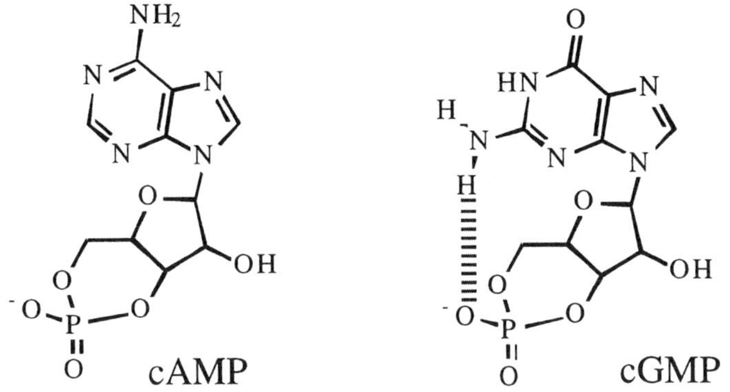

protein kinase A in the ligand binding domain [23]. However, the neighbor of positive arginine residue in the essential sequence of cyclic nucleotide binding is threonine in protein kinase G, instead of alanine in protein kinase A [Fig. 8(b)] [22]. Shabb et al. showed that threonine, which has a polar side chain, was essential for cGMP binding [24]. The side group of the threonine can extrude into the intramolecular hydrogen bonding in cGMP to destroy it in cGMP [Fig. 8(b)]. As a result, the anionic charge on the phosphate ester leaves it free for producing the charge interaction with the guanidinium portion of the arginine residue. They also showed that the mutation of Ala-334, which is in the neighboring position of arginine-335 in the cAMP-binding site of protein kinase A, to a threonine created a site with marked increase in cGMP affinity without changing cAMP affinity [24,25]. Thus, we synthesized 17mer peptide, CFGEIALVYNTPRTATV, (RTA peptide) in which alanine was exchanged to threonine (RAA → RTA) and also synthesized another 17mer peptide, CFGELAILYNSTRTASK, (PKG peptide) which has the sequence in protein kinase G corresponding to the RAA peptide sequence in protein kinase A. Figure 9 shows the effects of cAMP or cGMP on the redox currents of marker anion (ferrocyanide/ferricyanide redox couple) in each peptide-modified electrode. In the RAA peptide-modified electrode, cGMP did not affect the redox current of the marker anion practically. However, cGMP showed some electrochemical response in the RTA peptide-modified electrode, while the suppression of redox peak current by cAMP was similar to that in the RAA peptide-modified electrode. This indicates that the introduced threonine assisted cGMP binding to the modified peptide, as in the similar case of the protein kinase. The change of the selectivity to cGMP vs. cAMP was still smaller in the electrode than in the case of threonine-introduced mutant protein kinase A. This is probably because the oligopeptide on the electrode is exposed to water, weakening the hydrogen bonding between the threonine side arm and the guanine ring of cGMP, in contrast to the case of the protein kinase G, in which the threonine was located in a rather hydrophobic pocket. The PKG peptide-modified electrode also had a similar response in the presence of cGMP to the case of the RTA peptide-modified one. However, the response of cAMP was depressed compared with that in the RTA or RAA peptide-modified electrode. The difference in the amino acid sequence, other than threonine, between the RAA peptide and the PKG peptide may enhance the selectivity of cGMP against cAMP.

Above all, the results indicate that the mechanism for the guest recognition of each peptide, which was immobilized on the electrode, will be similar to that in the cyclic nucleotide–binding protein kinase.

VI. CONCLUSION

Second messengers are key molecules in the processing of cellular information. Thus, sensing them is very important, not only for understanding the intracellular signal transduction system but also for the diagnosis or validation of drug screening. However, the complicated structures of such messengers have obstructed the construction of convenient sensing systems, which need the selective ligands for those messengers, except for simple inorganic messengers like Ca^{2+}. We attempted to design an artificial ligand for cAMP, which is one of the most important second messengers, by learning from the molecular recognition

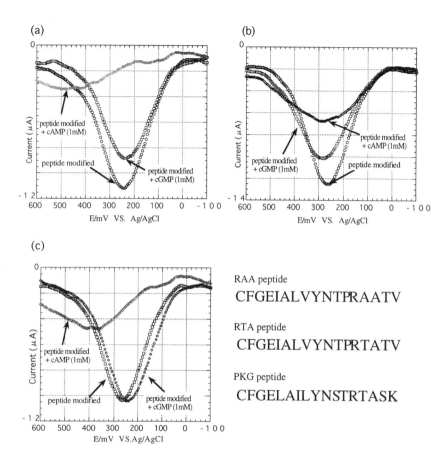

Figure 9 Differential pulse voltammograms of ferrocyanide/ferricyanide redox couple (5 mM) with the PKG peptide-modified electrode (a), RTA peptide-modified electrode (b), and RAA peptide-modified electrode (c) in the presence of cAMP or cGMP at 25°C. Experimental conditions are the same as those in Figure 6. Amino acid sequences of peptides used in these experiments are shown in the lower right.

of proteins and finally succeeded in the realization of a ligand selective for cAMP using a short peptide. The 17mer peptide, which was designed using essential subsites of the cAMP-binding domain in various cAMP-binding protein kinases families, retained the ability to recognize cAMP. Actually, a Au electrode that was modified with the peptide responded to cAMP with surprisingly high selectivity using an ion channel mechanism. Other studies using some related peptides suggested that the molecular mechanism of cAMP recognition is similar to that in protein kinase A.

The basic strategy we described here will be potentially useful for the design of artificial ligand to other second messengers. Living cells prepare various proteins for the recognition of each messenger. Thus, we will find valuable amino acid sequences for the ligand construction in their binding domain if adequate proteins are selected. Biosensor applications also may be suitable to the use of such peptide ligans in constructing sensing systems of second messengers, although further improvement will be required for the practical biosensor.

REFERENCES

1. Shortreed, M., Kopelman, R., Kuhn, M., Hoyland, B. (1996). Fluorescent fiber-optic calcium sensor for physiological measurements. Anal. Chem. 68(8):1414.
2. Blair, T. L., Yang, S. T., Smith-Palmer, T., Bachas, L. G. (1994). Fiber-optic sensor for Ca^{2+} based on an induced change in the conformation of the protein calmodulin. Anal. Chem. 66(2):300.
3. Takamatsu, T., Wier, W. G. (1990). High temporal resolution video imaging of intracellular calcium. Cell Calcium 11(2–3):111.
4. Tsien, R. Y., Rink, T. J. (1980). Neutral carrier ion-selective microelectrodes for measurement of intracellular free calcium. Biochim. Biophys. Acta 599(2):623.
5. Leybaert, L., Sneyd, J., Sanderson, M. J. (1998). A simple method for high temporal resolution calcium imaging with dual excitation dyes. Biophys. J. 75(4):2025.
6. Davies, E. V., Blanchfield, H., Hallett, M. B. (1997). Use of fluorescent dyes for measurement and localization of organelles associated with Ca^{2+} store release in human neutrophils. Cell Biol. Int. 21(10):655.
7. Grynkiewicz, G., Poenie, M., Tsien, R. Y. (1985). A new generation of calcium indicators with greatly improved fluorescence properties. J. Biol. Chem. 260:3440.
8. Montminy, M. (1997). Transcriptional regulation by cyclic AMP. Ann. Rev. Biochem. 66:807.
9. McCusker, R. H., Clemmons, D. R. (1998). Role for cyclic adenosine monophosphate in modulating insulin-like growth factor binding protein secretion by muscle cells. J. Cell. Physiol. 174(3):293.
10. Nguyen, P. V., Kandel, E. R. (1996). A macromolecular synthesis-dependent late phase of long-term potentiation requiring cAMP in the medial perforant pathway of rat hippocampal slices. J. Neurosci. 16(10):3189.
11. Roger, P. P., Christophe, D., Dumont, J. E., Pirson, I. (1997). The dog thyroid primary culture system: a model of the regulation of function, growth and differentiation expression by cAMP and other well-defined signaling cascades. Eur. J. Endocrinol. 137(6):579.
12. Bertolotto, C., Abbe, P., Hemesath, T. J., Bille, K., Fisher, D. E., Ortonne, J. P., Ballotti, R. (1998). Microphthalmia gene product as a signal transducer in cAMP-induced differentiation of melanocytes. J. Cell Biol. 142(3):827.

13. Fladmark, K. E., Gjertsen, B. T., Doskeland, S. O., Vintermyr, O. K. (1997). Fas/APO-1(CD95)-induced apoptosis of primary hepatocytes is inhibited by cAMP. Biochem. Biophys. Res. Commun. 232(1):20.

14. Leedman, P. J., Frauman, A. G., Colman, P. G., Michelangeli, V. P. (1992). Measurement of thyroid-stimulating immunoglobulins by incorporation of tritiated-adenine into intact FRTL-5 cells: a viable alternative to radioimmunoassay for the measurement of cAMP. Clin. Endocrinol. 37(6):493.

15. Kingan, T. G. (1989). A competitive enzyme-linked immunosorbent assay: applications in the assay of peptides, steroids, and cyclic nucleotides. Anal. Biochem. 183(2):283.

16. Adams, S. R., Harootunian, A. T., Buechler, Y. J., Taylor, S. S., Tsien, R. Y. (1991). Fluorescence ratio imaging of cyclic AMP in single cells. Nature 349(6311):694.

17. Hempel, C. M., Vincent, P., Adams, S. R., Tsien, R. Y., Selverston, A. I. (1996). Spatio-temporal dynamics of cyclic AMP signals in an intact neural circuitm. Nature 384(6605):166.

18. Higashi, H., Sato, K., Ohtake, A., Omori, A., Yoshida, S., Kudo, Y. (1997). Imaging of cAMP-dependent protein kinase activity in living neural cells using a novel fluorescent substrate. FEBS Lett. 414(1):55.

19. Katayama, Y., Ohuchi, Y., NakayamaA, M., Maeda, M., Higashi, H., Kudo, Y. (1997). Cyclic AMP detection by electrode modified with 17mer oligopeptide. Chem. Lett. 883.

20. Su, Y., Dostmann, W. R. G., Herberg, F. W., Durick, K., Xong, N-H., Ten Eyck, L., Taylor, S. S., Varughese, L. I. (1995). Regulatory subunit of protein kinase A: structure of deletion mutant with cAMP binding domains. Science 269(11):807.

21. Sugawara, M., Kojima, K., Sazawa, H., Umezawa, Y. (1987). Ion-channel sensors. Anal. Chem. 59(24):2842.

22. Shabb, J. B., Corbin, J. D. (1992). Cyclic nucleotide-binding domains in proteins having diverse functions. Biol. Chem. 267(9):5723.

23. Glass, D. B., Feller, M. J., Levin, L. R., Walsh, D. A. (1992). Structural basis for the low affinities of Yeast cAMP-dependent and mammalian cGMP-dependent protein kinases for protein kinase inhibitor peptides. Biochemistry 31:1728.

24. Shabb, J. B., Ng, L., Corbin, J. D. (1990). One amino acid change produces a high affinity cGMP-dependent protein kinase. J. Biol. Chem. 265(27):16031.

25. Shabb, J. B., Buzzeo, B. D., Ng, L., Corbin, J. D. (1991). Mutating kinase cAMP-binding sites into cGMP-binding sites. J. Biol. Chem. 266(36):24320.

14

Recombinant Photoproteins in the Design of Binding Assays

Jennifer C. Lewis, Agatha J. Feltus, and Sylvia Daunert
University of Kentucky, Lexington, Kentucky, U.S.A.

I. INTRODUCTION

Bioluminescence can be defined as the production of visible light through a chemical reaction occurring within a living organism. This important natural phenomenon is employed by many creatures for purposes of defense, mating, concealment, and the recycling of nutrients [1]. Hydrozoan coelenterates, a class of bioluminescent organisms, produce their luminescence through the presence of proteins known as Ca^{2+}-binding photoproteins [2].

This type of protein consists of an apoprotein, a chromophore, and molecular oxygen. In the presence of calcium ions, these proteins undergo a change in conformation that causes an intramolecular reaction and the subsequent emission of light. In some bioluminescent coelenterates, the production of blue light by the photoprotein is what one observes in the organism. However, in other coelenterates, the light emitted by the organism is green. This is because in the case of certain photoproteins, such as aequorin, a radiationless energy transfer occurs between the photoprotein and a green fluorescent protein (GFP) also present within the organism (Fig. 1) [3]. It is not clear yet why these GFPs are associated with certain photoproteins, except perhaps to increase the overall efficiency of light production [4].

There are seven photoproteins that have been isolated thus far, including thalassicolin (5), aequorin (6), mitrocomin (also known as halistaurin) (7), clytin (also known as phialidin) (8), obelin (9), mnemiopsin (10), and berovin (10). Four of these proteins—aequorin (11), clytin (12), mitrocomin (13), and obelin (14)—have been sequenced and cloned. These photoproteins are similar in

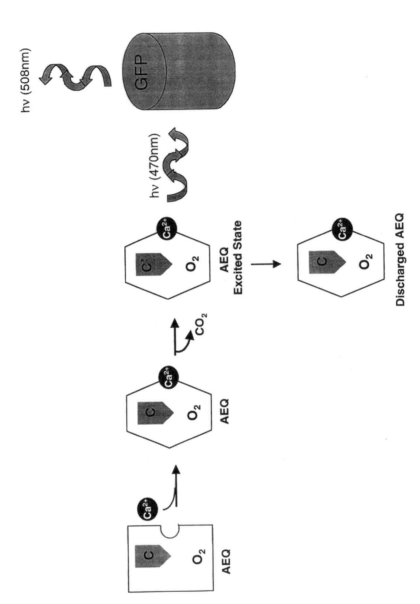

Figure 1 In vivo bioluminescence energy transfer between aequorin (AEQ) and the corresponding green fluorescent protein (GFP). Aequorin is activated by Ca^{2+}, causing excitation of the chromophore, coelenterazine (C), and leading to a radiationless energy transfer to GFP.

structure, each consisting of a relatively small apoprotein (21.4–27.5 kDa) that contains three calcium-binding sites ($K_D = 1$–10 µM) [3]. The calcium-binding sites are E-F hand motifs comprised of two α-helices separated by a β-pleated sheet. The amino acid sequence of these E-F hand structures is highly conserved among Ca^{2+}-binding proteins [15]. Each of the photoproteins also binds noncovalently an organic chromophore, coelenterazine, along with molecular oxygen. Upon the addition of calcium ions, the protein undergoes a conformational change that results in the oxidation of coelenterazine by the protein-bound oxygen, producing coelenteramide. The reaction also produces CO_2 and light ranging from 440 to 490 nm. The wavelength of emission of the photoprotein differs from one particular photoprotein to another [16]. The light is released as a flash lasting less than 10 s, with a quantum yield of 0.15–0.20 [3]. Although the reaction occurs as a single-turnover event, the photoprotein can be regenerated following the removal of the bound coelenteramide [17].

This family of photoproteins can be an attractive alternative to existing radioisotopic labels in analytical applications because they provide excellent sensitivity of detection while being free of the hazards associated with radioactivity. The detection sensitivity of these environmentally friendly protein labels is illustrated by the bioluminescent reactions of aequorin and obelin, which allow for their determination down to 1 tipomol (10^{-21} mol) [15]. Aequorin has also been shown to be quite stable as well. Indeed, this photoprotein retains its bioluminescence in a variety of buffers with a number of different additives. It can be stored in solution at 4°C for over a month while still retaining 85% of its original activity. Lyophilization of the protein allows for its storage up to one year [18]. Bioluminescent labels offer an advantage over conventional fluorescent tags when working with biological samples. This is because these samples usually contain a variety of fluorescent molecules that can cause significant background problems. Bioluminescence, on the other hand, is a relatively rare phenomenon in the biological kingdom; thus the problem of background signal is virtually eliminated [19]. Also, unlike some chemiluminescent labels that require highly alkaline conditions (pH > 9) for maximum activity, the photoproteins are active at physiological pH [20].

Thus far, aequorin has been the most widely used of the photoproteins in applications including immunoassays, nucleic acid probe–based assays, and extensively as a cellular calcium indicator. Some examples of binding assays employing aequorin as a label include the determination of amplified cytokine products [21], tumor necrosis factor-α [22], protein A [23], Forssman antigen [24], and prostate-specific antigen RNA [25]. Obelin has also been used in binding assays for the detection of large molecules, such as alfafetoproteins and IgG [26,27]. A majority of these assays have been performed in a noncompetitive assay format in which the photoprotein has been covalently coupled to large antigenic molecules or antibodies. The lack of reports in the literature on the use of aequorin and obelin in the determination of small molecules prompted us to investigate the feasibility of employing these proteins as bioluminescent labels in the development of assays for small biomolecules. This chapter will discuss the efforts of our group to develop competitive binding assays in which the photoprotein label has been attached to a small biomolecule analyte either through chemical or genetic engineering methods.

II. COMPETITIVE BINDING ASSAYS BASED ON CHEMICAL CONJUGATES OF PHOTOPROTEINS

In order to explore the feasibility of using photoproteins as labels for the determination of small biomolecules, a conjugate between aequorin and biotin was employed to develop competitive binding assays for biotin. Biotin is an important vitamin (vitamin H) found in the tissue and blood, which binds with high affinity ($K_a = 10^{14}$ M^{-1}) to the glycoprotein avidin. Avidin contains four identical subunits, each of which binds one molecule of biotin [28]. The aequorin–biotin (AEQ–biotin) conjugate was purchased from SeaLite Sciences (Norcross, GA) and contained 2.6 molecules of biotin attached per molecule of aequorin. This conjugate exhibited the same flash-type kinetics of the native protein, with a majority of the photons being released within 3 s after the addition of calcium ions. Chemical modification led to some loss of bioluminescence activity; however, the biotinylated photoprotein retained at least 70% of its original activity and was detected at subattomole levels [20].

The biotinylated photoprotein was used to develop both a homogeneous and a heterogeneous assay for biotin. A homogeneous assay format was possible due to the observation that, upon binding with avidin, the AEQ–biotin signal was inhibited. Both of these aequorin-based assays for biotin depend upon a competition between the photoprotein-labeled biotin and free biotin in solution for the binding sites on avidin. For the homogeneous assay, various concentrations of free biotin and a fixed amount of avidin were mixed in a test tube and incubated for 30 min. A chosen amount of AEQ–biotin was then added, followed by another incubation step of 30 min. Bioluminescence was measured on an Optocomp I luminometer after the injection of 100 mM $CaCl_2$ in 100 mM Tris-HCl, pH 7.5, buffer. A dose–response curve for biotin was generated by relating the inhibition of the bioluminescence signal of the AEQ–biotin conjugate with varying concentrations of free biotin in the sample. The detection limits obtained for this homogeneous bioluminescence assay were four orders of magnitude more sensitive than those reported for other homogeneous enzyme-based assays for biotin [20].

For the heterogeneous assay, avidin-coated microspheres were employed as the solid phase and mixed in a test tube along with equal volumes of biotinylated protein and varying concentrations of free biotin. The mixture was incubated for 30 min, and the phases were then separated. The solid phase was washed three times with buffer before the bioluminescence on the solid phase was triggered with Ca^{2+} [29]. The resulting dose–response curve can be seen in Figure 2. The AEQ–biotin dose–response curve generated for the heterogeneous assay demonstrates a "hook" effect, in which the curve descends back down at low concentrations of analyte. This effect can be explained by a positive cooperative interaction between adjacent binding sites on the avidin so that the binding of the first biotin molecule induces a conformational change in the avidin, making a second binding event more favorable. Indeed, further studies of the interaction of the AEQ–biotin conjugate with the immobilized avidin showed that his was likely. The "hook" effect shows a concentration dependence that is revealed when the amounts of both binder and conjugate are low. The biphasic shape of this dose–response curve does not preclude its use in quantitative analysis. In order to determine whether the signal from the sample corresponds to the as-

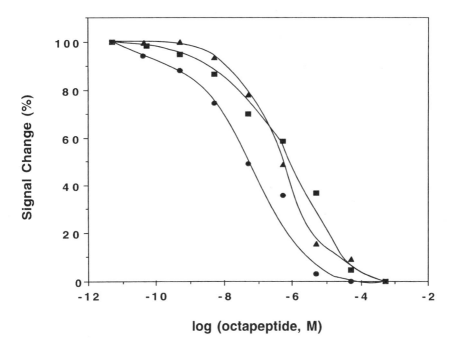

Figure 2 Dose-response curve for an octapeptide employing aequorin (●), obelin (▲), and GFP (■) as labels. Data is the average of ±1 standard deviation ($n = 3$). All error bars are less than 10%.

cending or to the descending portions of the curve, the sample must be spiked with a known quantity of biotin. The presence of the "hook" can be advantageous in terms of the detection limit of the assay when using the descending portion of the curve. Table 1 compares the detection limits obtained for biotin of three different photoprotein-based assays developed in our laboratory. It was found, as expected, that from the aequorin-based assays, the heterogeneous one has a lower detection limit than the homogeneous one and then the assay for biotin using GFP as a label [30].

The results of these assays demonstrate that the photoprotein aequorin can function effectively as a bioluminescent label in competitive binding assays for a small biomolecule employing chemical conjugation as a means to attach the analyte to the photoprotein label. Further, due to the inhibition obtained upon binding of the AEQ–biotin conjugate with avidin, a bioluminescent homogeneous assay was developed. In the case of the heterogeneous assay using the AEQ–biotin conjugate, we were able to achieve the most sensitive detection limit reported for biotin thus far. The detection limit, 1×10^{-15} M, corresponds to 100 zeptomole of biotin in the sample and should allow for miniaturization of the assay as well as for determination of biotin in small volumes (e.g., those corresponding to a single cell).

III. COMPETITIVE BINDING ASSAYS USING GENETICALLY ENGINEERED PHOTOPROTEINS

Gene fusion technology can be employed as an alternative method for the preparation of conjugates when the analyte of interest is a protein or a peptide. In this technique, the analyte is attached to the bioluminescent label at the DNA level through the manipulation of the genes encoding for the analyte and the photoprotein. The resulting product is a fusion protein in which the C-terminus of a peptide/protein has been attached to the N-terminus of another peptide/

Table 1 Detection Limits of the Photoprotein-Based Assays for Biotin

Conjugate	Detection limit,[a] M
AEQ–biotin (homogeneous)	1.0×10^{-14}
AEQ–biotin (heterogeneous)	1.0×10^{-15}
GFP-biotin	1.8×10^{-8}

[a]The detection limit refers to the concentration of biotin in the sample and was calculated using S/N = 2 or 3.

protein. Thus, by producing the labeled analyte as a fusion protein, a one-to-one homogeneous population of conjugates is obtained. This is advantageous in terms of assay development, since experimental and theoretical studies have shown that monosubstituted conjugates provide better assay performance [31].

The research in our laboratory has focused on the preparation of peptide–photoprotein conjugates for developing competitive binding assays for small peptides. Peptides are important analytes because they participate in a number of physiological processes as neurotransmitters and hormones [32]. Peptide assays commonly rely on a radioisotopic label, which requires special handling and disposal procedures [33]. Immunoassays for small peptides typically present a challenge in that the preparation of labeled conjugates must be performed in such a manner as not to interfere with the binding of the peptide to its corresponding antibody. This can be quite difficult to achieve with peptides that have an amino acid sequence where a large number of reactive groups are present. In these cases, chemical conjugation methods involving a reagent such as carbodiimide or glutaraldehyde may lead to a multisubstituted heterogeneous population of peptide analyte-conjugate. As already mentioned, it has been demonstrated that heterogeneous populations of analyte-conjugates lead to poorer assay performance and detection limits. Moreover, multisubstitution may either lower the activity of the protein label or hinder the recognition of the peptide by the antibody.

In the work presented here, a model octapeptide (Asp-Tyr-Lys-Asp-Asp-Asp-Asp-Lys) was selected to produce fusion proteins between aequorin and obelin. The particular octapeptide was chosen because of the large number of functional groups on the octapeptide and the relatively weak binding constant with its antibody ($K_a = 10^{6-7}$ M^{-1}), which is in contrast to the previously described assays for biotin using aequorin as a label. By fusing the gene encoding for the octapeptide to the genes encoding for the photoproteins, aequorin and obelin, one-to-one ratios of the octapeptide to the corresponding photoprotein were assured. Also, the peptide was site-specifically placed on a desired position of the bioluminescent label in a controlled fashion using this method. Another advantage of using gene fusion is that since the fusion proteins are produced from the same gene every time, each batch of conjugates is virtually identical, leading to greater lot-to-lot reproducibility.

In order to produce the octapeptide–photoprotein fusions, a series of expression vectors was constructed. As seen in Figure 3, separate vectors were constructed in which the gene encoding for the octapeptide was fused to the 5'-end of the DNA encoding for the individual apophotoproteins. Upon transformation into *E. coli*, the bacteria were induced with isopropyl-β-D-thiogalactopyranoside since the vector employed a *tac* promoter to produce the fusion proteins. After purification by anion exchange chromatography, the octapeptide–apoaequorin and –apoobelin fusion proteins were incubated with coelenterazine to yield the corresponding holoproteins.

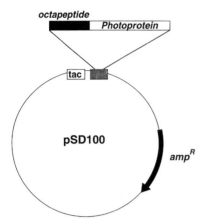

Figure 3   Generic plasmid used to express octapeptide fusion proteins for the development of competitive binding assays for the free octapeptide. The gene for the octapeptide is placed at the 5′-end of the gene of the photoprotein by employing standard recombinant DNA techniques. The *tac* promoter regulates the expression of the fusion protein through the addition of isopropyl-β-D-thiogalactopyranoside.

The assays for the octapeptide were conducted as follows: The immobilized antioctapeptide antibodies were incubated with varying concentrations of free peptide for 30 min; the octapeptide–photoprotein conjugates were added for an additional 30 min; the phases were separated, and the solid phase was washed to remove excess conjugate. The bioluminescence signal was then measured on the solid phase by injecting a luminescence-triggering buffer containing 100 mM Ca^{2+} to the tubes containing the octapeptide–aequorin (octapeptide–AEQ) and –obelin (octapeptide–obelin) [34,35]. Typical dose–response curves obtained with the two different photoprotein–octapeptide conjugates can be seen in Figure 4, along with a similar assay developed for the peptide using GFP as a label [36].

As the data shows, the curves are similar in shape but differ in the sensitivity of detection obtained for the free octapeptide. This difference is especially observed between the dose–response curves generated using the photoprotein labels (aequorin and obelin) in comparison to the fluorescent protein label (GFP). The GFP is a protein that contains an internal chromophore with a maximum excitation wavelength of 395 nm and a maximum emission wavelength of 509 nm [4]. The detection limit for each curve is given in Table 2. By using aequorin as a bioluminescent label rather than GFP, the detection limit was improved by one order of magnitude. The detection limit is also two orders of

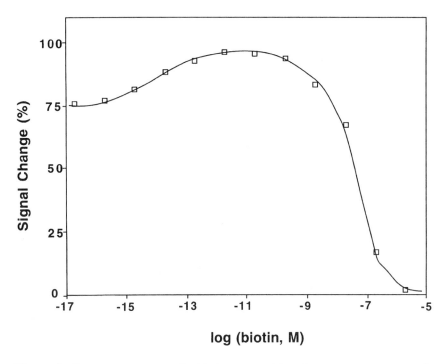

Figure 4 Dose–response curve for biotin generated in a heterogeneous assay mode using aequorin as the label. Data are the average of ±1 standard deviation ($n = 3$). All error bars are less than 10%.

Table 2 Detection Limits for the Octapeptide Using Different Labels

Conjugate	Detection limit,[a] M
Octapeptide–BAP	1×10^{-7}
Octapeptide–GFP	1×10^{-8}
Octapeptide–obelin	6.4×10^{-9}
Octapeptide–AEQ	1×10^{-9}

[a]The detection limit refers to the concentration of octapeptide in the sample and was calculated using $S/N = 2$ or 3.
Abbreviations: BAP, bacterial alkaline phosphatase; GFP, green fluorescent protein. The BAP assay used a fluorogenic substrate.

magnitude better than that obtained with an assay using a fusion protein of this octapeptide with the enzyme label bacterial alkaline phosphatase (BAP) [31]. These differences can be attributed to the individual characteristics of each label. Aequorin and obelin, which give the best detection limits, are the two photoproteins exhibiting flash-type bioluminescence kinetics resulting in virtually no background signal. The corresponding fusion proteins did not show any significant decrease in bioluminescence activity compared to that of the native proteins, with detection limits of approximately 1×10^{-14} M. The fluorescence of the octapeptide–GFP fusion protein was also comparable to that of the native protein, with a detection limit for the octapeptide–GFP of 2.8×10^{-10} M. In the case of BAP, the enzymatic activity was determined by using a fluorescent substrate. Even taking advantage of the high turnover number of BAP, the detection limit for the octapeptide is two orders of magnitude worse than that using the photoprotein–octapeptide fusion proteins. This can be attributed to the higher sensitivity achieved with the bioluminescent proteins.

One advantage of using these recombinant conjugates is the high amount of reproducibility they grant to the assay. When chemical coupling is used to produce a protein conjugate, it is often necessary to optimize the assay again to account for the change in activity of the newly prepared conjugate versus the old batch. In the case of the octapeptide–AEQ and octapeptide–GFP conjugates, three separate batches of protein were expressed and purified at different times. The bioluminescence activity of each was determined and compared to that of the other two batches. In the case of octapeptide–AEQ, all three batches demonstrated the same flash-type kinetics profile. The half-life of the bioluminescence decay was 0.68 ± 0.01 s for the three separate batches, which compares well to that of native recombinant aequorin (0.60 s). For the octapeptide–GFP, calibration curves performed on each lot of conjugate showed less than 10% deviation from batch to batch.

It is clear, therefore, that the use of gene fusions to produce conjugates results in a number of advantages. For example, N-terminal fusions of the photoproteins with a small peptide neither result in the loss of bioluminescence activity nor hinder the ability of the octapeptide to interact with its antibody. It also results in high lot-to-lot reproducibility for the fusions, eliminating the need to reoptimize the assay after preparing a new batch of conjugate.

IV. CONCLUSIONS

Our group has demonstrated that the naturally occurring photoproteins aequorin and obelin are highly effective labels in the development of competitive binding assays for small molecules. These assays are extremely sensitive because they take advantage of the flash-type kinetics of aequorin and obelin with their associated inherently low backgrounds. Both of these proteins offer the advantages of being safer to use compared to radioisotopic labels while also providing the opportunity to produce fusion proteins by recombinant methods. The fact that these proteins have been cloned and can be expressed in bacteria allows for their availability to the researcher in an almost limitless supply. Because these proteins can be detected down to very low levels using the bioluminescence signal they produce, it is possible to employ them as labels in the determination of important biomolecules in small-volume samples, even those approaching a single cell. We envision that these proteins will undoubtedly find use in the development of highly sensitive assays for a variety of analytes in the future. Moreover, these assays may find applications in the high-throughput screening of biopharmaceuticals.

ACKNOWLEDGMENTS

The authors would like to acknowledge the financial support provided by the National Institute of Health (GM47915), the Department of Energy (DE-FG05-95ER62010), and the National Science Foundation (IGERT program). SD is a Cottrell Scholar and a Lilly Faculty Awardee. We would also like to thank Drs. Sridhar Ramanathan, Emily Hernández, Allan Witowski, and Sergey Matveev for their contributions to this work, which are cited in References 20, 30, 31, 34, and 35.

REFERENCES

1. Rivera, H. N.; Patel, M. T.; Stults, N. L.; Smith, D. F.; Rigl, C. T. In: Campbell, A. K., Kricka, L. J., Stanley, P. E., eds. Biolumin. Chemilumin., Proc. Int. Symp. Wiley: Chichester, UK, 1994.
2. Tsuji, F. I.; Ohmiya, Y.; Fagan, T. F.; Toh, H.; Iouye, S. Photochem. Photobiol. 62:657, 1995.
3. Kendall, J. M.; Badminton, M. N. TIBTECH 16:216, 1998.
4. Cubitt, A. B.; Heim, R.; Adams, S. R.; Boyd, A. E.; Gross, L. A.; Tsien, R. Y. TIBTECH 20:448, 1995.
5. Herring, P. J. Mar. Biol. 53:213, 1979.
6. Shimomura, O.; Johnson, F. H.; Saiga, Y. J. Cell. Comp. Physiol. 62:XX, 1962.
7. Shimomura, O.; Johnson, F. H.; Saiga, Y. J. Cell. Comp. Physiol. 62:XX, 1963.
8. Levine, L. D.; Ward, W. W. Comp. Biochem. Physiol. 72B:77, 1982.
9. Campbell, A. K. Biochem. J. 143:411, 1974.
10. Ward, W. W.; Seliger, H. H. Biochemistry 13:1491, 1974.
11. Inouye, S.; Noguchi, M.; Sakaki, Y.; Takagi, Y.; Miyata, T.; Iwanaga, S.; Miyata, T.; Tsuji, F. I. Proc. Natl. Acad. Sci. USA 82:3154, 1985.

12. Inouye, S.; Tsuji, F. I. FEBS Lett. 315:343, 1993.
13. Fagan, T. F.; Ohmiya, Y.; Blinks, J. R.; Inouye, S.; Tsuji, F. I. FEBS Lett. 333: 301, 1993.
14. Illarionov, B. A.; Bondar, V. S.; Illarionova, V. A.; Vysotski, E. S. Gene 153:273, 1995.
15. Campbell, K. Chemiluminescence. Ellis Horwood: Chichester, UK, 1988.
16. Campbell, A. K.; Sula-Newby, G. In: Mason, W. T., ed. Fluorescent and Luminescent Probes for Biological Activity. Academic Press: San Diego, CA, 1993.
17. Ohmiya, Y.; Hirano, T. Chemistry Biology 3:337, 1998.
18. Flanagan, K.; Sanchez-Brambila, G.; Barnc, C.; Rivera, H.; Scheuer, B.; Stults, N.; Smith, D. F.; Hart, R. C.; Gray, J. In: Szalay, A. A., Kricka, L. J., Stanley, P. E., eds. Biolumin, Chemilumin., Proc. Int. Symp. Wiley: Chichester, UK, 1993.
19. Jackson, R. J.; Fujihashi, K.; Kiyono, H.; McGhee, J. R. J. Immunol. Methods 190: 189, 1996.
20. Witkowski, A.; Ramanathan, S.; Daunert, S. Anal. Chem. 65:1147, 1993.
21. Xiao, L.; Yang, C.; Nelson, C. O.; Holloway, B. P.; Udhayakumar, V.; Lal, A. A. J. Immunol. Methods, 199:139, 1996.
22. Erikaku, T.; Zenno, S.; Inouye, S. Biochem. Biophys. Res. Commun. 174:1331, 1991.
23. Zatta, P. F. J. Biochem. Biophys. Methods 32:7, 1996.
24. Stults, N. L.; Stocks, N. F.; Rivera, H.; Gray, J.; McCann, R. O.; O'Kane, D. O.; Cummings, R. D.; Cormier, M. J.; Smith, D. F. Biochemistry 31:1433, 1992.
25. Galvan, B.; Christopoulos, T. K. Anal. Chem. 68:3545, 1996.
26. Frank, L. A.; Illarionova, V. A.; Vysotski, E. S. Biochem. Biophys. Res. Commun. 219:475, 1996.
27. Frank, L. A.; Vysotski, E. S. In: Bioluminescence and Chemiluminescence: Molecular Reporting with Photons, Proceedings of the 9th International Symposium. Wiley: New York, 1996.
28. Gitlin, G.; Bayer, E. A.; Wilchek, M. Biochem. J. 242:923, 1987.
29. Feltus, A.; Ramanathan, S.; Daunert, S. Anal. Biochem. 254:62, 1997.
30. Hernandez, E. C.; Daunert, S. Anal. Biochem. 261:113, 1998.
31. Witkowski, A.; Daunert, S.; Kindy, M. S.; Bachas, L. G.; Anal. Chem. 65:1147, 1993.
32. Cooper, J. C.; Bloom, F. E.; Roth, R. H. The Biochemical Basis of Neuropharmacology. Oxford University Press: New York, 1996.
33. Tiong, G. K. L.; Olley, J. E. Clinical Experimental Pharmacol. Physiol. 17:515, 1990.
34. Ramanathan, S.; Lewis, J. C.; Kindy, M. S.; Daunert, S. Anal. Chim. Acta 369: 181, 1998.
35. Matveev, S. V.; Lewis, J. C.; Daunert, S. manuscript submitted for publication, 1998.
36. J. C. Lewis, J. Feliciano, S. Daunert. Anal. Chim. Acta, in press, 1998.

15
Particle Valency Strip Assays

Judith Fitzpatrick and Regina B. Lenda
Serex, Inc., Maywood, New Jersey, U.S.A.

Michael Munzar
Nymox Corporation, Maywood,New Jersey, U.S.A.

I. INTRODUCTION

We have developed a quantitative chromatographic strip assay platform [1], Lab Tab™, that does not require premeasurement or sample manipulation. The device provides assays of quantitative or semiquantitative laboratory-quality precision and accuracy on many bodily fluids in alternative settings in an easy-to-use format (Figure 1 illustrates dose response of the cotinine LabTab™). Utilizing this platform we have developed tests for cotinine and we are developing tests for other analytes.

LabTab™ utilizes a unique immunochemistry system that is neither a competitive nor a sandwich assay. LabTab™ relies on detection of the percent occupancy of antibody-binding sites on a particle, hereafter called *particle valency*, to indicate analyte level. The particle valency format is enabled by low-affinity binding, which is in turn enabled by the use of very low-affinity ligands, called *relands* [2,3].

In this chapter we describe the reland technology and the particle valency platform, and, to illustrate the unique benefits of the LabTab™ format, we present and discuss the performance characteristics of NicoMeter™, the first test to be commercialized in this format.

II. LOW-AFFINITY LIGANDS—
RELEASE LIGANDS (RELANDS)

Release assays in the reland format were first developed in 1991 [2,3]. These assays, which can be performed in homogeneous or heterogeneous format, utilize very low-affinity release ligands (relands) that are incubated with antibody to form a complex. The complex dissociates immediately upon contact with the analyte being measured, which has a higher affinity for the antibody than for the release ligand. Relands do not bind to the antibody under normal conditions, and are therefore not logical binding partners or ligands for the antibody. The essence of creating a release assay was to design a small low-affinity ligand (reland) from a set of analogs, one having less than 1% cross-reactivity and preferably less than 0.1% reactivity and an association constant of less than 10^4 M^{-1}.

Reland complexes are formed by incubating a high-specificity, monoclonal antibody with a great excess of reland (we routinely used millimolar concentrations of reland for long periods of time—often overnight or even throughout the assay).

Relands are small, generally less than 1000 molecular weight, and contact the paratope (epitope-binding region of the antibody) only through analyte-specific binding areas. Ideally relands have no functional charged groups. Release ligands are ligands having low association rates. They also have low dissociation rates. Most importantly, reland dissociation rates are greatly accelerated in the presence of analyte. We know that the dissociation rate is highly dependent upon the presence of analyte, since the dissociated reland does not reassociate under assay conditions, because it cannot compete for binding.

Different release assays have been described by others [4–6]. However, in these earlier cases analysis of the data indicates that the release ligand was a competitive ligand [7] and that the assays depended upon selecting an antibody with a high dissociation constant. These systems utilized large amounts of preformed complex and a large amount of analyte to effect release of a small percentage of ligand. They were time dependent—with time more ligand dissociates. Such test systems can be expected to show undesirable reactions to matrix. In contrast, Reland Assays exhibit stoichiometric release on a close to 1:1 ratio; equilibrate to a steady state within the first few moments; and exhibit characteristics that indicate remarkable insensitivity to matrix effects.

It is critical that the reland be small and form only analyte-specific bonds, because only then can the analyte specifically release the reland. When a reland of low molecular weight, such as an analog of cotinine, is attached to a protein carrier and binds to an anticotinine antibody, the area of contact between the hapten carrier and the complementarity-determining region of the antibody (CDR) is 600–900 A. This contact region involves 10–23 contact points, with 3–8 of these contributing most of the binding strength [8–11]. However, the area of contact between the hapten and the CDR is much less, on the order of 20% of the total area now contained between the two proteins [8,12,13]. Obviously this contact area is no longer available for diffusional access by analyte. Furthermore, as the two proteins sit, they generally undergo a process of accommodation [13–15]. Thus it becomes increasingly more difficult and eventually impossible to dissociate the proteins under nondenaturing conditions. This accommodation process represents rearrangement of each protein's tertiary structure to form a more complementary interface and involves the exclusion of water and the formation of other bonds. The formation of such other bonds would clearly not be expected to be analyte specific, and so it would not be expected that analyte could disrupt these bonds. Further, the existence of these other bonds significantly decreases dissociation rates, probably due to the increased avidity seen with the phenomenon of multiattachment [14,16–18].

Since it is critical that a reland be small and form no bonds with the antibody that are not analyte specific, it follows that this places constraints on any label attached to a reland: It too must be very small and ideally should not carry groups that could form significant bonds.

Using an Emit® format cotinine release assay [2,3] we were able to demonstrate that a release assay increased the range over 500-fold, from 0.05–2 µg/mL to 0.01–>1000 µg/mL. Range was increased by increasing reagents 27-fold. However, this increase in reagents did not increase background, which would lead to a decrease in sensitivity, but rather resulted in a fivefold increase in sensitivity. Further, the assay in this format showed greatly improved performance: Both C.V.s and cross-reactivity were reduced by half over the conventional format. Thus reland release assays are rapid, have very low background and increased precision, and unlike competitive assays have a large range and do not require limited amounts of reagents.

The characteristics of reland-type assays indicate that they constitute a new form of immunoassay that differs fundamentally from conventional assays, which are "basically limited to two approaches: (1) a competitive assay or limited-reagent assay, and (2) an immunometric, sandwich, or excess-reagent assay" [19]. The reland system is not competitive because it does not utilize limited reagent, and it is not a sandwich.

III. PARTICLE VALENCY ASSAYS

A. Background

The advantages of the reland system recommended it for adaptation to point-of-care testing. It might be expected to eliminate the need to manipulate or dilute samples, because it had a large range and was insensitive to matrix. It was rapid and demonstrated high precision and sensitivity, which meant that it might compensate for the technique-dependent problems seen with less rugged systems.

For point-of-care assays we required a format that could be read visually or in reflectance mode. The size constraint for reland and label made the release format difficult to adapt to a label detectable in the visual wavelength.

We met the requirements for a visual label by adapting the reland system to a chromatographic format. We had observed that it was possible to purify antibodies by low-affinity chromatography [2,20]. On this basis, we began our studies of the use of reland traps on chromatographic strips with gold particles as antibody label. Because we came to understand the critical role that valency played in this technology, we named the format *particle valency assays*.

B. Mechanism of Action of Particle Valency Assays

Particle valency assays involve two sets of reactions. The first reaction is an affinity reaction: A high-affinity monoclonal antibody interacts with the analyte and rapidly reaches endpoint. The second reaction is based on avidity and provides a method of interpreting or quantitating the results of this interaction by parsing of the particles based upon avidity. We shall use the word *affinity* to refer solely to the attraction of a ligand for an antibody-binding site, *avidity* to refer to a reaction that is predominantly a function of a multitude of other interactions, and the term *binding strength* to refer to a reaction that is dependent upon both avidity and affinity.

The first reaction, the binding of analyte to antibody, is based on affinity. Sample is applied to the strip and interacts with antibody on the particles. We generally use colloidal gold with particle diameter of about 20 nm. It can be calculated that antibody-coated particles of this diameter carry ~40 antibody molecules [21] or ~80 antibody-binding sites. Thus we may think of these particles as multivalent. (In actual fact a preparation of gold particles is not homogeneous in size and thus presents a population of valences. The theoretical valence of 80 represents the mean valence of the population.) In the diagrams that are intended to illustrate these phenomenon (Figure 2) we represent a binding site as a + sign and a ligand as − sign.

The addition of analyte to the population of particles results in the loss of binding sites on the particle; i.e., it changes the mean valence of the population of particles. The number of binding sites lost is directly proportional to the amount of analyte bound by the antibody on the particle. Thus the decrease in valence is directly related to the amount of analyte in the test sample.

In the next step the particles are displayed based on their valence (Figure 2). Increasing the number of contact points or valence increases the observed avidity; this phenomenon of stickiness is generally ascribed to a decrease in the dissociation rate [16,18]. The avidity of an antibody-coated particle greatly exceeds the affinity of any one antibody-binding site and is exquisitely sensitive to the valence or number of available or unbound antibody-binding sites.

To display the particles according to avidity we construct a series of traps of increasing binding strength. A trap is designed both to retain particles of a certain valence and to allow particles of lower valence to pass through. The traps actually function like a series of sieves. Particles are retained based on complementarity of binding strength; thus a high-avidity particle can be retained by a trap of very very low binding strength, a reland trap. Low-avidity or low-valence particles are retained by traps of higher and higher binding strength, which are constructed from high-affinity or competitive ligands. Thus loss of avidity, or stickiness, of the particle is compensated for by increasing the binding strength of the trap.

C. Construction of the Particle Valency Assay Strip

The LabTab™ strip is constructed of a Porex® membrane receiving zone upon which the antibody-coated gold particles are impregnated. This membrane overlaps a nitrocellulose membrane on which the traps are coated and that has at the distal end a green spot, which appears when adequate sample has traversed the strip and the test is done. The two membranes are sandwiched between top and bottom Mylar adhesive laminates in a manner that ensures that substantially the entire strip is encased within laminate [22]. This laminated packaging format of the strip facilitates quantitation without measurement by providing a defined test volume (Fig. 1).

When sample is applied to the strip, analyte in sample interacts with the antibody-coated gold particles and carries the particles to the nitrocellulose portion, which has "trap zones" coated sequentially up its length so that sample and mobilized gold flow across each zone sequentially upward from trap 1. From trap 1 upward, each successive trap has increased binding strength for the antibody-coated gold particles.

The antibody on the gold particles binds analyte in the sample, thus reducing the valency and avidity of the particle for the trap zones. The sample and mobilized gold conjugate continue to migrate up the dipstick, with gold conjugate binding to the trap zones successively from trap 1 upward, according to the valency of the particle population. If there is no analyte in the sample, the valency of the gold particles is unaltered and the high-valence particles bind to the lower-affinity, lower-numbered traps. If there is analyte in the sample, the valency of the gold particles is reduced, and particles bind to the higher-affinity, higher-numbered traps. Hence, the more analyte in the sample, the further the

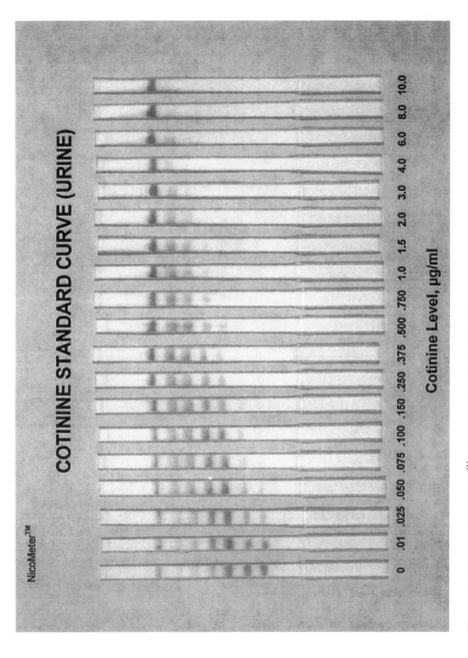

Figure 1 Prototype NicoMeter™ strips at various levels of cotinine.

population of gold particles migrates, because the migration distance of the particles is related to the amount of analyte in the sample.

One can see from this description that the strip varies fundamentally from other strips in that the immune reaction occurs before sample reaches the traps. The traps are designed to display the particles based on valence, which is a function of the amount of analyte in the sample.

D. Principles of Trap Construction

Construction of the trap materials is specific to each assay. In the case of the urine NicoMeter™ prototype (Fig. 1), the first trap that the particles pass through has very very low binding strength and is designed to trap only about 20% of the highest-avidity particles. The other 80% of the particles distribute themselves in the higher traps. In this manner we construct a cutoff. When the sample contains 100 ng/mL, the cotinine molecules bind to the population of particles, effectively decreasing the valence of all particles. The highest-avidity particles have their valence sufficiently altered to lose the ability to bind to trap 1 materials and migrate to trap 2: Likewise, the particles that bind to trap 2 in the absence of cotinine are now altered and migrate further to traps of higher binding strength (Fig. 2).

In order to bind a particle to a low-affinity trap, at least three conditions must be met. There must be a (1) dense display of ligand, (2) with which the particle comes in close contact over (3) a protracted period of time. These conditions are met by conjugating the ligand to a protein and coating the protein on the membrane at high density over a large area, typically 3- to 5-mm bands containing about 5 µg of protein. The laminated strip provides a means of slowing the flow and of ensuring that all fluid is channeled through the coated membrane pores. Visual examination of nonlaminated strips reveals that much of the fluid travels across the surface of the membrane, where it is not in intimate contact with the coating material. A wide coating band and lamination ensure that the particles come in close contact with the trap material over a sustained period of time. It takes a particle more than 20 seconds to traverse a trap.

Traps are constructed from epitope analogs, which are conjugated to carrier protein to form multivalent ligand complexes, which are immobilized on the membrane as "traps." The binding strength of a trap is a function of the intrinsic affinity of the ligand and avidity, which is a function of the density of the ligand on the surface of the membrane and the size of the protein. It is well known that increasing the density of ligand on protein can increase the observed binding strength or "functional affinity" [16]. However it is not as readily recognized that increasing the size of the ligand carrier increases binding strength.

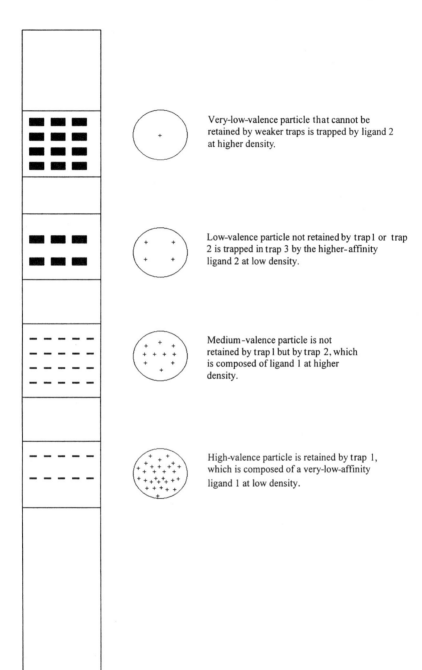

Very-low-valence particle that cannot be retained by weaker traps is trapped by ligand 2 at higher density.

Low-valence particle not retained by trap 1 or trap 2 is trapped in trap 3 by the higher-affinity ligand 2 at low density.

Medium-valence particle is not retained by trap 1 but by trap 2, which is composed of ligand 1 at higher density.

High-valence particle is retained by trap 1, which is composed of a very-low-affinity ligand 1 at low density.

We have demonstrated [23] a 10-fold increase in binding as the size of the particle is increased from IgG to latex-coated IgG.

Unlike competitive assays, the binding capacity of the trap is only very weakly a function of the protein coating concentration of the trap material. Traps are optimized to be coated at excess; that is, the concentration should be sufficiently high that a 50% decrease in trap-coating protein has no effect on performance. The amount of ligand in the trap exceeds the number of binding sites on the particle by 2–3 logs and so the system as constructed is relatively insensitive to variations in concentration of trap material.

The difference between particle valency and a competitive assay is that particle valency is not dependent on a limited amount of trap material or on a limited amount of antibody [24]. The strict limitations on the amounts of antibody and competitor and their ratio to one another are difficult to maintain over the life of the product: In manufacturing, low levels of reagents have to be carefully metered during impregnation of membranes, and further, since the ratios of antibody to competitor are critical for cutoff, these reagents hav to lose potency over time at the same rate.

E. Trap Composition of the Urine NicoMeter^{TM} Test Strip

Table 1 shows the composition of the traps utilized to construct the NicoMeter^{TM} assay.

1. Reland Traps

Trap 1 is designed to lose the ability to retain particles at a cotinine concentration of 100 ng/mL and contains the reland carboxyphenylethyl cotinine (CPC) conjugated to BGG at a conjugation ratio of 6:1. Trap 2, which contains the same reland at a twofold increase in conjugation ratio, can bind those particles displaced from trap 1 and does not lose the ability to retain particles until a concentration of over 0.25 μg/mL. Trap 3 contains the same reland at 25:1 and loses the ability to bind particles at >1000 ng/mL cotinine. This demonstrates the profound effect of avidity on trapping efficiency; i.e., for each doubling of ligand concentration we see an approximate twofold increase in binding

---

←

Figure 2 Principle of particle valency strip assay: The LabTab strip separates and displays particles based on valence. The traps act as sieves, retaining particles above a cutoff valence and allowing particles of lower valence to pass through: antibody-binding site (+); ligand 1 of low affinity (−); ligand 2 of higher affinity (■).

Table 1   Description of Traps for NicoMeter™ Urine

		NicoMeter™ urine
Trap 1	Reland	CPE
	Conjugation ratio to BGG	6.1
Trap 2	Reland	CPE
	Conjugation ratio to BGG	12:1
Trap 3	Reland	CPE
	Conjugation ratio to BGG	25:1
Trap 4	Reland	ICC
	Conjugation ratio to BGG	10:1
Trap 5	Reland	ICC
	Conjugation ratio to BGG	15:1
Trap 6	Reland/Ligand	ICC and C-COT
	Conjugation ratio to BGG	15:1 (ICC)
		60:1 (C-COT)
Trap 7	Immunogen	KLH-Cotinine

strength. Thus the system is very sensitive to the concentration of ligand on carrier but relatively insensitive to the total concentration of trap material.

Traps 4 and 5 utilize a reland of higher affinity for the antibody than CPC, isopropyl carboxy cotinine (ICC) at ratios of 10:1 and 15:1, respectively. Many proteins denature upon binding to solid surfaces [25]. We have observed that the relative affinities of ligands may change between a wet Elisa and a strip format.

2. Traps Composed of Competitive and Supercompetitive (Immunogen) Ligands

To achieve the desired binding strength, trap 6 utilizes a mixture of ICC at 15:1 and carboxy cotinine (C-COT) at 60:1. Carboxy cotinine is a competitive ligand. It may interact with the particle through a high-affinity interaction with a free antibody-binding site that may be partially buried or otherwise have its effective affinity compromised. This is discussed in Section V.

Trap 7 is the immunogen, cotinine conjugated to KLH. In our experience the affinity of the antibody for a hapten carrier immunogen is logs higher than for analyte; hence we refer to this trap material as *supercompetitive*. We will discuss the mechanisms by which this trap provides low-affinity binding in section V.

IV. PERFORMANCE OF NICOMETER™ PARTICLE VALENCY ASSAY

A. Configuration of the NicoMeter™ Strip

There are seven trap zones for the NicoMeter™ urine test (Figs. 1 and 3). If the antibody and traps are functional, the particles must bind at one of the traps; thus NicoMeter™ contains an intrinsic functionality control. When the test is not working, for example, when the pH is below 4 (Table 5), no color develops in any trap.

A LabTab™ test may be read visually or in a reflectometer. The visual thresholds are provided by the disappearance of a trap. At the first NicoMeter™ threshold of 100 ng/mL, trap 1 disappears and trap 2 becomes the lowest red level and the sample is classified as level 2, indicating a cotinine level of between 100 and 250 ng/mL. The strip configuration for visual reading is shown in Figure 3. Figure 4 illustrates the reflectance readings of a prototype NicoMeter™ strip. Note the significant change in particle distribution detectable by simple densitometry at 62 ng/mL of cotinine.

B. Performance of NicoMeter™

We will confine the comments to summarizing a few of the salient performance characteristics. There was 100% agreement on classification into smoker, non-smoker status when we correlated an Elisa method utilizing a 200-ng/mL cutoff with the urine NicoMeter with a 100-ng/mL cutoff. Correlation of actual Elisa cotinine levels to NicoMeter™ urine and saliva levels was $r = 0.95$ (Table 2). The Elisa utilized a polyclonal antibody.

The assay is comparatively unaffected by cross-reactants (Table 3) that commonly interfere in immunoassays for cotinine [26], common urine interferents (Table 4), and pH between 4.5 and 9 (Table 5).

V. DISCUSSION OF THE PHENOMENON OF LOW-AFFINITY BINDING

The ruggedness of the LabTab™ or particle valency format is due to the phenomenon of low-affinity binding, which is mediated through avidity. The multiplicity of contacts needed for the reaction probably provide for correction, and it is this redundancy factor that accounts for the superiority of the particle valency system over competitive and sandwich systems, which rely on one or two contacts for accuracy.

The phenomenon by which relands provide low-affinity binding is understandable in light of the current understanding of avidity. But it does not explain

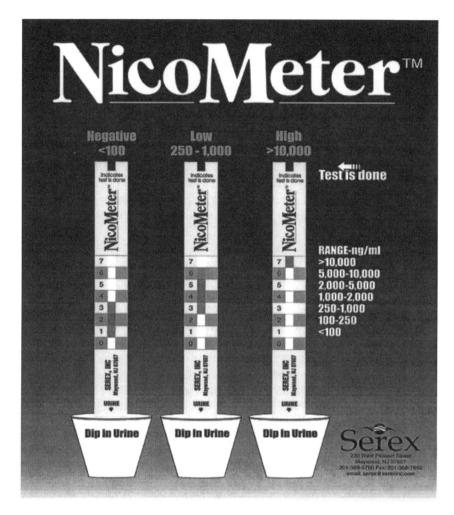

Figure 3 NicoMeter™ urine strip: Urine samples at cotinine levels of 0, 450, and 12,000 ng/mL were tested via NicoMeter™ strips. The design illustrates the expected appearance of the strips for these cotinine levels.

why and how zero-valence particles might be retained by traps synthesized from competitive and supercompetitive ligands.

One possibility is that by virtue of being a supercompetitive ligand it displaces cotinine bound to the zero-valence particle and binds the particle through a high-affinity interaction. While this may explain some of the binding

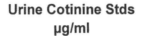

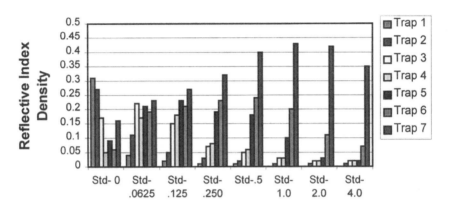

Figure 4 Densitometric reading of prototype urine NicoMeter™ strips: Urine samples at indicated cotinine levels were tested with NicoMeter™. The color of each trap was measured using a Gretag densitometer.

in this trap, examination of the strips indicates that >90% of gold reaching trap 7 is bound. This antibody, MAB #57G9.1, has an Elisa working titer of 1,250,000/mg. In the authors' experience, dissociation does not occur rapidly enough that a zero-valence particle would dissociate sufficient ligand in the less than the 1 minute that it takes a particle to pass through trap 7. After all, this particle does not bind an excess of the same hapten conjugated to BGG in trap 6. The possibility that binding is effected through displacement of the cotinine metabolite, hydroxycotinine, which has lower affinity for 57G9.1, is contraindicated by the observation that 10-μg/mL urine standards that contain only cotinine also bind to this trap.

An alternative explanation is that this antibody, which was raised to KLH–cotinine, contains in its CDR a binding pocket for the cotinine epitope and in addition a number of low-affinity contact residues in the CDR that "recognize" or are complementary to the surface of cotinine–KLH surrounding the cotinine epitope (we suggest calling this area *peritope*). We suggest that these peritope contacts would not be blocked by the binding of a small antigen like cotinine (MW 176) and that a multitude of these low-affinity secondary sites could exercise sufficient binding strength to retain the particles. The number of contact residues in the CDR of an antibody made with a KLH immunogen would be in the expected range of 10–23, and it would not be expected that the

Table 2 Comparison Between NicoMeter™ Urine and Saliva and CotiTraq®

CotiTraq® urine cotinine (ng/mL)	NicoMeter™ urine cotinine (ng/mL)						
	<100	100–250	250–1,000	1,000–2,000	2,000–5,000	5,000–10,000	>10,000
<100	40						
100–250	1	5	1				
250–1,000			1				
1,000–2,000				1			
2,000–5,000				1	3		
5,000–8,000					4	8	
8,000–10,000					1	12	6
>10,000						7	12

CotiTraq® saliva cotinine (ng/mL)	NicoMeter™ saliva cotinine (ng/mL)					
	<30	30–100	100–250	250–750	750–2,000	>2,000
<30 ng/mL	97					
30–100		5				
100–250			2			
250–750			1	2		
750–2,000					2	
>2,000						

103 urine samples and 109 saliva samples were tested in NicoMeter™ urine and saliva strip assays and in the CotiTraq Elisa kit (International Diagnostic Systems, St. Joseph, MI).

binding of cotinine would involve more than three to eight of the residues [8–11]. That means that there are potentially 7–20 contact points in the CDR of 57G9.1 available for interaction with cotinine-KLH, even when cotinine is bound. Thus the interaction between the zero-valence particle and the immunogen trap could be effected through a multitude of very-low-affinity reactions of the peritope with the CDR as well as the avidity of the particle for multivalent ligand. In support of peritope binding we observe that the binding at trap 7 is diffuse, like that seen with low-affinity interactions.

Further, we have left LabTab™ strips in the sample overnight, during which time there is some evaporation from the top so that cotinine-containing sample continues to wick up the strip: We have never observed any change in the distribution of the gold particles, indicating that free cotinine does not displace retained particles at any of the traps. It has been observed that due to the dual effects of affinity and avidity, multivalent interactions at solid surfaces are

Table 3 Cross-Reactivity Study (in Urine)

Cross-reactant	Level (μg/mL)	Visual reading (ng/mL)	% Cross-reactivity
Niacinamide	300	<10	<0.003
Nicotinic acid	300	<10	<0.003
Nicotinic hydrazide	300	<10	<0.003
Isonicotinic hydrazide	300	<10	<0.003
Isonicotinic acid	300	<10	<0.003
Iproniazide phosphate	300	<10	<0.003
Chlorpheniramine	300	<10	<0.003
	1000	<100	<0.03
Metyrapone	300	<100	<0.03
	1000	<100	<0.03
Nicotine	1	<10	<1%
	10	<100	<1%
	25	100–250	<1%
Trans-hydroxy cotinine	0.125	<100	~25%
	0.250	<100	~25%
	0.5	100–250	~25%
	1	250–1000	~25%
	2	250–1000	~25%
	4	250–1000	~25%

Each cross-reactant was spiked into negative urine pool at the indicated levels. Urine samples were assayed by NicoMeter[TM] urine and % cross-reactivity was calculated.

Table 4 Effect of Common Urine Constituents on NicoMeter[TM] Urine

Substance added	Spike level (μg/mL)	NicoMeter reading (100-ng/mL cotinine)	
		Expected	Actual
Glucose	≤500	100–250	100–250
Albumin	≤5000	100–250	100–250
Hemoglobin	≤50	100–250	100–250
Ascorbic acid	≤500	100–250	100–250

A negative urine pool spiked to 100 ng/mL cotinine was spiked to the indicated levels of potential interfering substances.

Table 5   Effect of pH on NicoMeter^{TM} Urine

| pH of Urine | NicoMeter^{TM} urine reading (ng/mL) | |
	Expected	Actual
2	100–250	No color in any trap— "Test result not valid"
3	100–250	<100
4	100–250	<100
4.5	100–250	100–250
5	100–250	100–250
6	100–250	100–250
6.8	100–250	100–250
8	100–250	100–250
9	100–250	100–250
10	100–250	250–1,000

A negative urine pool spiked to 100 ng/mL cotinine was adjusted to indicated pH with 1 M citric acid or 0.5 M sodium carbonate and tested.

virtually irreversible [16]. However, the particle arriving in trap 7 to interact with KLH–cotinine is not a multivalent receptor for cotinine. The antibody sites are saturated with cotinine and the fluid surrounding them at greater than 10 µg/mL certainly contains free cotinine. The antibody is of high affinity and surely has a low dissociation rate. Thus if there is dissociation it would only be limited and not sufficient to make the particle multivalent. If the particle is not multivalent, displacement should be possible and some of the particles retained in traps 6 and 7 should be released by free cotinine. The fact that additional cotinine does not displace gold particles in traps 6 and 7 indicates that the binding energy for the reaction may not be cotinine.

An observation that is explained by the peritope binding theory has been previously reported [20]. Briefly, it was demonstrated that a rabbit polyclonal antibody raised to the beta subunit of human chorionic gonadotropin (hCG) could be purified on a low-affinity column that consisted of sheep pituitary fractions containing LH, FSH, and TSH. The subunits of hCG, LH, FSH, and TSH are homologous [27]. Binding was sufficiently low that it could be disrupted by pH 5 elution buffer. We would propose that retention of the beta anti-hCG could be explained through peritope interactions that resulted because of shared structural features between the subunits of the sheep pituitary hormones and the immunogen, beta subunit of hCG.

VI. CONCLUSIONS

What is most remarkable about the LabTab™ system is its ruggedness. It is relatively insensitive to reagent quantities impregnated on the strip. Its performance is very accurate and consistent, even though it utilizes unmeasured quantities of the bodily fluids urine and saliva, which are generally considered problematic matrices. It is not affected by pH from 4.5 to 9. It shows no cross-reactivity >1% with any nicotine metabolite but hydroxycotinine, with which it shows 25% reactivity (this clone was selected for its ability to bind hydroxycotinine). It is not affected by any common interferents, even at very high levels.

Ruggedness is probably a function of redundancy. We believe that the redundancy in the phenomenon of avidity binding through low-affinity contacts confers ruggedness upon the LabTab™ system. Interestingly, the first response of the immune system to an invasion is a low- (10^3 M^{-1}) affinity interaction with antibody-coated cells in a system in which multiple interactions of low affinity produces reactivity while protecting from spurious response [28]. It would appear that, serendipitously, we have developed an assay format that is analogous to this phenomenon.

REFERENCES

1. J. Fitzpatrick, R. B. Lenda. Chromatographic immunoassay device and method utilizing particle valency for quantitation. PCT/US97/05077, March 20, 1997.
2. J. Fitzpatrick, R. B. Lenda. Differential binding affinities and dissociation assays based thereon. U.S. patent 5,527,686, June 18, 1996.
3. J. Fitzpatrick, R. B. Lenda. Receptor: Release Ligand (Reland) Complexes and Release Assays Using Said Reland and Methods and Kits Based Thereon. U.S. patent 5,710,009, Jan. 20, 1998.
4. A. Cocola, A. Orlandini, G. Barbarulli, P. Tarli, P. Neri. Release Radioimunoassay: Description of a new method and its application to the determination of Human Chorionic Somatomammotropin plasma levels. Analytical Biochemistry 99:121–128 (1979).
5. W. J. Freytag. Immunoassay wherein labeled antibody is displaced from immobilized analyte-analog. U.S. patent 4,434,236, Feb. 28, 1984.
6. J. A. Hinds, C. F. Pincombe, S. Smith, P. Duffy. Ligand displacement immunoassay—demonstration of its use for the measurement of serum phenobarbial and phenytoin. Clin. Chem. Acta 149:105–115 (1985).
7. W. J. Freytag, S. Chang. Heterogeneous immunoassay for digoxin using ouabain as a separation means. U.S. patent 4,551,426, Nov. 5, 1985.
8. D. R. Davies, E. A. Padlan, S. Sheriff. Antibody–antigen complexes. Annu. Rev. Biochem. 59:439–473 (1990).

9. L. Jin, B. M. Fendly, J. A. Wells. High-resolution functional analysis of antibody–antigen interactions. J. Mol. Biol 226:851–865 (1992).

10. R. F. Kelley, M. P. O'Connell. Thermodynamic analysis of an antibody functional epitope. Biochem. 32:6828–6835 (1993).

11. T. Clackson, J. A. Wells. A hot spot of binding energy in hormone–receptor interface. Science 267:383–386 (1995).

12. J. M. Nuss, P. B. Witaker, G. M. Air. Identification of critical contact residues in the NC41 epitope of a subtype N9 influenza virus neuraminidase. Proteins 15: 121–132 (1993).

13. J. M. Rini, U. Schulze-Gahmen, I. A. Wilson. Structural evidence for induced fit as a mechanism for antibody–antigen recognition. Science 255:959 (1992).

14. W. R. Tulip, V. R. Harley, R. G. Webster, J. Novotny. N9 neuraminidase complexes with antibodies Nc41 and NC10: empirical free energy calculations capture specificity trends observed with mutant binding data. Biochem. 33:7986–7997 (1994).

15. G. J. Wedemayer, P. A. Patten, L. H. Wang, P. G. Schultz, R. C. Stevens. Structural insights into the evolution of an antibody combining site. Science 276:1665–1669 (1997).

16. J. E. Butler. Perspectives, configurations and principles. In: Immunochemistry of Solid Phase Immunoassay (J. E. Butler, ed.). CRC Press, Boca Raton, FL, 1991, p. 16.

17. B. C. Cunningham, J. A. Wells. Comparison of a structural and a functional epitope. J. Mol. Biol. 234:554–563 (1993).

18. M. Stenberg, H. Nygren. Kinetics of antigen–antibody reactions at solid–liquid interfaces. J. Imm. Methods 113:3 (1988).

19. C. P. Price, G. H. G. Thorpe, J. Hall, R. A. Bunce. Disposable integrated immunoassay devices. In: Principles and Practice of Immunoassay, 2nd ed. (C. P. Price and D. J. Newman, eds.) Macmillan Reference, London, 1997, p. 581.

20. J. Fitzpatrick. Purification of antisera to beta human chorionic gonadotropin by a low-affinity chromatography technique. Clin. Chem. 32:1157 (1986).

21. P. Baudhuin, P. Van Der Smissen, S. Beauvois, P. J. Courtoy. Molecular interactions between colloidal gold, proteins, and living cells. In: Colloidal Gold: Principles, Methods, and Applications (M. A. Hayat, ed.), Academic Press, New York, 1989, p. 8.

22. F. V. Lee-Own, J. Fitzpatrick. An integrated packaging holder device for immunochromatographic assays in flow-through or dipstick formats. U.S. patent 5,500,375, March 19, 1996.

23. J. Fitzpatrick, R. B. Lenda. Chromatographic immunoassay device and method utilizing particle valency for quantitation, PCT/US97/05077, Fig. 6.

24. J. Fitzpatrick, R. B. Lenda. Method and device for detecting the presence of analyte in a sample, U.S. patent 5,451,504, Sept. 19, 1995.

25. M. H. V. Van Regenmortel. The antigen–antibody reaction in principles and practice of immunoassay. 2nd ed. (C. P. Price and D. J. Newman, eds.), Macmillan Reference, London, 1997.

26. G. Schepers, R. Walk. Cotinine determination by immunoassays may be influenced by other nicotine metabolites. Toxicology 62:395 (1988).

27. B. C. Nisula, G. S. Taliadouros, P. Carayon. Primary and secondary biologic activities intrinsic to the human chorionic gonadotropin molecule. In: Chrorionic Gonadotropin. (S. J. Segal, ed.) Plenum Press, New York, 1980, p. 25.

29. J. Banchereau, R. M. Steinman. Dendritic cells and the control of immunity, Nature 382:245–251 (1998).

16

"Smart" Materials for Colorimetric Detection of Pathogenic Agents

Quan Cheng
University of California Riverside, Riverside, California, U.S.A.

Raymond C. Stevens
The Scripps Research Institute, La Jolla, California, U.S.A.

I. INTRODUCTION

In cellular communication, receptors that are strategically localized in the cell plasma membrane recognize and respond specifically to the target molecules. Mimicking cell membrane biomolecular recognition poses a great challenge in materials chemistry research and opens the doors to innovation of new diagnostic and therapeutic methods for biomedical purposes. One effective approach has been engineering artificial cell membranes with desirable physical properties, i.e., optical or electrical "reporting" capability [1]. These so-called "smart" materials, similar in structure to the cell membrane of living cells, are able to transduce biological molecular recognition events occurring at the surface of the material into measurable signals. We are particularly interested in the artificial membranes of polydiacetylene (PDA) lipids and have been focusing on utilizing the engineered PDA materials to construct novel sensors. It has been shown that self-assembly of the amphiphilic diacetylenic molecules occurs by the same entropic driving force that results in the formation of biological cell membranes and vesicles [2]. Once the monomers are assembled into an ordered array, they can be polymerized by UV irradiation into a blue-colored polydiacetylene polymer [3–5]. The incorporated receptors in the PDA matrix bind the target materials at the surface of the materials. The biomolecular recognition triggers a chromatic phase transition in the engineered membranes, and thus provides colorimetric detection of the target molecules. Such a detection strategy allows molecular recognition and optical reporting to occur within a single macromolecular assembly. Featuring simplicity of design and good sensitivity, this approach offers a new and general method toward direct, one-step colorimetric detection of a variety of pathogenic agents [6].

II. DESIGN OF SUPRAMOLECULAR BIOSENSING ASSEMBLIES

The flexibility in the chemistry and the architecture of the self-assembling materials allows investigation of a variety of design strategies for the colorimetric sensors. Figure 1 shows the general sensor structure developed using engineered biomaterials. There are two major components linked together in the design: a biological sensing element that recognizes target molecules, and a physical transducer that ultimately translates molecular recognition into a measurable signal. The biosensing element may be receptors, enzymes, or antibody, while the signal transducer is the biochromic-ready PDA. Polydiacetylene matrices have been used in two molecular architectures so far: thin Langmuir–Blodgett (LB) films on solid glass support, and liposomes in solution. In addition to the two supramolecular architectures, two different approaches can be used to functionalize the surface of the assembly. In one case, the diacetylenic monomer lipid is derivatized directly with the appropriate receptor via synthetic coupling. This allows direct cross-linking of the "receptor lipid" with the surrounding PDA matrix. Binding affinity or ligand stability can be controlled by means of suitable modification of the receptor structure. Another approach avoids potentially complex synthetic steps. It has been shown that covalent cross-linking between the chromophore and the receptor is not essential to generate the chromatic transition on ligand binding; a receptor molecule can be noncovalently incorporated into the PDA matrix in a manner analogous to the heterogeneous mixing of molecules in cell membranes [6].

The "reporting" element polydiacetylenes come from polymerization of diacetylene lipids in the solid state by a 1,4 addition mechanism when irradiated by 254-nm ultraviolet (UV) light [3]. The resulting polymer is intensely blue, arising from the conjugated backbone that absorbs the visible light wavelengths. Color changes of polydiacetylenes have been known to occur in response to a variety of environmental perturbations, such as increased temperature [7], pH [8], or mechanical stress [9] (Fig. 2). UV-vis spectroscopy studies reveal that the blue-phase PDA yields an absorption maximum at ~630 nm, while the red form exhibits a peak absorption around 550 nm [10]. The precise mechanism of the blue-to-red color transitions is not completely understood yet, and most likely varies between different methods of inducing the transition (temperature,

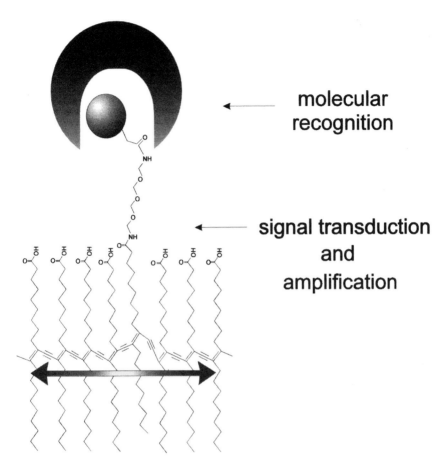

molecular recognition

signal transduction and amplification

Figure 1 Schematic illustration of the "smart" biosensor with engineered artificial cell membrane materials.

stress, pH, or affinity). It has been postulated that the blue-to-red color transition arises from changes in the conjugation length and bond angle of the polydiacetylene backbone [11]. Theoretical and experimental evidence suggests that small conformational changes in the polymer side chains affect the electronic properties of the polymer backbone [12]. Theoretical calculations predict that as little as a 5° rotation about the C—C backbone bond could account for the observed changes in the electronic structure of the backbone [13]. Here we show that biological interactions can be an effective driving force to induce the blue-to-red phase transition (biochromic induction).

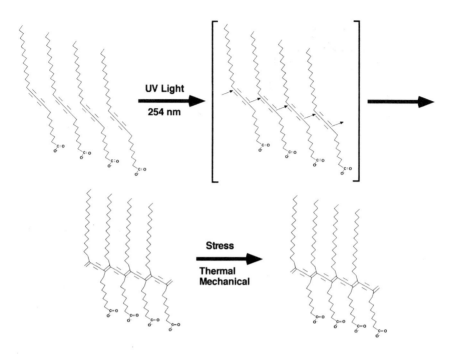

Figure 2 Mechanism of 10,12-pentacosadiynoic acid polymerization and color change.

III. COLORIMETRIC DETECTION OF NEUROTOXINS AND VIRUSES

As discussed previously, the lipid-linked receptors can be incorporated directly into the artificial macromolecular assembly to construct specific sensors. Gangliosides, a family of molecules that reside on the cell surface of neurons, provide a suitable system to demonstrate this approach. Gangliosides are located in the plasma membrane of cells and have a carbohydrate recognition group attached to the extracellular surface [14]. The lipid anchors the carbohydrate into the cell membrane. For our application, the lipid moiety allows incorporation of the molecule into the artificial PDA assemblies or liposomes. Two representative members of this family are the GT1b and GM1 gangliosides (Fig. 3, compounds 4, 5). The GM1 gangliosides, located on the surface of intestinal cells, are the primary target of cholera toxin (the toxin responsible for the disease cholera) [15]. The GT1b gangliosides are located at the neuromuscular junction and are the primary target of botulinum neurotoxin (the neurotoxin responsible for botulism) [16].

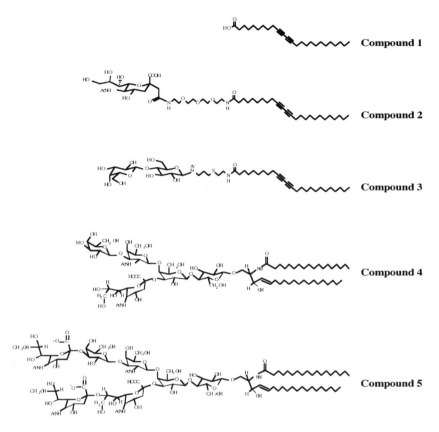

Figure 3 Lipids and lipid-linked cell surface moieties used in the design of colorimetric sensors of biologic agents. Compound 1 is the matrix lipid 10,12-pentacosadynoic acid (PDA). PDA derivatized with sialic acid (compound 2) or lactose (compound 3) is used as a "promoter" molecule in the sensor assembly. The gangliosides GM1 (compound 4) and GT1b (compound 5) are receptors used for molecular recognition.

The schematic diagram of a thin-film colorimetric sensor for neurotoxins is illustrated in Figure 4. The chromatic unit of this sensor is composed of PDA (Fig. 3, compound 1) and "promoter" molecule. The function of the "promoter" PDA is not fully understood, but it is essential to produce the chromatic transition in the toxin-binding experiments. We postulate that the "promoter" PDA lowers the activation barrier of the chromatic transition. The promoter probably changes lipid packing, altering the effective conjugated length of the backbone, or it may provide a connection between the nonconjugated receptor and the

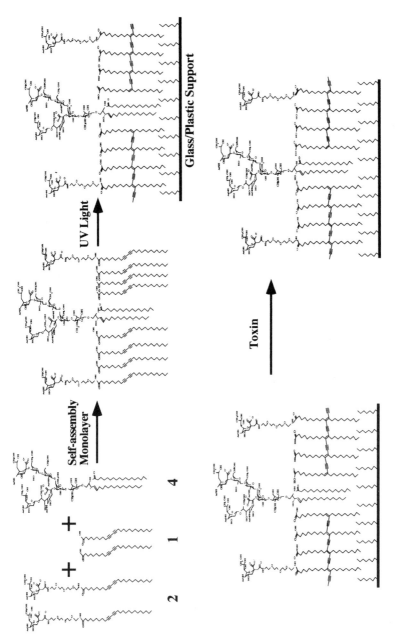

Figure 4 Construction of heterogeneously polymerized thin-film assemblies for the detection of toxins. Films were assembled from a starting solution of an organic mixed solvent (chloroform:methanol 2:1) containing 2–5% sialic acid– or lactose-derivatized PDA (compound 2 or 3), 90–93% PDA (compound 1), and 5% ganglioside GM1 or GT1b (compound 4 or 5). After polymerization, the film displays a steady blue color, but upon exposure to toxin the film turns red.

conjugated backbone, enabling the neurotoxin to induce the colorimetric transition. The promoter molecule used in these investigations is a sialic acid– or lactose-derivatized PDA lipid (Fig. 3, compounds 2, 3). It should be noted that in this case, the derivatized lipid is used to modify the film's optical properties and not as a molecular recognition site. The polydiacetylene bioassembly containing only sialic acid–derivatized PDA (or lactose-derivatized PDA) does not respond to the neurotoxins used in this study, indicating that there is insufficient interaction between the neurotoxins and the derivatized diacetylene lipid to induce the color change.

To self-assemble the most sensitive layers to detect toxin binding, typically a mole ratio of 90% PDA, 5% sialic acid–derivatized PDA, and 5% ganglioside lipid is used. If more than 5% ganglioside is used, polymerization is reduced to such an extent that the films are of poor optical quality, most likely due to steric hindrance of the solid-state polymerization. For films containing the lactose promoter lipid, it was found that too high a concentration of lactose-derivatized PDA (>5%) led to unstable films that turned red upon exposure to buffer solutions. In optimal conditions, the self-assembled monolayer of 2% lactose-derivatized PDA, 5% ganglioside, and 93% PDA resulted in a blue-to-red color change when the film is incubated specifically with cholera toxin.

The biosensors obtained through this scheme exhibit the characteristic blue-to-red color change and can be quantified by visible absorption spectroscopy (Fig. 5). For example, the blue-colored film has an absorption maximum of ~630 nm and a weaker absorption at ~550 nm. After incubation with the target analyte, a dramatic change in the visible spectrum occurs. The maximum at ~550 nm increases, with a concurrent decrease in the maximum at ~630 nm, and the film appears red. The color change can be quantified by calculation of the colorimetric response (CR) by measuring the relative change in the percentage of the intensity at ~630 nm relative to the intensity at ~550 nm [10].

To determine the sensitivity of the biosensors to target analyte, the response of the sensor (CR) as a function of analyte concentration was determined (Fig. 5c). It was found that the CR is directly proportional to the quantity of target analyte. For the GM1-containing biosensor, the colorimetric response to cholera toxin rises steeply at low toxin concentration, then levels out at higher concentration, indicating that the surface binding sites are saturated (Fig. 5c). The low detection limit corresponds to a sensitivity of approximately 1×10^{-10} M. The absolute sensitivity of the lactose-derivatized PDA doped film is slightly lower than that of films containing sialic acid promoter lipid, due to the higher background level in the presence of buffer only (CR = 7% for lactose-PDA; CR = 5% for sialic acid–PDA). Similar results are seen using the GT1b ganglioside biosensors for botulinum neurotoxin, and using the GM1 ganglioside biosensor for *E. coli* enterotoxin.

(a)

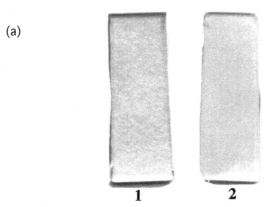

(b)

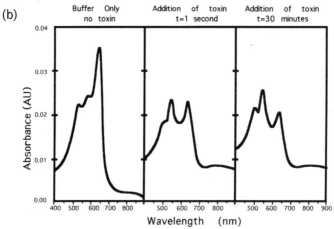

(c)

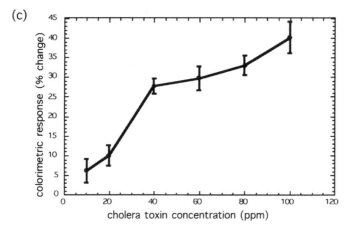

To demonstrate that incorporation of GM1 into the biosensor assembly did not compromise the GM1–cholera toxin interaction, the supramolecular array was self-assembled onto a gold chip, and the interaction was measured by surface plasmon resonance using a BiaCore 2000 instrument. The binding affinity (K_a) of cholera toxin to the GM1 biosensor was determined to be 3×10^{10} M^{-1} [17], in agreement with the published values observed in vivo [15]. This suggests that GM1 incorporated into the artificial membrane behaves similarly to GM1 on the surface of living cells.

To evaluate selectivity of the sensor material, a series of experiments was carried out to confirm that the functionalized polydiacetylene assemblies are specific to the biotarget. For example, *E. coli* cell lysate, bovine serum albumin (BSA), pertussis toxin, diphtheria toxin, and various buffers at different salt and pH conditions produce a background CR of approximately 5%; the highest background was seen using BSA. These results define the level of nonspecific adhesion and, therefore, the minimum detection limit. Low levels of toxin yield CRs that are significantly above the background level.

A much higher concentration of polymerized material can be achieved with liposome solutions, compared to monolayer assemblies, due to their greater cross-sectional density. This approach has the advantage of making the color change more visually striking and increasing the colorimetric response. The liposomes are prepared from starting monomers similar to those that would be used for thin-film assembly, and typically via a probe sonication method. The optical absorption properties of the liposomes are controllable to a certain extent by the polymerization time [18]. An influenza virus biosensor is described here as an example to demonstrate the construction of liposome-based sensor. The sialic acid–derivatized PDA, a wholly synthetic cell membrane-like structure, is used and cross-linked into the PDA matrix. Influenza virus binds to this assembly via the viral hemagglutinin (HA) lectin. The HA binds to terminal α-glycosides of sialic acid on cell surface glycoproteins and glycolipids [19,20], initiating cell infection by the virus [21]. The bifunctional sialic acid–derivatized PDA incorporates both the sialic acid ligand for viral binding and the diacetylenic

---

Figure 5 Colorimetric, spectrophotometric, and titration data for cholera toxin biosensor with the GM1 ganglioside. (a) The untreated GM1 sensor placed on silanized glass cover slides (left) is blue, but minutes after exposure to 40-ppm cholera toxin is red. (b) UV-vis spectra of 5% GM1, 5% sialic acid–PDA, 90% PDA sensor before (left) and after (middle, immediately after; right, 30 min after) exposure to 40-ppm cholera toxin. (c) Plot of colorimetric response of the biosensor used in (b) as a function of cholera toxin concentration, in ppm. Each point in the graph is the average value of four measurements, with the standard deviation as the error.

functionality in the hydrocarbon chain for polymerization. The carbon–glyco-side in this compound was designed into the structure to prevent hydrolysis by viral neuraminidase. Optimal sialic acid–derivatized PDA sensors are composed of 5–10% sialic acid lipid and 90–95% matrix lipid. The amount of virus that can be detected above the background is 8 HAUs (1 HAU is defined as the highest dilution of stock virus that completely agglutinates a standard erythrocyte suspension [22]; 8 HAUs corresponds to $\sim 8 \times 10^7$ virus particles [23]). It seems that the virus liposome sensors produce a higher response than the thin-film sensors. Typically, the liposome sensors have CR% values of $\sim 80\%$, relative to typical thin-film CR% values for virus and toxins of $\sim 30\%$. This may be a result of the greater accessibility of the ligand lipid in the liposome assembly, compared to the thin films, or the larger number of molecules in a liposome solution relative to a monolayer assembly on a solid support. A similar, liposome-based toxin sensor composed of PDA lipids with varied diacetylene position has recently been demonstrated by Charych and coworkers [24].

IV. COLORIMETRIC SENSORS FOR GLUCOSE

Colorimetric detection has been effective in the construction of sensors capable of detecting large pathogenic agents such as cholera toxin and influenza virus. In these two examples, the cell surface receptor was embedded or synthetically coupled to the polydiacetylene sensing interfaces. Upon binding, the target agents attempt to merge with, or insert into, the cell membranes. Relying on mechanical stress provoked by the toxin or virus itself, these sensors, however, are limited to detecting molecules capable of directly disrupting the PDA assembly. We extended the biosensing capability of the PDA-based sensors by utilizing the ligand-induced conformational changes of an enzyme (hexokinase) immobilized on the sensor surface. The conformational changes, caused by the binding of the small-molecule glucose to the enzyme-active site, are coupled to the polymeric backbone, ultimately providing detection of glucose colorimetrically [25].

Hexokinase is a ubiquitous metabolic enzyme that catalyzes the transfer of a phosphoryl group from ATP to glucose to form glucose-6-phosphate [26]. It is composed of 457 amino acids (MW ~ 51000), 17 of which are lysine residues located on the outside surface of the protein molecule. Upon binding glucose, the enzyme undergoes a large conformational change [27]. The two domains that form the active site move together in jawlike fashion to capture the glucose molecule. The movement of one domain relative to the other is approximately 8 Å, as determined by X-ray crystallography [28]. Coupling the conformational change of the enzyme to the chromatic unit of the PDA film is achieved through protein amine coupling. Figure 6 shows the architecture of

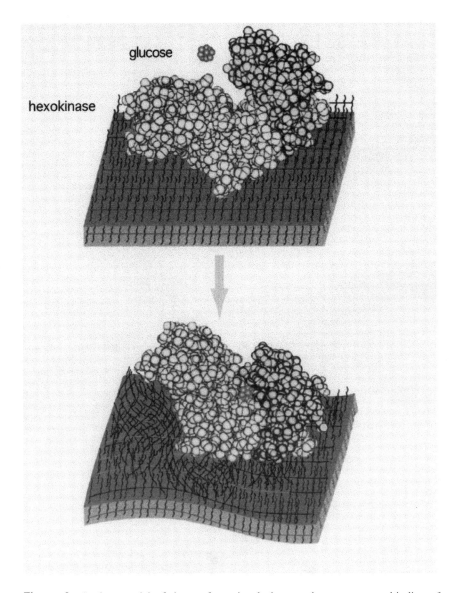

Figure 6 Surface model of the conformational changes that occur upon binding of glucose to the enzyme hexokinase. Upon binding glucose, the enzyme closes up around the substrate glucose. The two domains move approximately 8 Å closer to one another and rotate 12° relative to one another. The hexokinase is coupled to the derivatized diacetylene lipid through amine coupling to the free lysine residues of hexokinase. The dimensions of hexokinase are approximately 71 Å × 46 Å × 46 Å. The length of the lipid molecule is approximately 23 Å.

the hexokinase-conjugated PDA polymer on the solid substrate. The covalent immobilization of the hexokinase onto the surface of PDA monolayers occurs in a multimeric fashion (i.e., a single hexokinase molecule is cross-linked to multiple lipid molecules in the array). This approach is achieved through amidization between the protein surface lysine residues and the N-hydroxysuccinimide (NHS) head group of the derivatized PDA.

The preparation of stable PDA monolayer films before enzyme immobilization is critical for low background and enhanced reproducibility of the sensors. The Langmuir monolayer trough provides a method to measure film stability through the evaluation of the surface collapse pressure of the monolayers. We found that the mixed films appear to be much stabler than the monolayers consisting of one component, and thus more suitable for enzyme immobilization. For instance, the collapse pressure for 1:1 NHS-PDA/PDA monolayer at 5°C is 57 mN/m, while NHS-PDA and PDA monolayers collapse at 34 and 28 mN/m, respectively. Similar observations were reported in some fatty acid/ester isotherms [29]. It is suggested that interactions are more favorable in these mixed monolayers, presumably due to the optimal spatial arrangements that allow head groups of different size to pack closely.

Besides mechanical stability, the monolayers should possess desirable optical properties (i.e., high color intensity) to be suitable as sensors. Film quality—in this particular case, color intensity—was studied at different deposition pressures. It was found that films made at 40 mN/m gave the best transfer rate and color intensity. Therefore, the 1:1 NHS-PDA/PDA films obtained at this transfer pressure were selected for modification with hexokinase.

For the colorimetric measurements, the UV-vis spectra were first recorded in 0.1 M phosphate buffer (pH 6.5) and considered as background. Addition of glucose, or other sugar substitutes, occurred directly in the cuvettes. We found that addition of glucose provokes an immediate response, as reflected in the increase in peak at 550 nm. The response increases with time, reaching its peak at 60 min. The colorimetric response (CR) is 5.2, 13.7, and 17.1% for $t = 0.02$, 30, and 60 min, respectively. The color change is irreversible under the current study conditions. The selectivity of the glucose sensor was studied using sugar compounds structurally similar to glucose (Fig. 7). Addition of 10.0 mM sorbitol, galactose, and sucrose does not trigger the sensor, suggesting that the sensor is very specific to glucose. To further examine the mechanism of activation of the sensor, a PDA monolayer without immobilized hexokinase was tested. No significant response was observed, because the CR at $t = 60$ min is comparable to the background of the hexokinase-conjugated PDA monolayer (Fig. 7). This result demonstrates that glucose cannot by itself induce the color change in the PDA films. The presence of immobilized hexokinase is required to allow the sensor to respond to glucose.

It is worth noting that the CRs for glucose using hexokinase-immobilized

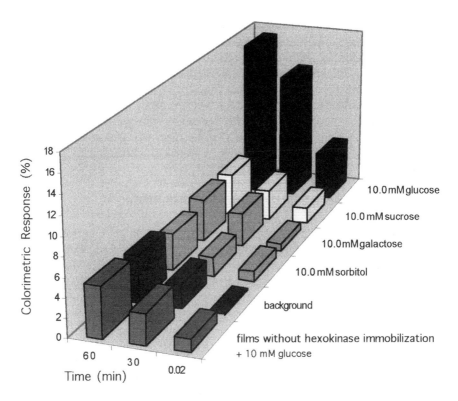

Figure 7 Colorimeric response (CR) of the hexokinase—immobilized PDA sensors for glucose and other compounds used as controls. All tests are made in 0.1 M phosphate buffer (pH 6.5). The last column on the left represents the glucose agitation on the PDA monolayers without immobilized hexokinase. The number of samplings (n) for the glucose is $n = 6$ and for the rest is $n = 3$.

PDA films are much smaller compared to those for cholera toxin and other neurotoxins. Aside from the fact that toxins and viruses are much larger ligands, there are probably differences in the mechanism of color change. Cholera toxin, for example, is a pentamer consisting of five binding domains and a translocation domain [30]. Cholera toxin's inducement of color change in PDA films may occur via two coherent steps: (1) The multiple interactions between the binding domains of the toxin and the receptor GM1 embedded in the PDA monolayers perturb the PDA array (by "tugging" at multiple sites in the array) and cause the chromatic transition; (2) the translocation domain may be further inserted into the membrane, similar to the entry of toxin into cells, disrupting the lateral interactions of the lipid head groups as well as the core of the PDA array. In contrast, the glucose sensor relies solely on the 8-Å conformational change of hexokinase, and this perturbation may be less severe than that resulting from the invasion of a toxin or virus. Therefore, to make the enzyme-linked PDA sensors more sensitive, additional forms of interactions and/or amplification should be added to the sensor design whenever they are approachable.

Although a number of more effective sensors for glucose are available, the choice of hexokinase and glucose as first targets serves as a demonstration that this type of sensor design is feasible; a protein conformational change can be used as a trigger mechanism for a low-cost solid-state sensor.

V. CONCLUDING REMARKS AND FUTURE WORK

Induction of colorimetric transition in polydiacetylenes by biological molecular recognition is a very recent phenomenon. Fundamental investigations on the optical properties and applications of these bioconjugated polymers in molecular electronics and sensors are now just beginning. However, the simplicity of design and litmus-type detection mechanism has gained the PDA assemblies considerable ground as popular prototypes of an attractive alternative in the detection of biological agents. In addition, the unique integration of a signal transduction component with biomolecular recognition may allow miniaturization of the device and eventually multichannel, simultaneous detection in a manner similar to that used in gene chip technology. Nevertheless, several concerns need to be addressed before massive, commercial sensors become available. These include overall sensitivity, inconsistency of the initial state, and film stability. Recent research in our lab has been directed at tackling the sensitivity problem by derivatizing the PDA lipids with favorable hydrophilic head groups. Significant improvements in liposome formation and color development have been obtained [31]. Stability study with a focus on monolayer morphology and domain formation for derivatized PDA was achieved with assistance of epifluorescent microscopy [32]. All the research seems to indicate that many exciting advances are expected as this field continues to grow. The marriage of colorimetric biomaterials with biological recognition elements has the potential of yielding enormous applications for a wide array of substrates using this basic sensor design.

REFERENCES

1. Charych, D.; Nagy, J. O. CHEMTECH 26:24, 1996.
2. Lipowsky, R. Nature 349:475, 1991.
3. Bloor, D.; Chance, R. R. Polydiacetylenes: NATO ASI Series E; Applied Science. Martin Nijhoff, 1985.

4. Day, D.; Ringsdorf, H. J. Polym. Sci. Polym. Lett. Ed. 16:205, 1978.
5. Tieke, B.; Lieser, G. J. Colloid Interface Sci. 88:471, 1982.
6. Charych, D.; Cheng, Q.; Reichert, A.; Kuziemko, G.; Stroh, M.; Nagy, J. O.; Spevak, W.; Stevens, R. C. Chem. Biol. 3:113, 1996.
7. Kuriyama, K.; Kikuchi, H.; Kajiyama, T. Chem. Lett. 1071, 1995.
8. Mino, N.; Tamura, H.; Ogawa, K. Langmuir 7:2336, 1991.
9. Rubner, M. F. Macromolecules 19:2129, 1986.
10. Charych, D.; Nagy, J. O.; Spevak, W.; Bednarski, M. D. Science 261:585, 1993.
11. Exarhos, G. J.; Risen, W. M. J.; Baughman, R. H. J. Am. Chem. Soc. 98:481, 1976.
12. Dobrosavljevic, V.; Stratt, R. M. Phys. Rev. B. 35:2781, 1987.
13. Orchard, B. J. & Tripathy, S. K. Macromolecules 19:1844, 1986.
14. Svennerholm, L. Life Sci. 55:2125, 1994.
15. Cuatrecasas, P. Biochemistry 12:3547, 1973.
16. Ledeen, R. W. In: Gangliosides: Structure, Isolation, and Function (Ed. Yu, R. K.). Plenum Press, New York, 1982.
17. Kuziemko, G. M.; Dtroh, M.; Stevens, R. C. Biochemistry 35:6375, 1996.
18. Spevak, W.; Nagy, J. O.; Charych, D.; Schaefer, M. E.; Gilbert, J. H.; Bednaski, M. D. J. Am. Chem. Soc. 115:1146, 1995.
19. Paulson, J. C. In: The Receptors (Ed. M. Conn). Academic Press, New York, 1985.
20. Wiley, D. C.; Skehel, J. J. Annu. Rev. Biochem. 56:365, 1987.
21. White, J.; Kielian, M.; Helenius, A. Q. Rev. Biophys. 16:151, 1983.
22. WHO Tech. Rep. Ser. Expert Committee on Influenza, 1953.
23. Mahy, J. W. B. Virology, A Practical Approach. IRL Press, Washington, DC, 1985.
24. Pan, J. J.; Charych, D. Langmuir 13:1365, 1997.
25. Cheng, Q.; Stevens, R. C. Adv. Mater. 9:481, 1997.
26. Kosow, D. P.; Rose, I. A. J. Biol. Chem. 246:2618, 1971.
27. Kraulis, P. J. J. Appl. Cryst. 24:946, 1991.
28. Bennett, W. S.; Steitz, T. A. Proc. Natl. Acad. Sci. USA 75:4848, 1978.
29. Birdi, K. S. Lipid and Biopolymer Monolayers at Liquid Interfaces. Plenum Press, New York, 1988, Ch 4, p. 57.
30. Merritt, E. A.; Sarfaty, S.; Van Den Akker, F.; L'Hoir, C.; Martial, J. A.; Hol, W. G. J. Protein Sci. 3:166, 1994.
31. Cheng, Q.; Stevens, R. C. Langmuir 14:1974, 1998.
32. Cheng, Q.; Fu, J. A.; Burkard, R.; Wang, W.; Yamamoto, M.; Yang, J.; Stevens, R. C. Thin Solid Films. In press.

17

Reagentless Diagnostics:
Near-IR Raman Spectroscopy

Irving Itzkan and Michael S. Feld
*Massachusetts Institute of Technology, Cambridge,
Massachusetts, U.S.A.*

Tae-Woong Koo
Intel Corporation, Santa Clara, California, U.S.A.

Andrew J. Berger
University of Rochester, Rochester, New York, U.S.A.

Gary L. Horowitz
Beth Israel Deaconess Medical Center, Boston, Massachusetts, U.S.A.

I. INTRODUCTION

Blood analyte concentrations are important information for making medical judgments. Glucose concentration is a critical indicator for diabetes; urea for kidney problems; cholesterol for cardiovascular problems; bilirubin for treating premature babies. Optical methods are relatively new techniques for blood analysis. In many optical methods, direct photon interaction with blood chemicals is measured, and thus reagentless blood analysis is possible [6].

II. RAMAN SPECTROSCOPY

The ability of Raman spectroscopy to perform blood analyte measurements was studied. Raman spectroscopy gives information about molecular vibrations by measuring the wavelength shift of a photon caused by inelastic scattering. Thus the Raman spectrum from a specific molecule is unique.

When an incident photon of frequency ω_i is directed on a sample, in most cases a photon of the same wavelength is emitted. In Raman scattering, the emitted photon gives up energy to a vibrational mode of the molecule and thus has a frequency ω_s, which is different from the frequency ω_i of the incident photon (Figs. 1 and 2). Although this is a rare event, with a probability of 10^{-6} to 10^{-8}, it can be readily measured by present-day sensitive equipment. The frequency shift $\Delta\omega$ equals the vibrational frequency of the molecule.

$$\Delta\omega = \omega_i - \omega_s$$

The spontaneous Raman spectrum is a linear combination of the spectra of each chemical component. This is important in quantitative analysis, because the linearity allows the use of linear multivariate calibration techniques. The calibration technique will be discussed later.

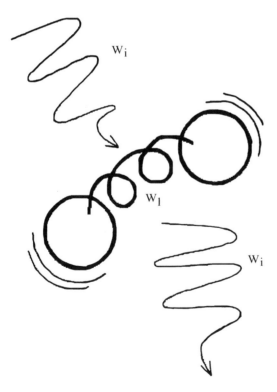

Figure 1 Schematic diagram of inelastic scattering.

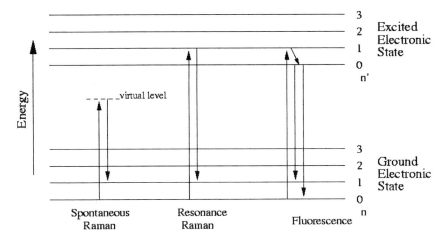

Figure 2 Idealized energy level diagram of electronic states in a molecular system. Levels (0, 1, 2, 3, . . .) in ground and first excited states represent vibrational levels.

A. Excitation Wavelength Selection: Near Infrared

There are four issues in selecting an optimal excitation wavelength for Raman spectroscopy. The first is fluorescence background generation. One of the challenges in applying a Raman technique is that the signal we are looking for is very small compared with the background. It is critical to minimize any fluorescence background and its associated shot noise. In biological systems, as a rule the nearer the excitation wavelength is to the visible, the bigger the fluorescence background; therefore, the further we can operate in the infrared, the better.

The second issue is penetration depth. Penetration depth is important for transcutaneous measurements as well as for determining sampling volume. If the penetration depth is short, the chemical signal for which we are looking may be from the wrong tissue. We are planning to apply this technique to transcutaneous measurements, so the penetration depth should be long enough to penetrate the depth of skin. The two major absorbers in the human body are water and hemoglobin. There is a wavelength "window" between 700 nm and 1300 nm in which the absorption of these absorbers allows for deep penetration (Fig. 3).

The third issue is the intensity of the Raman signal. The intensity of the Raman signal decreases with increasing excitation wavelength, approximately as λ^3 [3].

The fourth issue is detector sensitivity. The quantum efficiency of a charge-coupled device (CCD) array decreases at longer wavelengths. Silicon-based

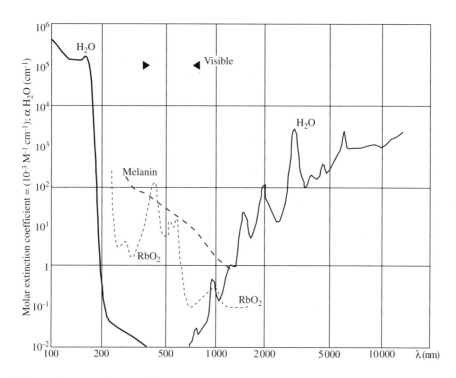

Figure 3 Absorption coefficients for water; molar extinction coefficients for hemoglobin and melanin.

CCD detectors cut off at about 1 μm. Thus, as the wavelength of the Raman signal approaches this value, it can be corrupted by readout noise.

We have chosen 830 nm as our excitation wavelength. This near-infrared wavelength generates a tolerable amount of fluorescence background and is in the low-absorption window, and the shifted Raman light is still below 1 μm. Therefore, the Raman signal intensity and the detector sensitivity make 830-nm excitation a near-optimum choice for biological studies.

III. EXPERIMENTAL SYSTEM

A schematic outline of the Raman system is shown in Fig. 4. The laser spectroscopic system consists of a laser source, delivery optics, collection optics, and a detector. For the laser source, a diode laser is operated at 830-nm wavelength

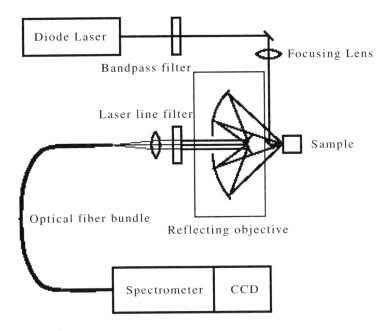

Figure 4 Schematic outline of the Raman measurement system.

in the continuous-wave (CW) mode. The delivery optics delivers the laser light from the laser source to the sample. A bandpass filter in the delivery optics path removes wavelengths other than the primary laser wavelength. A prism reflects and directs the laser beam to the sample. The collection optics collect the optical signal scattered and/or reflected by the sample and transmits the signal to the detector. A reflecting objective in the collection optics has a high numerical aperture and collects photons from a wide angle. Reflecting optics also have the advantage that they generate no Raman signal. The light emerging from the reflecting objective is filtered to block the laser wavelength, preventing generation of Raman signals in any subsequent component. The filtered light is focused onto the input end of the fiber bundle, which is arranged in a circular pattern, and transmitted through to the output end. The output end of the fiber bundle is arranged in a linear array that f-number-matching optics image onto the slit of the spectrometer. Within the spectrometer is a holographic grating that disperses the light, and the dispersed light is converted to an electrical signal by the CCD camera.

IV. EXPERIMENT

Each week a set of 8–11 blood samples was collected at Beth Israel Deaconess Medical Center for seven weeks, totaling 69 samples. Each sample was divided into two parts, one of which was centrifuged to obtain serum. Blood analyte measurements were performed on the serum samples by a hospital blood analyzer using immunoassay, and hematocrit was measured from the whole-blood part. Samples were kept at 4°C in a sterile air-capped environment to prevent the breakdown of glucose as much as possible.

Raman spectra were obtained for each pair of blood and serum samples, and each spectrum was exposed for 300 seconds at the laser power, 300 mW. The samples were stirred by a magnetic stirrer during the irradiation to keep the temperature uniform over the whole sample region, but no additional attempt was made to control the temperature.

V. ANALYTIC METHOD: MULTIVARIATE CALIBRATION TECHNIQUES

A typical spectrum gathered from a biological sample is a mixture of many overlapping spectra. Every spectral contribution from fluorescence, Raman, and infrared absorption/emission is additive. Extracting the concentration of one specific chemical component is a challenge, especially when strong background and severe noise are present. Multivariate calibration techniques are able to deal with such problems. There are various multivariate calibration techniques, but partial least squares (PLS) was chosen as most appropriate for these data sets [4–5,7,10].

PLS is an enhanced least-squares method, and thus assumes that any given spectrum is a linear superposition of component spectra. PLS requires a calibration set, or teaching set, of data to build a model. PLS considers an n-data-point spectrum as an n-dimensional vector. It compares this vector with the given chemical concentration level and finds those spectral components of the given chemical that have predictive value by means of a recursive algorithm. These are then used for predicting the unknown chemical concentration level in the prediction set.

A. Validity of Cross-Validation

Often cross-validation is used for calculating the prediction error and generating the overall prediction plot. The "leave-one-out" method is a typical cross-validation; it leaves out one data point for calibrating the model and then uses the model generated to predict the value of that data point. For example, when one measures N samples, one needs to repeat the calibration N times to get the prediction, each time taking a different sample as the object to be predicted and the rest of the spectra for calibration (Fig. 5).

Cross-validation maximizes the use of limited data sets. Ideally, N samples for cross-validation draw results similar to results with $(2N - 2)$ samples for "half-half" external validation; in either case, the calibration set is $N - 1$ samples.

Internal validation is basically not as robust as external validation. Cross-validation, however, can be accepted when done with close attention and inspection of the calibration model itself [9–10].

B. Limits

When one measures some physical value, it is measured in terms of a reference. Unavoidably, every concentration measurement has some amount of error in it. Thus every calibration set and prediction set contains measurement errors. By

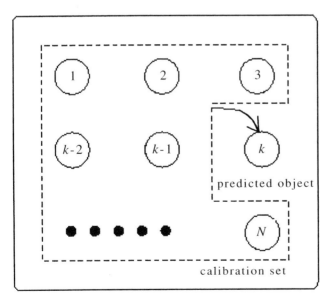

Figure 5 How cross-validation works. To predict a certain concentration in, for example, the kth spectrum, every spectrum other than the kth spectrum $(1, 2, \ldots, k - 1, k + 1, \ldots, N)$ is used to build the calibration model, which is then used to predict the concentration of the kth spectrum.

increasing the size of the calibration set, we can reduce the measurement error in the calibrated model. There is no way, however, to verify that the calibrated model is performing better than the reference technique, since the measurement error in the prediction set remains in the prediction error; even if a perfect model is obtained, the prediction error for validation would not be zero because of the measurement error in the prediction set:

$$\sigma_{total}^2 = \sigma_{reference}^2 + \sigma_{analysis}^2$$

where σ_{total} is the prediction error value from the analysis, $\sigma_{reference}$ is the measurement error of the reference technique, and $\sigma_{analysis}$ is the prediction error due to the analysis technique and the system.

The error we measure directly from the analysis is σ_{total}, and by knowing the measurement error of the reference technique we can estimate $\sigma_{analysis}$, the actual prediction error due to the calibrated model. Based on this, we carefully estimated the measurement error of the reference technique, and the prediction errors presented here should be compared to the measurement error of the reference technique.

VI. DATA PROCESSING

A. Spectral Range Selection

Multivariate calibration methods try to find mathematically the spectral components that are correlated with the species concentration. With the presence of a strong signal that varies distinctively from sample to sample, the algorithm may try to fit this strong signal, neglecting the variance of other regions. In addition, it is not logical to use a spectral range that does not contain the spectrum of the specific chemical component. With this reasoning, we chose the spectral range that is to be analyzed by the multivariate calibration algorithm. No special algorithm was devised for selecting the optimal spectral range. We iterated, adjusting the spectral range to minimize the prediction error by a trial-and-error method.

B. Cosmic Rays

A problem with CCD cameras is that cosmic ray signals degrade data (Fig. 6). Cosmic rays hit random pixels of the CCD array at random times with arbitrary intensity.

$\blacktriangleright$

Figure 6   A set of raw spectra of a biological sample before (top) and after cosmic ray filtering (bottom). Spike-shaped peaks are due to cosmic rays. A statistical algorithm was used to filter the cosmic ray.

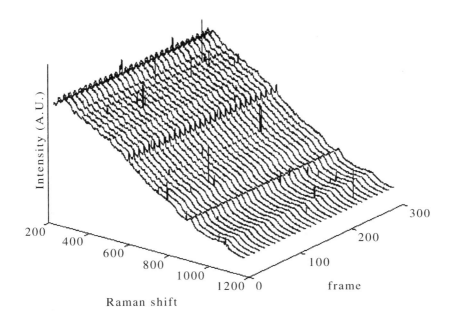

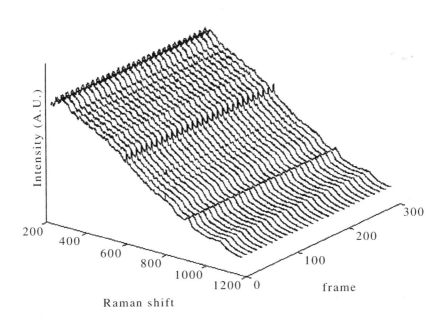

A solution for cosmic ray removal is to take spectral signals frame by frame. When a 300-second integration time was desired for a spectrum, 30 spectra of 10-second integration time each were collected. Each spectrum integrated over 10 seconds is called a *frame*. A statistical algorithm was used. The main concept of the cosmic ray filtering assumes that the spectrum does not change its intensity from frame to frame, other than due to noise and cosmic rays, and a sudden change in the spectrum is due to a cosmic ray.

Then we can mathematically express the intensity of one pixel:

$$I = S + N + c$$

where I is the intensity read by the detector, S represents the average signal, including laser, Raman signal, and fluorescence, N is the term representing the noise fluctuation, and c is the signal increase due to a cosmic ray.

Once given a statistically feasible number of frames, we can calculate the mean and the standard deviation of the set of pixel intensity in frames. The mean is mostly close to S. The standard deviation is mainly due to the noise n and cosmic rays c. The coefficient of standard deviation is used for deciding what percentile of the pixels are "normal." We varied the coefficient of the standard deviation, but mostly used the mean plus three standard deviations as the filtering criterion. Any pixel whose intensity is larger than this criterion was replaced with the average of the normal pixels in the other frames.

Cosmic ray filtering has one weakness in its assumption. The variation of the signal in one pixel gets bigger when there is an intensity change of the spectrum over the whole frame due to physical or chemical changes in the sample, such as chemical breakdown and temperature change. This increased standard deviation may make it difficult to detect cosmic rays by increasing the criteria, unless the cause is monitored.

VII. RESULTS

The prediction errors of seven analytes in serum and whole blood are listed in Table 1. Hematocrit, the volume percentage of red blood cells, is not available in serum. Note that the predictions in blood are poorer than those in serum. Predictions of clinical interest were not obtained for glucose and cholesterol in whole blood. This is due to additional sources of error in whole blood; the presence of more noise generates more Raman and fluorescence, resulting in interference and more background. The increased scattering reduces the penetration depth and hence the sampling volume by the current optical system. Thus, the noise from background added to the weaker signal intensity from reduced volume induces more error. More efficient signal collection at longer integration times should overcome these problems.

Table 1 Prediction Errors of Analytes in Serum and Blood

Analyte	Serum	Blood
Glucose	26 mg/dL	N/A
Cholesterol	12 mg/dL	N/A
Total protein	0.19 g/dL	0.37 g/dL
Albumin	0.12 g/dL	0.22 g/dL
Triglyceride	29 mg/dL	80 mg/dL
Urea	3.8 mg/dL	6.4 mg/dL
Hematocrit	N/A	1.5%

Figure 7 is the prediction of glucose in serum by PLS. The normal range of glucose in serum is 63–105 mg/dL [8]. Because the measurement of glucose is important to diabetics, a chart called the *Clarke Error Grid* has been developed for evaluating the glucose predictions of a measurement technique versus a reference technique [2]. Simply reporting a percent error or an absolute error is not useful for a clinician facing a treatment decision. The grid method provides a

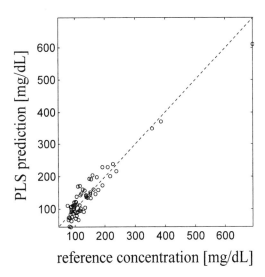

Figure 7 PLS prediction of glucose. Root-mean-square prediction error (RMSEP) is 26 mg/dL.

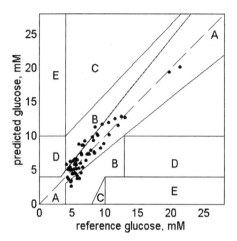

Figure 8 Glucose prediction plotted on Clarke's Error Grid. Note that the molar unit is used. One mM of glucose is equivalent to 18 mg/dL.

qualitative sense of how useful or harmful the glucose predictions would be to a diabetic in various stages of hyper- or hypoglycemia; boundary lines are not to be regarded as absolute. The data of Figure 7 is replotted on the Clarke Error Grid plot in Figure 8. Region A corresponds to a correct clinical decision based upon the Raman-predicted value; region B, a marginally acceptable clinical error in either direction; regions C through E, increasingly harmful incorrect decisions. For a method to be useful, most predictions should fall in the regions labeled A and B.

The prediction of total protein and albumin was comparable to that of the reference technique, and it was found that predictions of similar quality can be made with less integration time [1]. Protein is one major constituent of blood and serum [8] and thus the dominant Raman signal should be generated by proteins. The predictions of total protein, albumin, and other analytes are plotted in Figures 9 and 10.

VIII. CONCLUSION

Raman spectroscopy is shown to have the ability to measure blood analytes both in serum and whole blood. In serum, clinically acceptable accuracy was obtained with acceptable integration times. A future system will be redesigned to maximize the throughput and reduce the integration times for whole blood. These

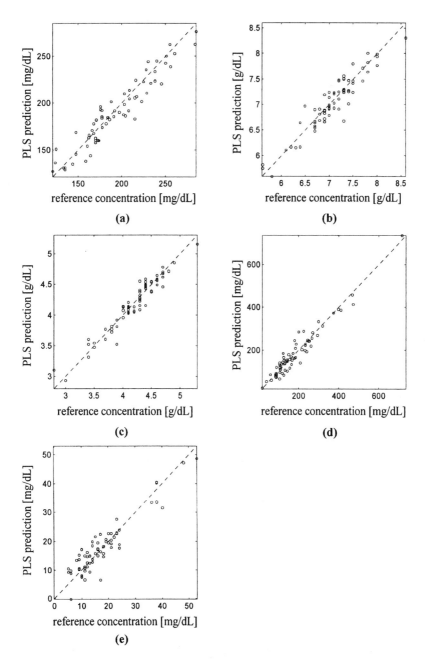

Figure 9 PLS predictions of analytes in serum: (a) cholesterol; (b) total protein; (c) albumin; (d) triglyceride; (e) urea (blood urea nitrogen).

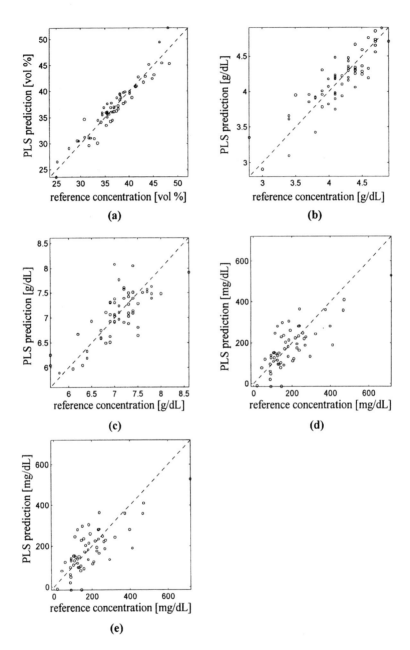

Figure 10 PLS predictions of analytes in whole blood: (a) hematocrit; (b) albumin; (c) total protein; (d) urea; (e) triglyceride.

promising results encourage further exploration of the Raman technique as a noninvasive blood analysis technique.

REFERENCES

1. A. J. Berger, T.-W. Koo, I. Itzkan, M. S. Feld. App. Opt. 38:12 (1999).
2. W. L. Clarke, D. Cox, L. A. Gonder-Frederick, W. Carter, S. L. Pohl. Diab. Care 10:5 (1987).
3. M. Diem. Introduction to Modern Vibrational Spectroscopy. Wiley-Interscience New York (1993).
4. P. Geladi, B. R. Kowalski. Anal. Chim. Acta 185 (1986).
5. D. M. Haaland, E. V. Thomas. Anal. Chem. 60 (1988).
6. T.-W. Koo, A. J. Berger, I. Itzkan, G. Horowitz, M. S. Feld. IEEE LEOS Newsletter 12:2 (1998).
7. R. Kramer. Chemometric techniques for quantitative analysis. Marcel Dekker, New York (1998).
8. C. Lenter. Geigy Scientific Tables: Physical Chemistry Composition of Blood Hematology Somatometric Data. Ciba-Geigy, Basel, Switzerland (1985).
9. A. Lorber, B. R. Kowalski. J. Chemometrics 2 (1988).
10. H. Martens and T. Næs. Multivariate Calibration. Wiley, New York (1989).

18
Noninstrumented Quantitative Devices Using Detection Film Built on Woven Fabric

Wai Tak Law
PortaScience, Inc., Moorestown, New Jersey, U.S.A.

I. INTRODUCTION

Traditionally, a diagnostic assay system is based on wet chemistry in which the absorbance produced in a reaction mixture is read with an instrument. In dry-phase format either the color is read visually and compared to a color chart (qualitative test), or the reflectance from the matrix is read with an instrument. The wet-chemistry systems are usually designed for fast-throughput, highly automated applications performed in hospital and reference laboratories [1]. The dry-phase strips, using either a dip stick format or reagent strips, are designed for point-of-care use in the physician's office or at home [2]. There are also noninstrumented dry-phase analytical devices aimed at the point-of-care applications [3–4], but they either give qualitative results or require multiple-step user intervention. There is a need for a simple noninstrumented device that can produce permanent quantitative results with no operator intervention other than the initial deposit of blood sample. We describe here an analytical platform that is capable of doing that. The platform is based on filtration and precipitation technology coupled with a detection film built on woven fabric. Our experience indicates that this platform is adaptable to a multiple number of clinical, enzymatic, and immunochemical assays.

II. THE PLATFORM

Figure 1 is an expanded view of the individual components in the ENA·C·T platform. There are a total of 13 components in the ENA·C·T total cholesterol device [5]. In addition to the base, the components may be categorized into

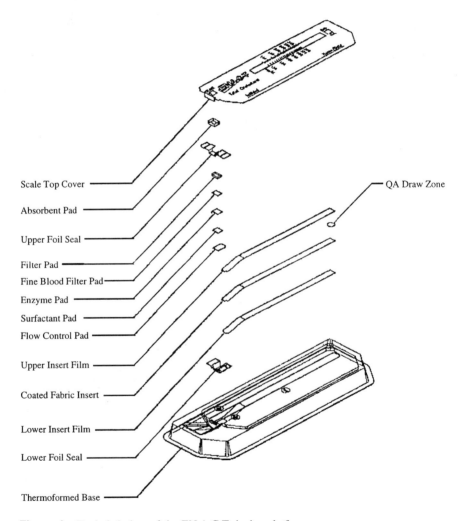

Scale Top Cover

Absorbent Pad

Upper Foil Seal

Filter Pad

Fine Blood Filter Pad

Enzyme Pad

Surfactant Pad

Flow Control Pad

Upper Insert Film

Coated Fabric Insert

Lower Insert Film

Lower Foil Seal

Thermoformed Base

QA Draw Zone

Figure 1   Exploded view of the EN·A·C·T device platform.

three groups: (1) a stack of pads performing functions such as filtering, flow control, and providing a site for enzymatic reactions; (2) a cover with a printed scale for easy reading of the result, one end of which is bent to provide capillary suction to draw the whole-blood sample into the stack of pads; and (3) a strip of detection film based on woven fabric sandwiched between two plastic layers, the end of the strip being encoded with chemicals that signal the completion of the assay. The components are assembled in a completely automated, computer-controlled manufacturing process that allows overall continued quality assurance through a feedback control.

To perform a test, finger-stick blood is obtained from an appropriately prepared individual using a single-use lancet [6]. Blood is added to the sample well of the device until the "start window" on the top cover turns red (i.e., after at least 80 µL of whole blood has been added). This event signals that blood has been transferred to the absorbent pad and that a sample of sufficient volume has been obtained. No further user intervention is required until the QA draw-zone window turns green, after which the length of blue color zone is read in concentration units.

To ensure plasma transport from the sample well, which receives the whole-blood sample, through to the QA draw zone at the end of the device, the device uses a gradient of increasing surface energy established along the path of liquid flow. To further enhance flow through the device, the design minimizes the resistance to flow, particularly in the front section, for which a stack of special filters was developed. These filters accommodate the use of blood within a wide range of hematocrit (HCT) values and lipid concentrations. Other diverse functions of the filters are: separation of erythrocytes from plasma, addition of enzymes and detergents to the resulting plasma with complete mixing, retention of the plasma solution sufficiently long to ensure complete conversion of choles-terol and cholesterol esters into cholesternone and hydrogen peroxide, and sub-sequent release of the reacted plasma into the measurement area of the detection zone. The filters are fastened in place by a hot-melt-coated aluminum foil seal activated remotely by a radio frequency sealer. This sealing process ensures that plasma flows through the filters rather than around them.

Plasma leaving the filter stack is directed into the detection zone. In this zone, a hydrogen peroxide–sensitive dual-component dye system is coated onto a fabric that is sandwiched between two plastic foils. This creates an enclosed flow channel through which the plasma travels, its hydrogen peroxide content generating a quantitative, visible color signal that is converted directly into con-centration units via a scale printed on the cover of the device. The end of the detection zone connects with the QA draw zone, where another cholesterol-converting reaction occurs with exogenous cholesterol. This verifies the stability of key components in the reagent system now dissolved in the plasma sample.

A. The Measuring Channel and Detection Zone

The measuring channel is formed by heat-sealing the upper and lower polyeth-ylene insert support films into a sandwich around a coated, very precisely woven fabric (polyester PES 105/52; Saati Corp., Stamford, CT). The measuring chan-nel thus formed is illustrated in Figure 2. The surface energies of the support films and the coated plastic sheets are optimized with thin polymer coatings to ensure controlled flow rates and to minimize bubble formation inside the chan-nel. The coatings on the woven fabric were created by a multistep process to maximize the shelf life of the product. The first coat is applied with horseradish peroxidase in a buffer with stabilizers and a binder. The horseradish peroxidase is the catalyst that speeds up the oxidative dye reaction with hydrogen peroxide. The second coat contains the sodium salt of 3-methyl-6-carboxy-2-benzothiazol-inone hydrazone (CMBTH) [7] and a polymer in isopropyl alcohol. CMBTH is the free component of the dye compound that has to be physically separated

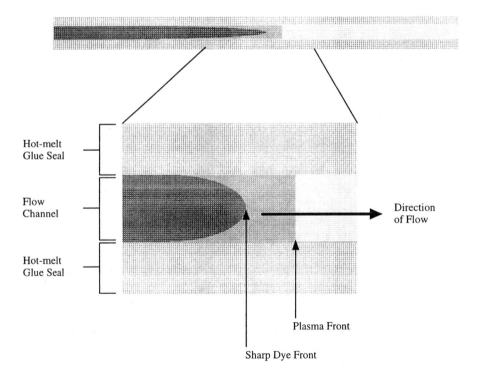

Figure 2 Heat-sealed flow channel created by sandwiching a precision woven fabric between two plastic laminate sheets.

from the peroxidase to keep the enzyme stable at room temperature. An alcohol solvent is used to ensure minimum mixing of the two coatings during the coating and drying process. The third coat has derivatized aniline dye covalently linked to silica particles (<3 μm in diameter) embedded in an acrylin/polyethylene copolymer. The immobilized dye component ensures a sharp color endpoint on the measurement bar. Finally, an optional fourth coating of waterproofing can be applied to fine-tune the surface energy of the coating. These coatings are applied in a tightly controlled process with optimized humidity and temperature using an automated coating machine.

III. MATERIALS AND METHODS

A. Reagents

Cholesterol oxidase (EC 1.1.3.6), cholesterol esterase (EC 3.1.1.13), and horseradish peroxidase (EC 1.11.1.7) are purchased from Toyobo, Osaka, Japan; pancreatic cholesterol esterase was purchased from Diagnostic Chemicals, Oxford, CT. We prepared the sodium salt of 3-methyl-6-carboxy-2-benzothiazolinone hydrazone (NaCMBTH) at ActiMed. Sodium cholate, sodium chloride, lactose, and hydroxylamine hydrochloride are from Aldrich Chemical Co. Milwaukee, WI. Lectins, lithium heparin, Pipes buffer, and bovine serum albumin are from Sigma Chemical Co., St. Louis, MO.

B. Components of the Device

The base of the device is made of a polyester thermoformed into a shape. It can accommodate the placement of all structural elements for the analytical process. The surface of the sample well, an integral part of the base, is rendered hydrophilic by treatment with corona discharge followed by spray-coating with polyacrylic acid containing a heparin derivative. The absorbent pad is made of loosely woven Orlon (polyacrylonitrile) or polyester material, and the reagent pads are of glass fiber materials of defined porosity. The flow delay pad is made of nitrocellulose membrane [8]. The stack of pads is sealed in place by a combination of two seals formed with hot melt (National Starch Co., Bridgewater, NJ)–coated aluminum foil (activated by heat generated remotely by radio frequency sealer). The seals prevent the flow of plasma around the pads and direct the flow of the plasma through the pads. The measuring channel is formed by heat-sealing the upper and lower polyethylene insert support films into a sandwich around a coated, very precisely woven fabric (polyester PES 105/52: Satti Corp., Stamford, CT). The top cover of the device is a polyester sheet with silk-screen design and markings of the concentration scale printed on the top.

Windows in the top cover allow a view of the top of the absorbent pad and of the QA zone during the analysis.

IV. EXAMPLES OF APPLICATIONS OF THE ENA·C·T PLATFORM

A. Total Cholesterol

In the ENA·C·T total cholesterol assay, the absorbent pad and the filtration pads underneath are for retention of the red cells while allowing the plasma to pass through to enzyme and surfactant pads. The enzyme pad is constructed from glass fiber material, which has a large surface area, and the enzyme reagent contains porous bulking agents that trap a large number of air pockets within the pad. The enzyme pad is impregnated with cholesterol esterase and cholesterol oxidase, which catalyzes the oxidation of cholesterol, producing hydrogen peroxide. Supplemental reagents and additives, such as sodium cholate, hydroxylamine hydrochloride, sorbitol, and buffer, are added to the enzyme-enriched plasma as it enters the surfactant pad. The flow-control pad ensures sufficient time for the reactions to complete and precisely times the flow of H_2O_2-containing plasma into the film insert. The film insert contains horseradish peroxidase and an appropriate dye that change color on reaction with H_2O_2, producing a color bar whose length is proportional to the amount of H_2O_2 in the plasma.

The dynamic range of the ENA·C·T total cholesterol test was established to be 1,200–3,600 mg/L using the Abell–Kendall method [9]. The precision of the test devices was evaluated at four clinical sites, with two controls containing cholesterol concentrations near the medical decision points. The results ranged from 2.11% CV to 5.04% CV. Heparinized whole-blood precision studies were also performed, and the results are shown in Table 1.

The accuracy of the test devices was established by direct comparison with the Abell–Kendall method in clinical sites. The results from 198 clinical samples showed a correlation coefficient of .932, where ENA·C·T = 0.976 *

Table 1 Within-Run Precision of Total Cholesterol Assay with Heparinized Whole Blood ($n = 10$)

	Sample 1	Sample 2	Sample 3
Mean, mg/L	1,600	2,240	2,740
Std. dev., mg/L	54	97	77
CV, %	3.38	4.31	2.83

Abell–Kendall + 79.3. The average bias in this comparison over the analytical range of 1,200–3,600 mg/L was 1.35%.

B. LDL

The ENA·C·T direct LDL test incorporates the proven immunoseparation feature in the ENA·C·T device platform, but eliminates the clumsy centrifugation step necessary in the laboratory-based assay. In the ENA·C·T direct LDL cholesterol assay, antibodies against ApoE and ApoA$_1$ are embedded in the absorbent and filtration pads, respectively. Together, they precipitate the HDL and VLDL fractions in less than five seconds, allowing only the LDL fraction to pass through to the enzyme pad, where the enzymatic reactions begin. Thus these two pads are adapted to serve multiple purposes: filtering of erythrocytes and precipitation of unwanted cholesterol fractions. Since only the LDL fraction enters the enzyme pad, the length of the color bar is proportional to the LDL concentration in the plasma. The number of components in the direct LDL test is exactly the same as the total cholesterol test shown in Figure 1. The basic difference is that the absorbent pad in the direct LDL device contains nucleating particles and anti-ApoE antibody, and the filtration pad contains anti-ApoA$_1$ antibody.

To perform the assay, finger-stick blood is deposited into the sample well of the device until the "start window" on the top cover turns red. The blue color bar is then read directly from the printed calibration on the top cover after the QA zone changes to a green color. Because triglycerides, up to 8,000 mg/L, do not interfere with this direct LDL test, no fasting is required prior to the administration of the test.

The ENA·C·T direct LDL test has a dynamic range of 600–2,400 mg/L. The total precision of the direct LDL devices has been evaluated by running whole-blood samples in-house. The precision of samples between 1,000 and 1,600 mg/L ranges from 3.3% CV to 5.1% CV. The accuracy of the devices was established by comparison to the Genzyme N-geneous [10] as well as to the reference beta-quantitation ultracentrifugation methods [11]. The ENA·C·T method was found to be comparable to the two reference methods, with an average correlation coefficient of .94 and a mean bias of −3.8%.

C. HDL

Similar to the approach of the LDL assay, the ENA·C·T HDL cholesterol assay has appropriate nucleating agents and dextran sulfate embedded in the absorbent pad as well as in an extra pad placed underneath the filtration pad. These reagents precipitate the LDL and VLDL fractions, leaving only the HDL to pass on to the enzyme pad to undergo the enzymatic reactions to generate H_2O_2. The length of the color bar would thus be proportional to the HDL concentration in the plasma. Prototype devices have been demonstrated, giving a satisfactory correlation coefficient of .947 against clinical values obtained with a Cholestech LDX analyzer [12]. The precision of these devices was 4.9% CV to 9.0% CV, and the dynamic range was 250–1,000 mg/L.

D. Coagulation Assays and Immunoassays

Prototypes using the ENA·C·T platform for clotting assays and immunoassays have been demonstrated in our laboratories. The unique feature of a noninstrumented device providing a quantitative measurement with a one-step procedure has once again been demonstrated.

V. CONCLUSION

In summary, we have developed a truly one-step disposable system that is read like a thermometer, is quantitative, and is as accurate and precise as instrumented methods. The system is easy to use, requires no technical expertise, can be performed anywhere, and typically produces results in less than 20 minutes. The ENA·C·T platform is easily adaptable for use with other analytes, as illustrated by several working prototypes that have been demonstrated for total cholesterol, LDL, HDL, PT, and other assays.

REFERENCES

1.   Kaplan LA. Clinical Chemistry, Theory, Analysis, Correlation. St. Louis: Mosby, 1996.
2.   Price CP, Hicks JM. Point-of-Care Testing. Washington, DC: AACC Press, 1999.
3.   Allen MP, et. al. Clin Chem 36:1591, 1990.
4.   Johnston JB, Palmer JL. Clin Chem 38:1066, 1992.
5.   Law WT, et al. Clin Chem 43:384, 1997.
6.   Ramel UA. US Patent 5,366,470, 1994.
7.   Nikolyukin Y. US Patent 5,710,012, 1998.
8.   Gibboni DJ. US Patent 5,447,689, 1995.
9.   Abell LL, et al. J Biol Chem 195:357, 1952.
10. Nader R, et al. Clin Chem 44:1242, 1998.
11. Belcher JD, et al. Methods for Clinical Laboratory Measurement of Lipid and Lipoprotein Risk Factors. Washington, DC: AACC Press, 1991.
12. Kafonek SD, et al. Clin Chem 42:2002, 1966.

19

A Survey of Structural and Nonreactive Components Used in the Research, Development, and Manufacture of Solid-Phase Medical Diagnostic Reagents

Myron C. Rapkin
UriDynamics Inc., Indianapolis, Indiana, U.S.A.

I. INTRODUCTION

Developing a solid-phase diagnostic reagent is a process that requires:

> An understanding of the test principle and the ways in which the test principle interacts with the analyte being measured, the biological fluid that contains it, and the structural and nonreactive components.
>
> A means of obtaining the structural and nonreactive components, in appropriate quantities, when the diagnostics industry is regarded as a small consumer compared to other industries.
>
> A strategy for developing and coping with the heat, light, humidity, and mechanical stresses products encounter in manufacturing, in the distribution system, and in the hands of end users.

Table 1 compares some general attributes of wet and dry reagents [1]. Table 2 highlights the characteristics of some methods for manufacturing dry reagents [2], and Table 3 lists components widely used in solid-phase diagnostic devices [3].

Table 1 General Attributes of Reagent Systems

	Wet	Dry
Mathematics	Beer's law	Kubelka–Monk
		Williams–Clapper
Sample size	Milliliters	Microliters
Shelf life	Days–Months	2–3 Years
Package	Bulky	Compact
Nonreactive components	0–2	2–4
Buffer	Hard	Soft
Production equipment	Simple	Complex
Sample pretreatment	Separation, dilution	Varies
User training	Moderate	Minimal
Answered obtained	Instrument	Instrument or visual
Instrumentation cost	$$$	$
Instrumentation size	Benchtop +	Handheld
Response time	5–120 minutes	Instant to 2 minutes

Source: Ref. 1.

II. THE MATRIX: PAPER

Many solid-phase devices for testing urine and other aqueous fluids rely on a filter paper or cellulosic matrix to carry the active ingredients [4]. Novices in the field of product development are apt to assume that the matrix is inert and does not affect the stability of the reagent system. Table 4 lists 20 parameters in paper that affect the stability and performance of solid-phase test systems [5]. Table 5 shows the thickness of some commonly available α-cellulose filter papers and the extent to which a single parameter will vary [6,7].

The data in Table 6 was gathered during the investigation of a problem in which a colorimetric reagent was developing too much color. After considerable investigation the problem was traced to lot-to-lot variance in the paper matrix. A panel of raw material tests was developed to prevent reccurence of this particular problem [8]. The caveat inherent in this solution is that manufacturers will not necessarily conform to specifications imposed by a single, small-volume customer. The primary sources for α-cellulose filter papers are listed in table 7.

III. THE MATRIX: MEMBRANES

The trend to smaller sample volumes, primarily for analytes in blood, has made synthetic membranes the matrix of choice for many devices [10]. Also, the unique property of nitrocellulose membranes to bind antibodies noncovalently

Table 2 Systems for Manufacturing Dry Reagents

	Lyophili- zation	Tableting	Impregnation	Coating	Printing
Cycle time	Days	Seconds	Minutes	Minutes	Seconds
Scrap rate	Aprox. 5%	Approx. 10%	Edges	Edges	>5%
Material prepar- ation	Dispense	Dry, blend	Mix	Mix	Mix
Changeover	Slow	Complex	Cleanup	Cleanup	Cleanup
Products	Reagents Controls	Reagents	Reagents Controls	Reagents	Reagents
Uniformity	Variable	Variable	Variable	Consistent	Consistent
Stress in manu- facturing	Low	Heat Pressure	Heat Some denatur- ation by solvents	Minimal heat Some denatur- ation by solvent	Minimal heat Some shear and solvent dena- turation
Used in	Chemistry Urinalysis Hematology Immunology	Chemistry Urinalysis FOBT	Chemistry Urinalysis Immunology Microbiology FOBT	Chemistry Immunology Coagulation	Immunology FOBT Chemistry Sensors
Drawbacks	Long cycle	Very low relative humidity needed	$$ Capital equipment	$$ Capital equipment	Special equipment
Finishing opera- tions	Labeling Packaging	Bottling Labeling Packaging	Lamination Converting Slitting Bottling Labeling Packaging	Converting Slitting Bottling Labeling Packaging	Bottling Labeling Packaging

Source: Ref. 2.

has made them popular for immunoassay devices. When paper is used as a matrix in a diagnostic device, it is almost always α-cellulose derived from cotton. Membranes, however, may be made of 100% of a single polymer or blends of several different polymers [11,12] and, as expected, have their own set of chemical and physical parameters that affect stability and performance of the final product. In addition to carrying reagents, membranes can transport, separate, and immobilize reagents and fluids for testing. Table 8 lists properties that must be considered when building a diagnostic device [13]. An indication, shown in Figure 1, of the increasing interest in membrane-based diagnostic devices was obtained by a Boolean search of U.S. patents over a 10-year period

Table 3 Nonreactive Components Used in Dry Reagents

Matrix	Packaging
Papers	Bottles
Membranes	Caps
Coatings	Labels
Adhesives	Carton
Silicones	Inserts
Acrylics	Pouches
Rubber	Functional materials (see Table 17)
Hot melts	"Inert" ingredients
Support	Surfactants
Plastic	Polymers
Cardboard	Solvents
Desiccants	Water
Silica gel	Organic, polar
Molecular sieves	Organic, nonpolar
Clays	
Blends	

Source: Ref. 3

[14]. Manufacturers of membranes used in solid-phase diagnostic devices are listed in table 9.

IV. THE MATRIX: COATINGS

Papers and membranes are both existing elements that may be selected for use in a diagnostic device. Coatings, however, are formulated by the developers of those devices. Like membranes, coatings may be composed of one polymer or blends of polymers in solution or latex suspensions. In many cases coatings may be used to modify properties of membranes and papers [16,17]. Table 10 lists

Table 4 Paper Properties[a]

Uniformity	Bursting strength	% Soda soluble	Freeness
Basis weight	Absorption	% Alcohol soluble	Color
Thickness	Tensile strength	pH	Whiteness
Density	% Alpha cellulose	Trace elements	Porosity
Smoothness	Copper number	Fiber size distribution	Capillary rise

[a]Definitions of terms and assay procedures for all properties available from TAPPI in Atlanta, GA.
Source: Ref. 5.

Table 5 Thickness of Some Filter Papers Used in Solid-Phase Chemistries

Manufacturer	Product	Thickness (mils)
Whatman	1	7
	3mm	13
	31ET	15
	54	5
	17	20
Schleicher & Schuell	470	20
	597	7
	903	12
	2043	14
Ahlstrom	204	11
	222	15
	237	14
Mead	469	18
Buckeye	S-10	10

Source: Ref. 6.

some general types of coatings [18]. Table 11 lists factors developers need to be familiar with when applying coatings [19].

V. MATERIALS: PLASTIC SUPPORT

Most solid-phase diagnostic devices use some type of plastic as a support or handle for the reagent. The selection process for the plastic material is usually

Table 6 Measurement of Physical Properties of Paper to Predict Reagent Performance

Lot No.	Porosity (sec)	Capillary rise (cm)	Burst strength (lb/sq. in.)	Absorbance (mL H_2O)	Basis weight (mg/sq. cm)	Pass/fail performance
1	3.0	2.5	24.0	16.4	94.55	Pass
2	3.0	2.6	25.4	17.0	94.46	Pass
3	2.6	2.6	26.5	14.8	93.60	Pass
4	2.1	2.8	26.4	14.8	93.60	Pass
5	2.5	2.7	26.0	16.4	92.80	Pass
6	1.7	3.1	15.3	17.4	92.50	*Fail*
7	2.3	2.8	19.2	14.9	93.20	Pass

Source: Ref. 8.

Table 7 Primary Sources of Filter Papers

Whatman Paper Ltd.	Ahlstrom Inc.	Schleicher & Schuell Inc.
9 Bridwell Place	122 W. Butler Street	10 Optical Ave.
Clifton, NJ 007014	Mt. Holly Springs, PA 17065	Keene, NH 03431
Tel: 800-441-6555	Tel: 800-326-1888	Tel: 800-437-7003
URL: *www.whatman.com*	URL: *www.ahlstrom.com*	URL: *www.s-and-s.com*

Source: Ref. 9.

handled in an off-hand or casual manner, however. Table 12 lists problems encountered with plastic support materials during the development of various solid-phase diagnostic devices [20]. Many manufacturers of plastic sheeting can be located by consulting the Thomas Register in hard copy or online at *www.thomasregister.com.*

VI. MATERIALS: ADHESIVES

When the components of a diagnostic device are joined together in manufacturing, there are two primary methods in use: adhesives and sonic welding. The four principal types of adhesives are rubber, acrylic, silicone, and hot-melts. The caveat concerning adhesives is not to assume adhesives are inert and nonreactive. Actually, adhesives contain many components that may react with the reagents in a short period of time or during storage or shipping. Table 13 lists

Table 8 Membrane Properties

Pore size
Pore size distribution
Anisotropy
% Open area
Tensile strength
Binding capacity
Thickness
Elongation
Opacity
Whiteness
Capillarity
Extractables

Source: Ref. 13.

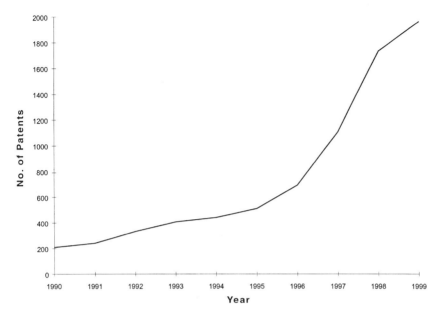

Figure 1   Number of U.S. membrane-based diagnostic device patients, 1990–1999

the components found in adhesives [21]. Table 14 gives sources for adhesives [22].

VII.   MATERIALS: DESICCANTS

Desiccants are not an integral part of any test device, but most solid-phase devices need a desiccant to provide acceptable shelf life. Desiccants are available as pellets, permeable bags, or plastic tubes or molded in plastic or impregnated in paper. Sizes available range from 1-gram to 1-pound bags that protect

Table 9   Sources of Membranes

Millipore	Schliecher & Schuell	Micron Separations	Pall-Gelman
P.O. Box 255	P.O. Box 2012	P.O. Box 1046	600 S. Wagner Road
Bedford, MA 01730	Keene, NH 03431	Westborough, MA 01581	Ann Arbor, MI 48103
Tel: 800-225-1380	Tel: 800-245-4024	Tel: 800-444-8212	Tel: 734-665-0651

Source: Ref. 15.

Table 10 Types of Coatings Used in
Diagnostic Devices

Water soluble
Organic soluble
Cellulose derivatives
Waterborne latex
Epoxy
Urethane

Source: Ref. 18.

product during intermediate storage. The chemical types of desiccant [23] are
listed in Table 15. Some sources [24] of desiccants are listed in Table 16.

VIII. FUNCTIONAL MATERIALS

Functional materials are a catchall category of materials used for avoiding specific problems or imparting special properties to a diagnostic device. Table 17
the types of functional materials available [25].

IX. TROUBLESHOOTING

Even when the most rigorous research and development have gone into a device,
problems such as auto-oxidation, discoloration, and poor stability or performance can occur. Unfortunately, the process of tracking down the cause of a
problem tends to be unique to that particular problem. The grid in Table 18 is
a general approach to facilitating that process [26].

Table 11 What Developers Need to
Know About Coatings

Potlife
Viscosity
Tack
Evaporation rate
Adhesion to substrate
Integrity of coating

Source: Ref. 19.

Table 12 What Can Go Wrong with the Plastic Support?

Coating or adhesive does not adhere
Too flexible
Haze develops in transparent material
Material fractures when cut
Resin contains component that interferes in chemistry
Shrinks when exposed to heat
Attacked by solvents
Supplier discontinued product
Lot-to-lot variance (e.g., thickness, color)
Splices caused production equipment to jam
Not available in less than truckload quantities
Material produces dust when slit
Plasticizer migrates
Curling
Incompatible with steps in manufacturing process (sonic welding, die cutting, coating)
Material stretches under tension
Solvent out-gassing

Source: Ref. 20.

Table 13 Components of Adhesives

Component	Example
Binder	Starch, P.V. Butyral
Solvents	MIBK, Cellosolve
Diluents	Highly volatile organics
Catalysts	NH_4Cl, peroxides
Hardeners	Paraformaldehydes
Fillers	Clay, wood pulp
Extenders	Wheat or soy flour
Preservatives	Cu or Hg salts, phenols
Fortifiers	Resorcinols
Carrier	Tissue paper, film, foil

Source: Ref. 21.

Table 14   Sources for Adhesives

LecTec Corp.	Scapa Tapes	Adhesives Research
10701 Red Circle Drive	111 Great Pond Drive	P.O. Box 100
Minnetonka, MN 55410	Windsor, CT 06095	Glen Rock, PA 17327
Tel: 612-933-2291	Tel: 800-801-0323	Tel: 800-445-6240
Fax: 612-933-4808	Fax: 800-688-7000	Fax: 717-235-8320
T.H. Glennon	General Adhesive & Chemical	Sharnet
109 Methuen Street	6100 Centennial Blvd.	175 Ward Hill Avenue
Lawrence, MA 01843	Nashville, TN 37209	Ward Hill, MA 01830
Tel: 508-682-3888	Tel: 615-367-7833	Tel: 508-372-7783

Source: Ref. 22.

Table 15   Types of Desiccants

Silica gel
Molecular seives
Clays
Blends

Source: Ref. 23.

Table 16   Sources of Desiccants

MultiSorb Technologies Inc.	United Desiccants	ADCOA Inc.
325 Harlem Road	101 Christine Drive	1269 Eagle Vista Drive
Buffalo, NY 14224	Belen, NM 87002	Los Angeles, CA 90041
Tel: 716-824-8900	Tel: 800-989-3374	Tel: 800-228-4124
Fax: 716-824-4091	Fax: 505-864-9296	Fax: 310-532-5404

Source: Ref. 24.

Table 17 Types of Functional Materials

Antioxidant	Background dye	Opacifier
Antistat	Coupling agent	Solubilizer
Biocide	Defoamer	Stabilizer
Binder	Film former	Thickener
Chelant	Humectant	UV absorber

Source: Ref. 25.

Table 18 Troubleshooting Grid

	Mixing	Process	Storage	Assembly	Packing	Transit	Misuse
Heat							
Light							
Thermal cycling							
Moisture							
Shake							
Drop							
Contamination							
Incompatibility							

Source: Ref. 26.

REFERENCES

1. Myron C. Rapkin and Arthur M. Usmani. Polymer News 22:402–403, 1997.
2. Myron C. Rapkin and Arthur M. Usmani. Polymer News 22:402–403, 1997.
3. Myron C. Rapkin. Where to Find It: Locating Materials Used to Make Solid Phase Diagnostic Reagents. Presented at American Association of Clinical Chemistry, 1999.
4. U.S. Patent 4,013,416.

5. Myron C. Rapkin. Practical Aspects of Paper. Presented at Miles Laboratories Science Forum, October 1981.

6. Myron C. Rapkin. Practical Aspects of Paper. Presented at Miles Laboratories Science Forum, October 1981.

7. R.D. Kremer and Myron C. Rapkin. Selecting Alpha Cellulose Filter Papers for Use in Dry Chemistry Test Strips. Presented at Southern Cellulose Conference, New Orleans, 1994.

8. Myron C. Rapkin. Practical Aspects of Paper. Presented at Miles Laboratories Science Forum, October 1981.

9. M. Rapkin, "internet search; keyword filter paper" www.altavista.com, 3 Jun 99.

10. J.L. Rudolph et al. A new microporous membrane for diagnostic immunoassays. Biotechniques 9(2):218–223, 1990.

11. Israel Cabasso. Membranes. In: ECT. 3rd ed. vol. 9, pp. 509–579, SUNY Syracuse.

12. Arthur M. Usmani. Medical diagnostic reagents. In: ECT. 4th ed. Vol. 16, pp. 88–107, Bridgestone/Firestone.

13. Joseph Lee. Characteristics of Microporous Membranes and Their Applications. Presented at AACC, 1986.

14. M. Rapkin, "Boolean search, www.USPTO.gov, keyword membranes, solid phase" 10 Jun 99.

15. M. Rapkin, "Internet search, www.dogpile.com, keyword, membrane" 10 Jul 99.

16. Eric Diebold, Myron Rapkin, and Arthur M. Usmani. Chemistry on a stick. Chemtech 21:464–471, 1991.

17. U.S. Patent 5,260,195.

18. Arthur M. Usmani, Biotechnology symposium, Atlanta, 1992.

19. M. Rapkin. Technical data. Technovations, Indianapolis, IN, 1996.

20. Myron Rapkin. Collected Papers, vol. 1 "Dry Chemistry Reagents" articles 26–40.

21. "Adhesives" in ECT, Vol. 1, pp. 445–466, by Alphonsus V. Pocius, 3M Corp.

22. M. Rapkin, "Internet search, www.thomasregister.com, keyword adhesives 25 Jul 99.

23. Myron Rapkin. Collected Papers, vol. 1, "Dry Chemistry Reagents," articles 63–65.

24. M. Rapkin, "internet search, www.thomasregister.com, keyword desiccent" 25 Jul 99.

25. M. Rapkin. Technical data. Technovations, Indianapolis, IN, 1997.

26. Myron C. Rapkin. Work in progress.

20

Current Status and Future Prospects of Dry Chemistries and Diagnostic Reagents

Richard Kordal
University of Cincinnati, Cincinnati, Ohio, U.S.A.

Naim Akmal
The Dow Chemical Company, South Charleston, West Virginia, U.S.A.

Arthur M. Usmani
Altec USA, Indianapolis, Indiana, U.S.A.

I. INTRODUCTION

Biosensors are relatively new to the field of diagnostic reagents. Despite advances in biosensors, dry chemistry dominates and may continue to dominate as the primary choice of analyte detection in body fluids, e.g., blood. The main reason is economics. Dry reagents are less expensive than biosensors, in both developmental and manufacturing costs. Essentially, biosensors are analytical sensing devices for quantitatively measuring specific body analytes, e.g., blood glucose.

In the early 1960s, a promising approach to glucose monitoring was developed in the form of an enzyme electrode that used oxidation of glucose by the enzyme glucose oxidase (GOD) [1]. At that time, it was anticipated that the enzyme electrode would replace dry reagent for glucose determination. Dry chemistry as we know it today was in its infancy at that time. The enzyme electrode approach was incorporated into a few clinical analyzers for blood glucose determination.

Since then, third- and fourth-generation blood glucose biosensors that utilize a mediator to shuttle the electrons have emerged, and they should continue to emerge into the marketplace.

343

Usmani and coworkers have comprehensively described the history, chemistry, and technology of dry chemistry earlier [2–7]. Currently three types of dry chemistry for blood glucose are available: impregnated dry reagents coated with a membrane to which red blood cells will not adhere, coating film, and discrete multilayered coatings. All of them are based on aqueous systems. Nonaqueous systems have also been researched and developed by us. Additionally, both wiping and nonwiping strips are available. In wiping strips, excess blood is removed manually, whereas in the more popular nonwipe method, capillary action or some other mechanism removes excess blood.

Any diagnostic coatings or impregnation must incorporate all reagents necessary for the reaction. Dry-chemistry systems are used in physicians' offices and hospital laboratories and by millions of patients worldwide. They are used for routine urinalysis, blood chemistry determinations, and immunological and microbiological testing. The main advantage of dry-chemistry technology is that it eliminates the need for reagent preparation and many other manual steps common to liquid reagent systems, resulting in a greater consistency and reliability of test results. Furthermore, dry chemistry has a longer shelf stability, and we thereby find a reduction of reagent waste. Each test unit contains all reagents and reactants necessary to perform assays.

In this chapter we present a brief history of medical diagnostic reagents along with their chemistry, technology, current status, and new trends. For completeness, newer emerged or emerging technologies will be covered.

II. DRY CHEMISTRY

A. History

Insulin became available in 1922, increasing the demand to determine urine glucose. In 1940, dry tablet for glucose determination in urine appeared on the market. Eli Lilly and Miles Laboratory independently developed enzymatic impregnated urine strips around 1956. A significant step occurred in 1964 when Miles introduced the first wiping blood glucose strips based on chemical impregnation and utilizing ethyl cellulose membrane to wash off or wipe off excess blood and red blood cells. The strips were visually read. The handheld light reflectance meter became available in the late 1960s. The greatest advance in biomedical diagnostic reagents occurred in the early 1970s, when Boehringer Mannheim in Germany researched and developed the coating-film type of diagnostic chemistry. Coating films have since become the dominant format. The multilayered coating type, as typified by Ektachem of Kodak/J&J, became available in the early 1980s. Medisense/Abbott introduced the first electrochemical biosensor based on a glucose oxidase enzyme electrode around 1985. A significant milestone was the introduction of the first user's friendly nonwipe One-

Touch LifeScan/J&J technology in 1987. Roche Diagnostics Corporation introduced the first GDH-based biosensor in mid-1995.

B. Market Evolution

The development of colorimetric dip sticks or test strips enabled point-of-care (POC) testing. Main applications include whole-blood glucose testing by diabetics as well as pregnancy, fertility, and cholesterol testing at home. In the physician's office, infectious diseases, e.g., strep, can be tested. Urinalysis and tests for drugs of abuse (DOA), cardic markers, infectious diseases, and cancer are performed in hospitals and clinical laboratories.

C. Diabetes

The incidence of diabetes has reached significant proportions in the Western world and is growing at an alarming rate in the rest of the world. Methods for diagnosis and care are well developed, though still below where it should be in the Western world. In the rest of the world, both diagnosis and management of the disease are only marginal. The social and economic impact of diabetes in the United States is over $100 billion.

Management and treatment of Type I (insulin dependent) and some Type II diabetics involves self-monitoring of blood glucose together with self-administration of insulin to mimic the body's response in adjusting blood glucose levels. This testing system consists of a test strip, either dry chemistry or biosensor, that can be read by meter. Roche, Johnson and Johnson, Abbott, and Bayer are major marketers of such strips and meters.

Over 16 million Americans are diabetic. About 8 million are undiagnosed. The three major types are insulin-dependent diabetes mellitus (IDDM—Type I), noninsulin-dependent diabetes mellitus (NIDDM—Type II), and gestational diabetes. Treatment for Type I consists of insulin shots or spray, proper diet, and exercise. For Type II, the treatment may include insulin but preferably glucose-lowering drugs, diet, and exercise.

Death by diabetes in the United States occurs at a rate of about 400,000 per year. Diabetics are prone to heart disease, peripheral vascular disease, stroke, retinopathy, renal disease, and neuropathy. About 6 million hospital days can be attributed to diabetes. Emergency room visits due to the disease total over 600,000. The institutional cost for diabetes is over $40 billion, plus over $8 billion for outpatient care. The total direct and indirect cost of this disease in the United States is now over $100 billion a year.

The World Health Organization predicts that by 2025 or so, an estimated 300 million people worldwide will become diabetic, primarily in the developing nations of the world. No doubt, the disease will challenge and impact the social and economic situation.

D. Quantification

Noninstrumented quantification methods, although reliable, are semiquantitative. These include colorimetric matching to color blocks, e.g., pH papers and ChemStrip bG of Roche Diagnostics. Examples of chromatographic strips are ActiMed's Cholesterol EnACT for blood glucose and Enzymatics Q.E.D. salvia alcohol test. Micral of Roche for semiquantitative determination of microalbumin is an example of an immunostrip. Qualitative tests involve plus/minus readings, e.g., E.P.T. pregnancy test and Roche DOA. A threshold qualitative with a greater cutoff level are cardic markers by Roche Diagnostics.

Instrument-based quantitative measurements are useful at home and in physicians' offices, hospitals, and clinical laboratories. Home pocket-size reflectance meters come with or without visual backup. Roche AccuCheck Easy and J&J SureStep have visual backup, whereas J&J One Touch has no visual backup. An example of a quantitative instrument type of test useful in a physician's office is the Reflotron System of Roche. Hospital-based instruments for urinalysis utilizing the Roche ChemStrip 10 SG multianalyte urine dipsticks can determine nitrite, pH, protein, glucose, ketones, urobilinogen, bilirubin, blood, leukocytes, and specific gravity. Response Biomedical Corporation uses a rapid analyte measurement platform (RAMP) for a quantitative immunochromatographic test device.

E. Types of Test Strips

The diagnostic strip can be paper impregnated with chemicals, e.g., pH paper; the impregnated membrane-coated type (Bayer), combination materials with capability for wicking, chemistry, absorbent sink, separation components (Roche Reflotron); single-layer coating-film type (Roche ChemStrip bG); and multilayer thin coating film (Ektachem). Future materials include the Gamera compact-disk (CD)–based system that incorporates a laboratory within a CD and contains reaction chambers and fluidic channels. The spinning of the CD drives fluid movement.

The basic components of a typical dry reagent that utilizes reflectance measurement are a base support material, a reflective layer, and a single-layer or multilayer reagent. The base layer serves as a base for building the dry reagent and usually is a thin, rigid thermoplastic film. The reflectance layer reflects light to the detector not absorbed by the chemistry and is typically made from white-pigment-filled plastic film, coating, foam, membrane, paper, and

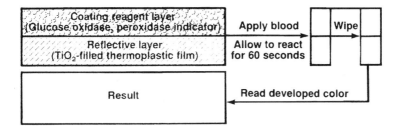

Figure 1 Single-layer coating-film type of dry chemistry.

metal foil. The reagent layer contains the integrated reagents for a specific analyte.

An example of a singled-layer coating-film that effectively excludes red blood cells is shown in Figure 1. The emulsion type of coating contains all the reagents for a specific analyte (e.g., blood glucose), is coated onto a lightly titanium dioxide–filled thermoplastic film, and then dried. The enzymatic coating contains, in addition to enzymes and indicator, buffer for pH adjustment, color-ranging antioxidant, and coalescing solvent. Paper-impregnated dry chemistry differs by having a reagent-impregnated paper layer under a film membrane, as shown in Figure 2.

The special construction using combination materials is shown by the Roche Reflotron (Fig. 3). The separation layer retains the red blood cells. The auxiliary reagents eliminate interfering substances. The treated plasma then passes into and fills the fiberglass transport layer. When the instrument presses, the transport layer contacts the reagent layer and the biochemical reaction begins. After a few minutes' interval, controlled by the magnetic code, the intensity of the color signal is measured. Calibration of the result is then made by a test-specific and lot-specific function curve contained in the magnetic code.

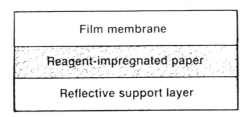

Figure 2 Impregnated-paper dry chemistry.

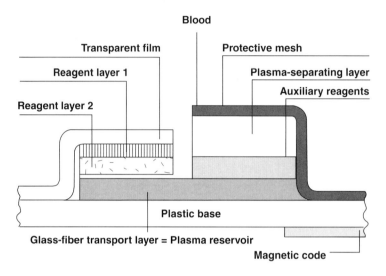

Figure 3   Special-construction dry chemistry.

A typical multilayer thin-coating dry reagent for determining blood urea nitrogen (BUN) is shown in Figure 4. It consists of a spreading and reflective layer that spreads the sample containing BUN uniformly. The first reagent layer is a porous coating film containing the enzyme urease and 8.0 pH buffer. Urease reduces BUN to NH_3. A semipermeable membrane coating allows NH_3 to permeate while excluding OH^- from the second reagent layer. The second layer is composed of porous coating film containing a pH indicator in which the indicator color develops when NH_3 reaches the semipermeable coating film. Typically, such reagents are on a slide, 2.8 cm $\times$ 2.4 cm, and the spreading layer is about 100 μm thick.

F.   Chemistry and Technology

Enzymes are essential in dry chemistry. In a typical glucose-measuring dry reagent, glucose oxidase (GOD) and peroxidase (POD) enzymes, along with a suitable indicator, e.g., tetramethylbenzidine (TMB), are dissolved and/or dispersed in a latex or water-soluble polymer. The enzyme-containing coating is applied to a lightly pigmented plastic film and dried to a thin film. The coated plastic, cut to about 0.5 cm $\times$ 0.5 cm, is the basic dry reagent. The user applies a drop of blood and allows reaction with the strip for 60 s or less. The blood is wiped off manually or alternatively automatically in nonwipe strips. The developed color is then read.

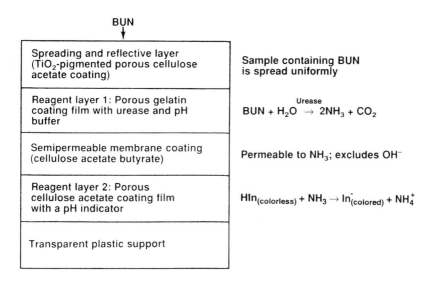

Figure 4 Multilayer-coating dry chemistry.

Dry-chemistry reagent diagnostic tests are used to determine metabolite concentration and activity in a biological matrix, e.g., blood and urine. The reactive components, i.e., enzymes and indicator, are usually present in excess, except for the analyte, to ensure that the reaction goes to completion quickly. Other enzymes or reagents are also used to drive the reactions in the desired directions. Glucose and cholesterol are the most commonly measured analytes. Glucose concentrations that deviate from the normal, i.e., hypo- or hyperglycemia, are important clinical indications of disease.

Glucose is measured by conversion to gluconic acid and hydrogen peroxide using glucose oxidase. Hydrogen peroxide is then coupled to an indicator, for example, tetramethyl benzidine, by the enzyme peroxidase. The rapidly developed color is then measured at or around 660 nm. The biochemical reactions are shown in Figure 5a.

There is a strong correlation between high levels of cholesterol and heart disease. Cholesterol esters, present in blood serum, can be quantitatively saponified by cholesterol esterase into free cholesterol and fatty acids. Free cholesterol is oxidized by cholesterol oxidase, in presence of oxygen, to choles-4en-3one and hydrogen peroxide. There are several indicator peroxidase systems that may be used to detect hydrogen peroxide, e.g., tetramethylbenzidine or oxidation of 4-aminoantipyrine followed by coupling with phenol to form a compound that could be read at 490 nm (see Fig. 5b). For additional reading on cholesterol

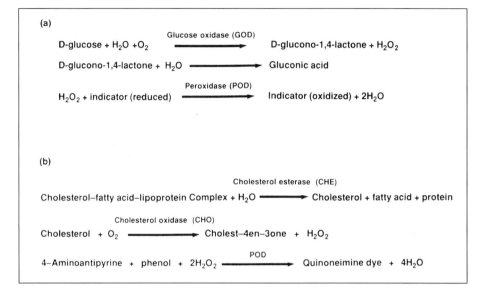

Figure 5 Reactions in glucose and cholesterol determinations.

testing, readers may wish to refer to Chapter 18, "Noninstrumented Quantitative Devices Using Detection Film Built on Woven Fabric," in this book.

The developed color is measured by using reflectance spectroscopy or by visually comparing the reacted strip to a preprinted color chart. Dry-reagent test kits are generally available as disposable thin strips, either coated or impregnated, and mounted onto a plastic support or handle. The most basic diagnostic strips thus consist of a paper or plastic base, polymeric binder, and reacting chemical components consisting of enzymes, surfactants, buffers, and indicators. Diagnostic coatings or impregnation must incorporate all reagents necessary for the reaction. The coatings can be single-layer or multilayer in design. A few of the common metabolites analyzed by diagnostic test kits are bilirubin, blood urea nitrogen, calcium, cholesterol, creatinine, glucose, hemoglobin, ketones, phosphorus, theophylline, total protein, triglycerides, urea, lactate, and uric acid.

Polymeric materials account for more than 95 wt% of most dry chemistry strips and must be selected carefully. We have provided a strong fusion of polymer chemistry with biochemistry that has provided better understanding and resulted in improved dry chemicals and biosensors. Even stronger fusion of polymers and biochemistry is required. Other researchers are encouraged to fill this gap.

The polymer binder incorporates the system's chemical components either as a coating or by impregnation. The reagent matrix must be carefully controlled to mitigate nonuniformity in the reagent concentrations due to improper mixing, settling, or nonuniform coating thickness. Aqueous-based polymer latex, e.g., acrylics, polyvinyl acetate homo- and copolymers, styrene acrylic, polyvinyl propionate homo- and copolymers, ethylene vinyl acetate, lightly cross-linkable acrylics, and polyurethane dispersions can be used in dry chemicals. Water-soluble polymers have low molecular weight in comparison to latex. They are used, however. Examples of useful water-soluble polymers are polyvinyl alcohol, polyvinyl pyrrolidone, and hydroxyethyl cellulose. Usmani and coworkers have researched and developed a new class of hydroxyethyl methacrylate–rich copolymers that are solvent based and have hydrogel character. These polymers give excellent chemistries due to their stabilization of the enzymes, outstanding thermostability, and excellent capability for ranging [8]. Despite their superiority, these new diagnostic polymers have not found commercial acceptability.

III. BIOSENSORS

The history, chemistry, technology, and applications of biosensors are described elsewhere in this book (see Chapter 3). Commercial electrochemical biosensors, specifically amperometric types, have been successful.

Researchers are now applying photolithography and silicon micromaching used in the integrated circuit (IC) industry to develop miniature biosensors.

IV. GROWTH AREA AND THE FUTURE

One of the areas projected to grow the fastest is gene probe and chip technology. The current market of about $150 million is expected to grow to about $2 billion by 2004. By 2005, this market may exceed $2.7 billion. Some recent developments in genosensors are discussed briefly in the following paragraphs.

Sequenom is developing a fully integrated DNA-chip-based diagnostic system. The front end is sample preparation, the back end is TOF-MS signal detection. SpectroChip 250 location DNA microarray on silicon comprises the middle. The application is genotyping, with a throughput of 10,000 genotypes per day.

Clinical Microsensors is developing point-of-contact diagnostic devices based on direct electronic detection of DNA–DNA hydridization. Cephid's microfabricated DNA-capture chip utilizes micromachining and precision injection-molding to develop miniaturized diagnostic devices. Zeneca/SKB is researching micromachined amplifiers for PCR.

The GeneChip of Affymetrix is utilizing semiconductor fabrication techniques to develop a gene detection system with very large arrays containing DNA probes. Packard Instrument, Motorola, and the Argonne National Laboratory have joined forces to develop an advanced biochip for medical diagnostics. In a future book, leading experts will describe their genobiosensor work.

V. CONCLUSIONS

We have described the current status and future prospects of biomedical diagnostic reagents. Electrochemical sensors, biosensors, and DNA chips are a few of the new applications of medical diagnostics. There is a pressing need for development of less invasive or noninvasive technologies. Monitoring of blood glucose has been very useful in managing diabetes so far. However, there are other diabetes-related analytes, such as cholesterol, triglyceride, and fructosamine, that should be monitored. What is needed is a strip capable of quantifying these analytes using minute amounts of whole blood and produced at a reasonable cost. No doubt, such a strip will certainly be welcomed by diabetics worldwide.

Electrochemical sensors have made their way into the glucose diagnostic field. The DNA chip will revolutionize the field in the next few years, however.

REFERENCES

1. L. C. Clark, C. Lyons. Ann NY Acad Sci 102:29 (1962).
2. A. M. Usmani. Medical Reagents. In: Kirk-Othmer Encyclopedia of Chemical Technology. 4th ed. Wiley, New York, 1995.
3. A. M. Usmani. Chapter 1, In: A. M. Usmani, N. Akmal, eds. Diagnostic and Biosensor Polymers. ACS Books, Washington, DC, 1994.
4. E. Diebold, M. Rapkin, A. M. Usmani. ChemTech 21:462 (1991).
5. A. Burke, J. DuBois, A. Azhar, A. M. Usmani. ChemTech 21:547 (1991).
6. M. T. Skarstedt, A. M. Usmani. Polymer News 14:38 (1989).
7. W. J. Schrenk, A. M. Usmani. In: H. Mark, R. B. Seymour, eds. History of Coatings. Elsevier, New York, 1990.
8. A. Burke, A. F. Azhar, J. DuBois, A. M. Usmani. J Appl Polymer Sci 47:2083 (1993).

21

Water-Soluble Phospholipid Polymers as a Novel Synthetic Blocking Reagent in an Immunoassay System

Shujiro Sakaki, Yasuhiko Iwasaki, and Nobuo Nakabayashi
Tokyo Medical and Dental University, Tokyo, Japan

Kazuhiko Ishihara
The University of Tokyo, Tokyo, Japan

I. INTRODUCTION

For detecton or quantification of an analyte (a very small amount of physiological activity matter), immunological measurements can be effectively used. In the immunological measurements, the enzyme-linked immunosorbent assay (ELISA) method for the measurement of antigen using an immobilized antibody and antibodies conjugated with enzyme (enzyme–antibody conjugate) is known as a sandwich immunoassay technique [1–2]. This method's principle, presented in Figure 1, is very widely used because it can be applied easily with high sensitivity.

The use of enzyme as a label molecule has a lot of advantages over the use of the other kind of label molecules in both immunohistochemistry and immunoassay. In immunohistochemistry, enzyme–antibody conjugate permits localization and demonstration of cellular antigens in relation to tissue structures via optical microscope and electron microscope [3–5]. However, in the ELISA method, nonspecific adsorption of enzyme–antibody conjugate to solid phase considerably decreases the reliability of the measurement. Accordingly, in the

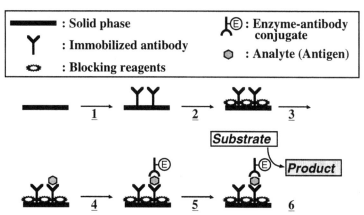

1. Add antibody solution to prepare immobilized antibody.
   And then wash to remove non-immobilized antibody.
2. Add a blocking reagent solution to cover adsorption points of antibody
   and restrain non-specific adosorption.
3. Add a analyte solution for immobilized antibody / analyte reaction.
   And then wash.
4. Add a enzyme-antibody conjugate solution for analyte / enzyme
   antibody conjugate reaction.
   And then washing to remove non-reacted enzyme-antibody conjugate.
5. Add a substrate solution for enzyme / substrate reaction.
   (Absorbance is increased in proportion to the amount of analyte.)
6. Absorbance is measured.

Figure 1 Principle of the enzyme-linked immunosorbent assay (ELISA) method.

sandwich method, a blocking reagent is necessary to restrain nonspecific adsorption of enzyme–antibody conjugate; this is the primary purpose of the blocking reagent. In Table 1, immunological measurement methods needing blocking reagent are summarized. Actually, when polystyrene [poly(St)] particles are used as solid phase, rabbit antibody is used as immobilized primary antibody, bovine serum albumin (BSA) is used as a blocking reagent, and antibody conjugated with horseradish peroxidase (HRP–antibody conjugate) is used as enzyme–antibody conjugate, it is known that 0.10–0.11% of the added HRP–antibody is nonspecifically adsorbed to the poly(St) particles [6–8]. In the sandwich method using immobilized antibody, after preparation of the solid-phase immobilized antibody, the other protein that has no influence on the immunological

Table 1 Immunological Measurement Methods Needing Blocking Reagents

Radioimmunoassay (RIA)
Enzyme-linked immunosorbent assay (ELISA)
Western blot technique
Immunospecific tissue staining
Immunospecific staining for electromicroscope
Flow cytometry

and enzymatic reaction is added to cover the adsorption point of the antibody. Another purpose (the second purpose) of the blocking reagent is stabilization of immobilized antibody. When the immobilized antibody is not stable, the reproducibility of the biological assay will be decreased. In general, BSA, ovalbumin, casein, and serum (containing proteins) are used as blocking reagents for the prevention of nonspecific adsorption and the stabilization of immobilized antibody. The last purpose (the third purpose) of the blocking reagent is stabilization of enzyme–antibody conjugate. When the enzyme–antibody conjugate is not stable, the reproducibility and reliability of the ELISA method are lowered. Accordingly, in the sandwich method using the enzyme–antibody conjugate, the other protein that has no influence on these immunological and enzymatic reactions is added to maintain the immunological activity of the enzyme–antibody conjugate. Typically, poly(St) particles and anti-(human growth hormone)immunoglobulins are used as a solid phase and an immobilized antibody, respectively, and BSA is added into antibody conjugated with horseradish peroxidase (HRP–antibody conjugate) solution to prevent denaturation of HRP–antibody conjugate [9]. In general, BSA, ovalbumin, casein, and serum (containing proteins) are used as blocking reagents for the prevention of nonspecific adsorption and the stabilization of immobilized antibody and enzyme-antibody conjugate. However, these blocking reagents made of protein have serious problems, that is, denaturation after a long preservation period, when they are frozen and melted over and over, heating, and autolysis. The purpose of this study is to develop a novel synthetic blocking reagent for ELISA.

The polymers having phospholipid polar groups, 2-methacryloyloxyethyl phosphorylcholine (MPC) polymers, are well known for suppression of protein adsorption [10] and protein denaturation [11]. In this study, water-soluble amphiphilic PMSt was examined as the blocking reagent in the ELISA method.

II. MATERIALS AND METHOD

A. Synthesis of Water-Soluble Phospholipid Polymer

MPC was synthesized by the method reported previously and was purified by recrystallization from acetonitrile [12]. Styrene and t-butyl peroxy pivalate were commercial reagent grade. Other reagents were extrapure commercial grade. The random copolymer of MPC and St, PMSt, was prepared via a conventional radical polymerization technique in ethanol using t-butyl peroxy pivalate as an initiator. The chemical structure of PMSt was confirmed with ^{1}H-NMR (JNM-EX270, JEOL, Tokyo, Japan) in D_2O. Gel permeation chromatography (TSKgel G400PW$_{XL}$ and TSKgel G300PW$_{XL}$, TOSOH, Tokyo, Japan) was used to estimate the number-average molecular weight (Mn) and the weight-average molecular weight (Mw) of the PMSt in 20 mM sodium phosphate buffer (pH 7.4) with poly(ethylene oxide) standards. The chemical structure of the PMSt and synthetic results are shown in Figure 2 and Table 2, respectively.

B. Measurement of the Amounts of Nonspecific Adsorbed Enzyme–Antibody Conjugate

Poly(St) microtiter plate (Nunc Maxisorp F96, Nunc, Roskilde, Denmark) was used as a solid phase, anti(mouse IgG)goat IgG (Lampire Biological Lab, Pipersville, PA) was used as an immobilized antibody, mouse IgG (Lampire

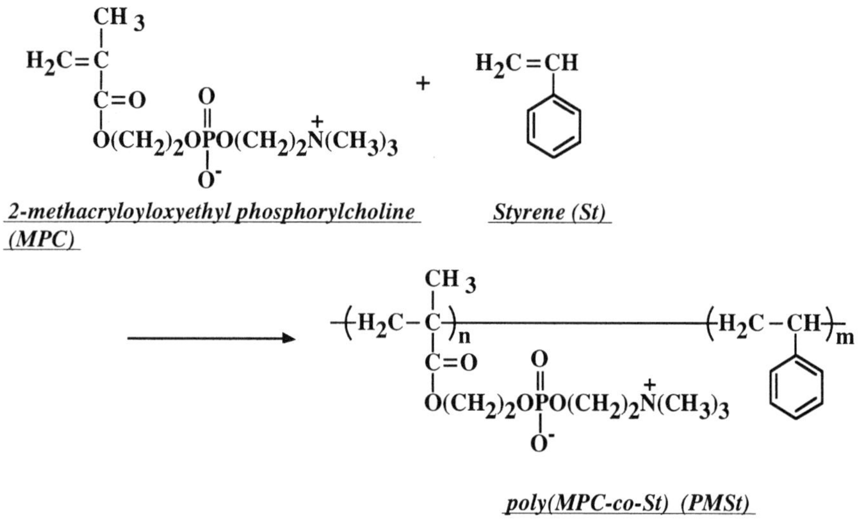

Figure 2 Chemical structure of PMSt.

Table 2 Synthetic Results of Poly(MPC-co-St) (PMSt)

Code	Mole fraction of MPC		Yield (%)	$Mn \times 10^{-5c}$	$Mw \times 10^{-5c}$	Mw/Mn^c
	In feed[a]	In copolymer[b]				
PMSt-1	0.50	0.62	85.0	1.0	1.6	1.6
PMSt-2	0.70	0.69	85.0	1.5	5.9	3.9

[a]PMSt-1: [monomer] = 1.0 mol/L, [t-butyl peroxy pivalate] = 0.003 mol/L; PMSt-2: [monomer] = 2.0 mol/L, [t-butyl peroxy pivalate] = 0.005 mol/L; polymerization was carried out at 60°C for 6 hr in ethanol.
[b]Unit mol fraction of MPC for copolymer and estimated by ^{1}H-NMR in D_2O.
[c]Estimated by GPC with poly(oxyethylene) standard, Mn and Mw represent the number- and the weight-average molecular weights, respectively.

Biological Lab, Pipersville, PA) was used as an antigen, and anti(mouse IgG)-goat IgG conjugated with horseradish peroxidase (HRP–IgG conjugate) (Wako, Osaka, Japan) was used as an enzyme–antibody conjugate. BSA (Sigma, St. Louis, MO) and casein (from bovine milk, Sigma, St. Louis, MO) were commercial reagent grade and used without further purification. o-Phenylenediamine hydrochloride (OPD) (Wako, Osaka, Japan) was used as a substrate of HRP. The preparation of antibody-immobilized solid phase, 100 µL of 10-µg/mL anti(mouse IgG)goat IgG solution (100 mM sodium phosphate buffer, pH 7.4) was pipetted into each well of the microtiterplate, and then the microtiterplate was sealed with adhesive strip and incubated at 4°C overnight. After incubation, anti(mouse IgG)goat IgG solution was aspirated from each well. To remove unimmobilized anti(mouse IgG) goat IgG, the microtiterplate in each well was washed with 300 µL phosphate-buffered saline (PBS, pH 7.4). The washing process was repeated four times. After washing, to prepare a microtiterplate blocked by blocking reagents, one of the PBS solutions containing 0.1 wt% PMSt, 1.0 wt% BSA, and 1.0 wt% casein was pipetted into the wells (300 µL/each well), and then the microtiterplate was sealed with adhesive strip and incubated at 4°C overnight. After incubation the solutions were removed from each well, and then the microtiterplate was washed with PBS four times. For measurement of the amount of nonspecific adsorption of HRP–IgG conjugate, the following process was carried out. The HRP–IgG conjugate solution was diluted PBS containing 0.5 wt% BSA (dilution was 1:10,000). One hundred microliters of diluted HRP–IgG conjugate solution was pipetted into each well, and then the microtiterplate was sealed with adhesive strip and incubated at 4°C overnight. After incubation the diluted HRP–antimouse IgG solution was aspirated from each well, and then the microtiterplate in each well was washed with PBS four times. To prepare substrate solution, 6 mg OPD was dissolved with 15 mL aqueous solution containing 50 mM Na_2HPO_4, 24 mM citric acid, 0.006% H_2O_2. One hundred microliters of the OPD solution was pipetted into well and incubated at 25°C for 10 min. After incubation, to stop the reaction 50 μL of 2N H_2SO_4 was pipetted into each well. Absorbance at 492 nm was measured via microtiterplate reader (MPRA-4i, TOSOH, Tokyo, Japan).

C. Effect of PMSt on Initial Sensitivity for Assay

After the microtiterplate that was blocked by blocking reagents was stored at 40°C for 20 days, to measure the activities of immobilized antibody, 100 μL of 1.0-μg/mL mouse IgG solution dissolved in PBS containing 0.5 wt% BSA was pipetted into the well, the microtiterplate was sealed with adhesive strip and incubated at 4°C overnight. The IgG solution was removed from each well, and then the microtiterplate was washed with 300 μL of PBS four times. The same operation was then carried out as for the measurement of amounts of nonspecific adsorbed enzyme-antibody conjugate.

D. Effects of PMSt on Immunological Activities of Enzyme–Antibody Conjugate

To prepare antibody-immobilized solid phase, 100 μL of 10-μg/mL anti(mouse IgG)goat IgG solution (100 mM sodium phosphate buffer, pH 7.4) was pipetted into each well of the microtiterplate, and then the microtiterplate was sealed with adhesive strip and incubated at 4°C overnight. After incubation, anti(mouse IgG)goat IgG solution was aspirated from each well. The microtiterplate in each well was washed with 300 μL of PBS four times. To prepare the microtiter plate blocked by BSA, 300 μL of PBS containing 1.0 wt% BSA was pipetted into each well, and then the microtiter plate was sealed with adhesive strip and incubated at 4°C overnight. After incubation, the solutions were removed from each well, and then the microtiter plate was lyophilized to maintain the activities of immobilized antibody. The lyophilized microtiter plate was in a refrigerator until used or applied to the next step. For the measurement of the immunological activities of HRP–IgG conjugate, the following process was carried out. For reaction between the immobilized antibody and mouse IgG (which was used as antigen), 100 μL of PBS containing both 1.0 μg/mL mouse IgG and 0.5 wt% BSA was pipetted into each well, and the microtiter plate was sealed with an adhesive strip and incubated at 4°C overnight. The solution was removed from the well, and then the microtiter plate was washed with PBS four times. The HRP–IgG conjugate solution was diluted with PBS containing various blocking reagents (PMSt, casein, or BSA) (dilution rate was 1:10000). The final concentration of PMSt was 0.1 wt% and 1.0 wt%, that of casein and BSA was 1.0 wt%. One hundred microliters each of the diluted HRP–IgG solutions containing various blocking reagents were pipetted into each well, and then the microtiter plate was sealed with an adhesive strip and incubated at 4°C overnight. After incubation, the HRP–IgG conjugate solution was aspirated from each well, and then the microtiter plate was washed with PBS four times. The same operation was then carried out as for the measurement of amounts of nonspecific adsorbed enzyme–antibody conjugate.

E. Measurement of Immunological Activities of HRP–IgG Conjugate

The diluted HRP–IgG solutions containing various blocking reagents were stored at 25°C for a period of 37 days. To measure the immunological activities of HRP–IgG conjugate by the ELISA method, the same operations were carried out as for the effects of PMSt on the immunological activities of HRP–IgG conjugate.

III. RESULTS

A. Synthesis of Water-Soluble Phospholipid Polymer

Table 2 summarizes the results of the copolymerization of MPC with St. The copolymerization proceeded homogeneously in ethanol. The chemical structure of PMSt was confirmed with ^{1}H-NMR. That is, the peaks assigned to α-CH$_3$ (0.95 ppm), —N$^+$(CH$_3$)$_3$ (3.1 ppm) and —C$_6$H$_6$ (7.2 ppm) were observed. From the ratio of the integration of the —N$^+$(CH$_3$)$_3$ peak and the —C$_6$H$_6$ peak, the mole fraction of MPC was determined. The PMSt obtained was soluble in water, PBS, and ethanol.

B. Measurement of Amounts of Nonspecific Adsorbed Enzyme–Antibody Conjugate

Figure 3 shows the amount of nonspecific adsorption of HRP–IgG conjugate. In comparison with BSA and casein used as a blocking reagent, PMSt as a blocking agent had almost the same level of function as for nonspecific adsorption ($p < 0.01$).

C. Effect of PMSt on Initial Sensitivity for Assay

Figure 4 shows the effect of the blocking reagent on the ELISA method. When measurement of the amount of non-specific adsorbed enzyme–antibody conjugate, PMSt, BSA, and casein had almost equal ability for prevention (Fig. 3).

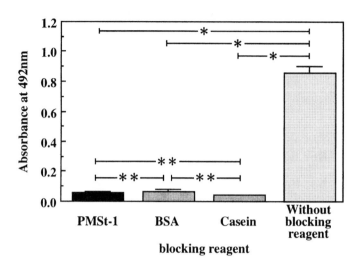

Figure 3 Amount of nonspecific adosorption of HRP-IgG conjugate. Concentration: [PMSt-1] = 0.1 wt%, [BSA] = 0.01 wt%, [casein] = 0.01 wt%, average ± SD ($n = 4$), *: $p < 0.01$, **: $p > 0.01$.

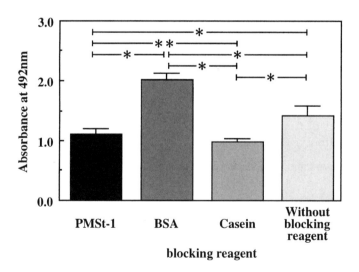

Figure 4 Effect of blocking reagent on initial sensitivity for assay. Concentration: [PMSt-1] = 0.1 wt%, [BSA] = 0.01 wt%, [casein] = 0.01 wt%, average ± SD ($n = 6$), *: $p < 0.01$, **: $p < 0.01$.

However, in the case of the measurement of activities of immobilized antibody using mouse IgG as antigen, BSA had higher responsibility as compared with other blocking reagent ($p < 0.01$). The difference between PMSt and casein was not significant ($p > 0.01$).

Figure 5 shows the remaining activities of immobilized antibody. When the BSA and casein were used as blocking reagent, the immunological activity decreased about 50% over 20 days. However, in the case of PMSt, the activity remained at approximately 100%. It is already reported that the proteins adsorbed on the MPC maintained their secondary structure. The character appears when the antibody is immobilized on the surface. In this study, we used poly(St) microtiterplate as solid phase to compare blocking agents. With another combination of solid phase, PMSt will sufficiently prevent nonspecific adsorption.

D. Effects of PMSt on Immunological Activities of Enzyme–Antibody Conjugate

Figure 6 shows the absorbance of product by the reaction between the enzyme (HRP) and the substrate (OPD) for 10 min. The maximum wavelength of the absorption spectrum of products is at 492 nm, so absorbance at 492 nm is proportional to the amount of product. When the absorbance at 492 nm was compared with 1.0 wt% BSA solution used as blocking reagent, that of PMSt solu-

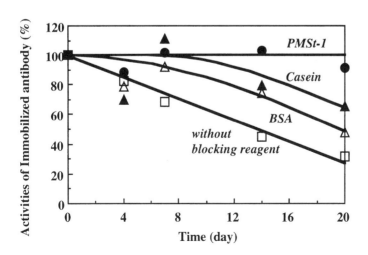

Figure 5   Stabilization of immobilized antibody. PMSt-1: ● (0.01 wt%); casein: ▲ (0.1 wt%); BSA: △ (0.1 wt%), without blocking reagent: □.

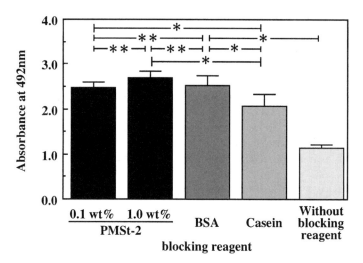

Figure 6 Amount of product by enzyme–substrate (HRP–OPD) reaction. Concentration: [PMSt-2] = 0.1 wt% and 1.0 wt%, [BSA] and [casein] = 0.1 wt%, average ± SD ($n = 6$), *: $p < 0.01$, **: $p > 0.01$.

tions with 0.1 wt% and 1.0 wt% concentrations were almost equal ($p < 0.01$). However, in the case of the 1.0 wt% casein solution, the absorbance decreased to about 80% as compared with the BSA case ($p > 0.01$). Moreover, in the case of diluted HRP–IgG solution without the blocking reagent, the absorbance was decreased to about half as compared with that of the solution containing 1.0 wt% BSA ($p > 0.01$).

E. Measurement of Immunological Activities of HRP–IgG Conjugate

Figure 7 shows the remaining immunological activities of HRP–IgG conjugate. After they stand at 25°C, in casein of 1.0 wt%, with BSA solutions used as blocking reagent and in the absence of the blocking reagents, the immunological activities decreased to about 5% of their initial value after 37 days. In the case of 1.0 wt% casein solutions, the immunological activity decreased to about 30% of its initial value after 37 days. However, in case of 0.1 wt% PMSt solutions, the activity remained at 74% of its initial value. Moreover, when the 1.0 wt% PMSt solution was applied, the immunological activity remained at 92% of its initial value even after 37 days.

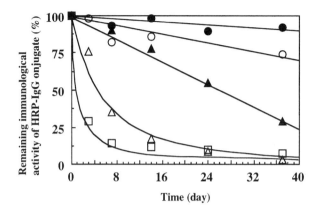

Figure 7 Remaining imunological activities of HRP–IgG conjugate. PMSt-2: ○ (0.1 wt%), ● (1.0 wt%); BSA: △ (1.0 wt%); casein: ▲ (1.0 wt%), without blocking reagent: □.

IV. DISCUSSION

The goal of this research is to develop a novel synthetic blocking reagent for ELISA in place of blocking reagent made of protein. In both immunohistochemistry and immunoassay, the enzyme–antibody conjugate and the proteins that have no influence on the immunological and enzymatic reaction are widely used as stabilizer of enzyme–antibody conjugate [1–5,9]. However, these protein stabilizers have serious problems, that is, denaturation after a long preservation period, when they are frozen and melted over and over, heating, and autolysis, and then there is danger of cross-reaction and biohazard.

It was already reported that the MPC polymer functions for reduction of the amount of absorbed protein and suppression of conformational change of the protein [10,11]. Protein was used as a blocking reagent with the function of preventing the nonspecific adsorption of enzyme–antibody conjugate, stabilizing the immobilized antibody, and stabilizing the enzyme–antibody conjugate. Therefore, we examined PMSt as the blocking reagent in the immunoassay system.

Figure 3 shows the amount of nonspecific adsorption of HRP–IgG conjugate. As compared with BSA and casein used as a blocking reagent, PMSt as a blocking agent had almost the same level of function as nonspecific adsorption ($p < 0.01$). Without immobilized antibody (only microtiterplate), when HRP–IgG solution was pipetted into wells treated with these blocking reagents, PMSt also showed equal function (data was not shown). This is because the hydrophobic units in PMSt could adsorb on microtiterplate surface immobilized of the anti(mouse IgG)goat IgG, and the MPC units prevented nonspecific adsorption of HRP–IgG conjugate.

Figure 4 shows the effect of the blocking reagent on the ELISA method. However, in the case of measurement of activities of immobilized antibody using mouse IgG as antigen, BSA had higher responsibility compared with the other blocking reagents. This result indicated that blocking reagents could attach the gaps not only between immobilized antibodies but on the immobilized antibody itself. Thus, if the hydrophilic-hydrophobic nature of immobilized antibody were to change, the responsibility would be changed.

Figure 5 shows the remaining activities of immobilized antibody. When the BSA and casein were used as blocking reagent, the immunological activity decreased about 50% over 20 days. However, in the case of PMSt, the activity remained at approximately 100%. It is already reported that the proteins adsorbed on the MPC maintained their secondary structure [11]. The character appears when the antibody is immobilized on the surface. In this study, we used poly(St) microtiterplate as solid phase to compare blocking agents. With another combination of solid phase, PMSt will sufficiently prevent nonspecific adsorption.

As shown in Figure 6, compared with the amount of product from the enzyme–substrate (HRP–OPD) reaction using 1.0 wt% BSA solution as blocking reagent, the amount of product using 0.1 wt% PMSt solution and 1.0 wt% PMSt solution was almost the same ($p < 0.01$). This is because the PMSt did not inhibit the reaction between antibody and antigen and the reaction between enzyme and substrate and prevent nonspecific adsorption of enzyme–antibody conjugate onto the polyethylene surface of test tubes and pipette during measurement. Without blocking reagent, the amount of product was about half as compared with 1.0 wt% BSA solution used as stabilizer ($p > 0.01$). This was due to the nonspecific adsorption of enzyme–antibody conjugate.

Figure 7 shows the remaining immunological activities of HRP–IgG conjugate. By using the 0.1 wt% PMSt solution, the immunological activities of HRP–IgG remained at 74% of their initial value; and by using the 1.0 wt% PMSt solution, the activities of HRP–IgG remained at 92% of their initial value, even after 37 days. The concentration of PMSt is an important factor in maintaining the immunological activity of HRP–IgG conjugate. It was already reported that the surface tension of aqueous solution of random poly(MPC-co-n-butyl methacrylate (BMA)) (poly(MPC-co-BMA)) depended on the polymer concentration, and it was then reported that the fluorescence intensity of both 8-amino-naphthalene-1-sulfonate (ANS) and 1-anilinonaphthalene (AN) solutions containing poly(MPC-co-BMA) became strong with a decrease in MPC mole fraction in the poly(MPC-co-BMA) [13]. The two different fluorescent dyes, ANS and AN, were used as extrinsic probes for the hydrophobic region in water [14]. When these dyes exist in a hydrophobic region of polymers, the enhancement of the fluorescence quantum yield and a shift of emission maximum toward the blue are observed [15]. Properties in water of the PMSt cannot be measured using ANS and AN because the PMSt have styrene groups. The PMSt can be bound to the hydrophobic cleft of HRP–IgG conjugate because the PMSt has the same tendency as poly(MPC-co-BMA).

It was already reported that the proteins adsorbed onto the MPC surface maintained their nature secondary structure [11]. Using the PMSt solution as blocking reagent, the same stabilization effects also appear.

We used HRP and OPD for labeling the antibody and substrate of HRP, respectively. If there are other combinations of the enzyme and substrate, PMSt will have enough functions to maintain the immunological activities of enzyme–antibody conjugate. When differential scanning calorimetric analysis of the protein solution was carried out, the peaks based on the thermal denaturation of proteins are observed at about 55–65°C [16]. However, PMSt solutions without protein did not show any peak in this temperature range. Moreover, when the protein solution is frozen and melted over and over again, the protein will be denatured and then appear as aggregation or precipitate of protein. On the other hand, no characteristic changes of PMSt are observed from its being frozen and melted repeatedly. The proteins (BSA and casein) have a danger of cross-reaction and biohazard because BSA and casein are made of bovine serum and bovine milk, respectively, containing another protein. In the case of PMSt, there is no cross-reaction and no danger of biohazard because PMSt is a synthetic polymer not containing another protein. From these results, it is concluded that the PMSt is superior to proteins as a blocking reagent and is an effective reagent for the immunoassay system.

ACKNOWLEDGMENTS

The authors are grateful to the members of the NOF Corporation, Tokyo, Japan—Dr. Kenshiro Shuto, Mr. Satoshi Yamada, and Mr. Ryota Ando—for their useful comments on this work.

REFERENCES

1. B. H. Anderton, R. C. Thorpe. New methods of analyzing for antigens and glycoproteins in complex mixtures. Immunol. Today 2:122–127, 1980.
2. G. B. Wisdom, Enzyme-Immunoassay. Clin. Chem. 22:1243–1255, 1976.
3. M. Osborn, R. E. Webster, K. Weber. Individual microtubules viewed by immunofluorescence and electron microscopy in the same PtK2 cell. J. Cell Biol. 77:R27–R34, 1978.

4. A. G. Farr, P. K. Nakane. Immunohistochemistry with enzyme labeled antibodies. A brief review. J. Immunol. Method. 47:129–144, 1981.
5. L. Orci. The insulin factory: a tour of the plant surroundings and a visit to the assembly line. Diabetologia 28:528–546, 1985.
6. E. Ishikawa, M. Imagawa, S. Hashida, S. Yoshitake, Y. Hamaguchi, T. Ueno. Enzyme labeling of antibodies and their fragments for enzyme immunoassay and immunohistochemical staining. J. Immunoassay 4:209–327, 1983.
7. E. Isikawa, M. Imagawa, S. Hashida. Ultrasensitive enzyme immunoassay using fluorogenic, luminogenic, radioactive and related substrates and factors to limit the sensitivity. Develop. Immunol. 18:219–232, 1983.
8. M. Imagawa, S. Yoshitake, Y. Hamaguchi, E. Isikawa, Y. Niitsu, I. Urushizaki, R. Kanazawa, S. Tachibana, M. Nakazawa, H. Ogawa. Characteristics and evaluation of antibody–horseradish peroxidase conjugates prepared by using a maleimide compound glutaraldehyde and periodate. J. Appl. Biochem. 4:41–57, 1982.
9. E. Ishikawa, S. Hashida, S. Kato, Y. Imura, H. Imura. Sensitive enzyme immunoassay of human growth hormone for clinical application. A review. J. Clin. Lab. Anal. 1:238–242, 1987.
10. K. Ishihara, N. P. Ziats, B. P. Tierney, N. Nakabayashi, J. M. Anderson. Protein absorption from human plasma is reduced on phospholipid polymers. J. Biomed. Mater. Res. 25:1397–1407, 1991.
11. K. Ishihara, H. Nomura, T. Mihara, K. Kurita, Y. Iwasaki, N. Nakabayashi. Why do phospholipid polymers reduce protein absorption? J. Biomed. Mater. Res. 39: 323–330, 1998.
12. K. Ishihara, T. Ueda, N. Nakabayashi. Preparation of phospholipid polymers and their properties as polymer hydrogel membranes. Polym. J. 22:355–360, 1990.
13. K. Ishihara, T. Tsuji, Y. Sakai, N. Nakabayashi. Synthesis of graft copolymers having phospholipid polar group by macromonomer method and their properties in water. J. Polym. Sci. A, Polym. Chem. 32:859–867, 1994.
14. M. Ikemi, N. Odagiri, S. Tanaka, I. Shinohara, A. Chiba. Hydrophobic domain structure of water-soluble block copolymer. 2. Transition phenomena of block copolymer micelles. Macromolecules 15:281–286, 1982.
15. S. Ghosh, M. K. Basu, J. S. Schweppe. Interaction of 1-amino-8-naphthalene sulphonate with human serum low-density lipoprotein. Biochem. Biophys. Acta. 337: 395–403, 1974.
16. J. W. Donovan, R. A. Beardslee. Heat stabilization produced by protein–protein association. Differential scanning calorimetric study of the heat denaturation of the trypsin–soybean trypsin inhibitor and trypsin–ovomucoid complex. J. Biol. Chem. 250:1966–1971, 1975.

22
Biocompatible Phospholipid Polymers for Prevention of Unfavorable Bioreactions on the Surface of Medical Devices

Kazuhiko Ishihara
The University of Tokyo, Tokyo, Japan

Yasuhiko Iwasaki and Nobuo Nakabayashi
Tokyo Medical and Dental University, Tokyo, Japan

Michiharu Sakakida
Kumamoto University School of Medicine, Kumamoto, Japan

Motoaki Shichiri
Kikuchi Medical Doctor's Association Hospital, Kumamoto, Japan

I. INTRODUCTION

A biocompatible surface is important, not only for blood-contacting medical devices, but also for subcutaneously implanted diagnostic devices. Hemodialysis is one of the most important methods for blood purification [1]. The properties required for a hemodialysis membrane are an excellent ultrafiltration rate, permeability by solutes, mechanical strength, and blood compatibility. Many synthetic polymer membranes have been investigated to raise the efficiency of dialysis; however, cellulose membranes are still used worldwide for 50% of hemodialysis. Although the cellulose membrane has both good permeability and mechanical strength, its blood compatibility must be further improved for better hemodialysis [2]. Thus, it is necessary to infuse an anticoagulant such as heparin during hemodialysis to prevent coagulation. Moreover, the cellulose membrane induces significant activation of the complement system due to strong interactions between the membrane surface and complement proteins [3].

Recently, microdialysis system is developed and applied to the monitoring of low-molecular weight biosubstances in living organisms [4]. This system needs a semipermeable hollow-fiber probe to separate the target biosubstances from proteins. The measurement has to be performed precisely for a long period and should not affect the host by causing chronic inflammation, infection, or pain. Implantation of a foreign material in living organism causes an inflammatory response that involves complex interactions between specific cells and molecular mediators. The grade, intensity, and pathological consequences of the inflammation, however, depend on the coating materials. Therefore the surface biocompatibility of the hollow-fiber probe must be improved for applying the system to long-term continuous monitoring. In treatment of diabetes, the artificial endocrine pancreas is a promising clinical device [5]. The most sensitive and critical function of the artificial endocrine pancreas is measuring glucose concentration, either in vivo by the needle-type enzymatic glucose sensor, or ex vivo using the microdialysis method.

We have found that polymers with a phospholipid polar group, 2-methacryloyloxyethyl phosphorylcholine (MPC, Fig. 1) copolymerized with hydrophobic monomers such as n-butyl methacrylate showed improved blood compatibility [6–10]. The amount of plasma protein adsorbed on the MPC polymer from human plasma was drastically reduced with an increase in the MPC mole fraction in the polymer [8,9]. These results clearly indicated that the MPC moieties in the polymer play an important role in improved blood compatibility. It has been reported that the MPC polymer could modify on the surface of the cellulose dialysis membrane and hollow fibers [11–15]. The MPC polymer-modified membrane suppressed protein adsorption, platelet adhesion, and complement activation when it contacted whole blood without anticoagulant.

We considered that if the cellulose hollow fiber modified with the MPC polymer for the hemodialyzer can be applied as the microdialysis probe, long-term monitoring of glucose in situ will be realized as shown in Figure 2. The

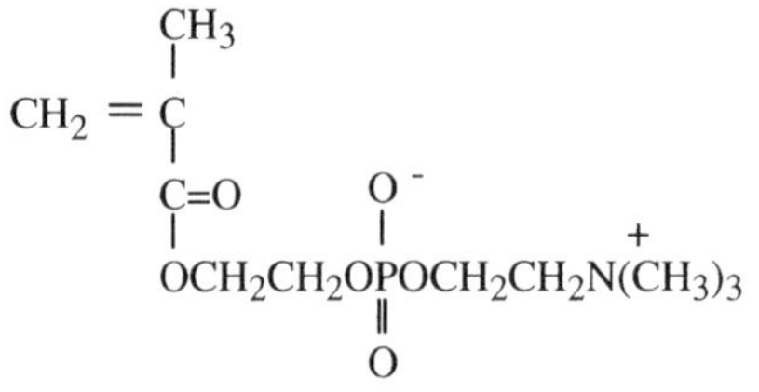

$$CH_2 = \overset{\displaystyle \overset{CH_3}{|}}{\underset{\displaystyle \underset{\displaystyle OCH_2CH_2O\overset{\displaystyle \overset{O^-}{|}}{\underset{\displaystyle \underset{O}{\|}}{P}}OCH_2CH_2N(CH_3)_3^+}{\underset{|}{C=O}}}{C}$$

Figure 1 Chemical structure of MPC.

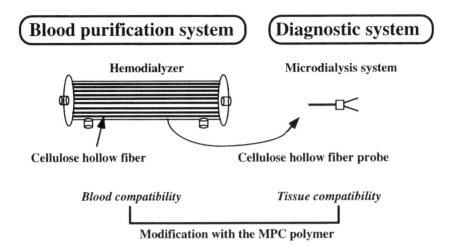

Figure 2 Cellulose hollow fibers for biomedical devices.

tissue compatibility of the microdialysis probe was investigated after the coating with the MPC polymer.

II. MATERIALS AND METHOD

A. Materials

MPC was synthesized by the method reported previously [6]. The water-soluble graft polymer constituted of cellulose and poly(MPC), MPC-grafted cellulose (MGC, Fig. 3), was synthesized by the method described previously [13]. The regenerated cellulose hemodialysis membrane was obtained from Enka, A.G. (Wappertal-Barmen, Germany). The thickness of the membrane was 20 μm. The cellulose hollow-fiber probes for the microdialysis method were obtained from Eicom, Kyoto, Japan, the outer diameter was 0.22 mm, the implanted length was 15 mm, and the molecular cutoff was 5×10^4.

B. Coating of the MGC on Cellulose Membrane

The coating of the MGC on the cellulose membrane was carried out using a 0.5 wt% aqueous solution of the MGC. The cellulose membrane was immersed in the solution for 3 min; the membrane was removed from the solution and dried under atmospheric conditions for 2 hr and then dried in vacuo for 15 hr. The

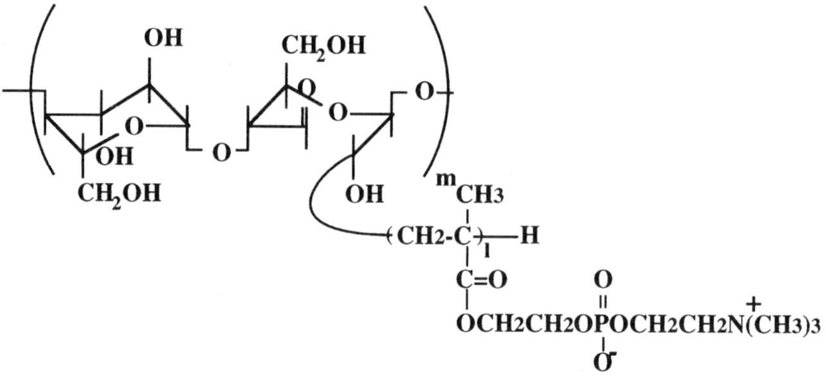

Figure 3 Chemical structure of water-soluble cellulose grafted with poly(MPC) (MGC).

surface of the membrane was characterized with an X-ray photoelectron spectroscope (XPS, ESCA-200, Scienta, Uppsala, Sweden).

C. In Vitro Blood-Contacting Test

The citrated whole blood of rabbit was immediately centrifuged for 15 min at 750 rpm to obtain citrated platelet-rich plasma (PRP) [7].

The cellulose membrane and that coated with the MGC were interposed between two parts of a separable acrylic well 1.5 cm in diameter for cell culture. A phosphate-buffered solution (PBS, pH 7.4, ionic strength 0.15) was poured into the well to equilibrate the membrane surface. After 15 hr, the PBS was removed and 1 mL of PRP was poured into the well and kept for 180 min at room temperature. After removal of the PRP, the membrane was rinsed twice with PBS and immersed into PBS containing 2 wt% glutaraldehyde to fix the adhered platelets. The membrane was freeze-dried and coated with gold to observe the surface using a scanning electron microscope (SEM, JEOL JSM-5400, Tokyo, Japan).

D. Preparation of Cellulose Hollow-Fiber Probe Covered with the MGC

The microdialysis sampling system was purchased from Eicom, Kyoto, Japan. The principle of this monitoring system is that of dialysis. An illustration of the system is shown in Figure 4. The hollow-fiber probe was implanted in the subcutaneous tissue and perfused with physiological saline solution at a

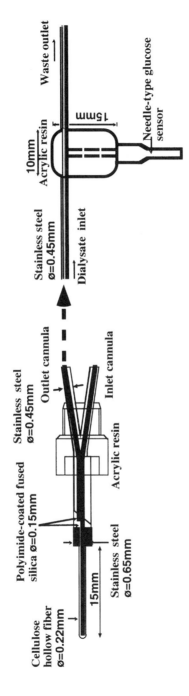

Figure 4 Schematic representation of microdialysis system composed of cellulose hollow-fiber probe (left) and flow cell unit with sensor (right).

rate of 120 μL/hr. The saline solution comes to the hollow fiber, and dialysate comes directly to the glucose electrode. Glucose concentration in the dialysate is determined continuously with a needle-type glucose sensor extracorporeally.

The surface of the hollow-fiber probe was covered with MGC via solution-dipping with 0.5 wt% aqueous solution of MGC.

Before in vivo application, all implants—the hollow-fiber probes—were sterilized in ethylene oxide gas (40°C, 4 hr) and visually inspected.

E. Measurement of Subcutaneous Glucose Concentration Using Microdialysis System

Continuous subcutaneous tissue glucose monitoring in healthy and diabetic volunteers was carried out. The cellulose hollow-fiber probe was connected via a connecting tubing to a microdialysis unit that incorporated a flow cell with a needle-type glucose sensor for extracorporeal sensing, a micro-roller pump, a saline reservoir, and a waste bag. Sensor currents are then transmitted to the glucose monitoring system. Subcutaneous tissue glucose concentrations are digitally displayed continuously on this monitoring system. Hyperglycemia or hypoglycemia is signaled by the sound of an alarm. In this experiment, a cellulose hollow-fiber probe was inserted into the subcutaneous tissue of the abdomen, and the perfusion rate was selected at 120 mL/hr.

F. Implantation of Cellulose Hollow-Fiber Probe in Subcutaneous Tissue

Rats were anesthetized with a barbiturate, but only a local anesthesia was used for the human volunteers. Under sterile conditions a needle catheter unit was used as a tunnel to implant the hollow-fiber probes (by 22-gauge catheter). The catheter was inserted subcutaneously and the implant was placed into the catheter. The implant was left situated freely in the subcutaneous tissue after the catheter was withdrawn. The ends of the hollow fiber or sensor were fixed to the skin with tape to keep the implant in position and to avoid mechanical pressure and tension inside the tissue. In the case of the rat experiments, a plastic cover was seen above the implanted hollow fibers to protect the material and to avoid premature removal by the rat.

Hollow-fiber probes in a rat were located dorsally left and right of the spinal column. Two or four hollow-fiber probes were implanted; half of the samples were MGC-coated hollow-fiber probe, whereas the other half of the implants were original cellulose hollow-fiber probe. At determined intervals the hollow-fiber probes are extracted, with surrounding tissue, from the rats. Rat tissue was embedded in paraffin and stained with hematoxylin-eosin. The other half of the hollow-fiber probes were embedded in Epon 812.

In each human volunteer, two hollow-fiber probes were inserted in the abdomen. For comparing biological reactions to different materials individually, the surface of one of the hollow-fiber probes comprised cellulose while the other was coated additionally with MGC. After 1, 7, and 14 days the hollow-fiber probes were perfused with physiological saline (0.9%) and connected to a glucose sensor. The hollow-fiber probes were pulled out carefully after 7 or 14 days and the specimen was prepared for microscopic observation.

III. RESULTS AND DISCUSSION

A. Cellulose Membrane Coated with the MGC

We tried to prepare MGC and applied them as coating materials on the cellulose membranes.

As shown in Figure 5, when MGC was immobilized on the surface of the cellulose membrane from an aqueous solution by drying, the cellulose backbone in the MGC could act as a fixation site for the poly(MPC) chains on the surface because of the strong affinity due to hydrogen bonding between the base cellulose and the cellulose backbone. That is, the cellulose backbone could orient to the base cellulose membrane selectively and the poly(MPC) chains could spread out when blood contacts membrane. Since the treatment process includes only coating and drying, it is an easy process to improve blood compatibility on the cellulose membrane.

Coating with the MGC on cellulose membrane surface was confirmed by

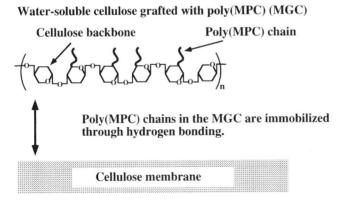

Figure 5. Concept of immobilization of poly(MPC) chain on cellulose membrane by coating with MGC.

XPS and phosphorus analysis based on the MPC moiety in the MGC. The amount of MGC on the surface was about 50 $\mu g/cm^2$. The MGC coated on the surface did not elute when the membrane was washed with distilled water sufficiently. The permeability of low-molecular-weight solutes through the cellulose membrane modified with the MGC did not change compared to the original cellulose membrane. The tensile strength of the cellulose membrane also did not change after coating with the MGC. Therefore, the coating of MGC on the cellulose membrane did not show any adverse effect on membrane performance.

Figure 6 shows an SEM view of cellulose membranes after contact with PRP for 180 min. It can be seen that the number of adherent blood cells on the original cellulose membrane were decreased dramatically by coating with MGC. In earlier studies, we showed that the MPC moiety on the polymer membrane was important to suppress protein adsorption and platelet adhesion [8,9,11–13]. Protein adsorption of membranes for medical use influences the performance of membranes with regard to permeability and selectivity. Therefore, we consider that the cellulose membrane covered with the MGC may maintain permeability of solute when the membrane is exposed in the bloodstream. From these results, it can clearly be said that the MGC is a suitable material for modification of the surface of the cellulose dialysis membrane, which requires blood compatibility, biocompatibility and permeability of solute.

B. Continuous Glucose Monitoring Subcutaneously Using Microdialysis System

As shown in Figure 7, with the original cellulose hollow-fiber probe, the linear regression line between apparent subcutaneous tissue glucose concentrations and blood glucose concentrations obtained on the fourth day was not significantly

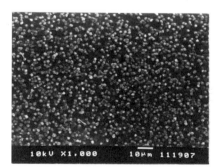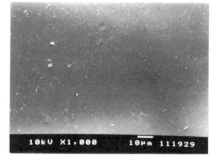

Figure 6   SEM picture of cellulose membrane (left) and that coated with MGC (right) after contact with PRP for 180 min.

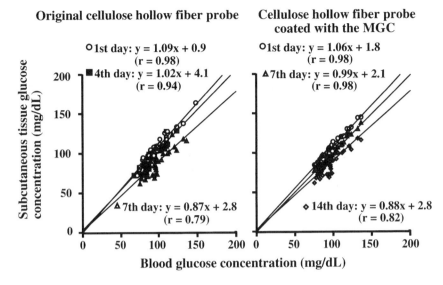

Figure 7   Linear regression analysis between subcutaneous tissue glucose concentrations measured by extracorporeal glucose monitoring system and blood glucose concentrations determined by glucose oxydase method in healthy subjects.

different from that obtained on the first day; however, the regression line obtained on the seventh day was significantly different from that obtained on the first day, demonstrating that apparent subcutaneous tissue glucose concentrations were lower than blood glucose concentrations. On the contrary, with cellulose hollow-fiber probes covered with MGC, a highly significant correlation between apparent subcutaneous tissue glucose concentrations and blood glucose concentrations was observed during seven days of monitoring. But the regression line obtained on the 10th or 14th day was significantly different from that obtained on the first day. By introducing the in vivo calibration technique corrected with fasting blood glucose levels every morning after seven days of continuous monitoring, subcutaneous tissue glucose concentrations measured by this monitoring system again correlated with glycemic excursions for 14 days.

D.   Tissue Compatibility of MPC-Polymer-Modified Cellulose Hollow-Fiber Probe

Figure 8 presents optical microscope pictures of cellulose hollow-fiber probe with and without MGC coating. After 11 days of implantation, the inflammatory reactions of the tissue surrounding the cellulose hollow-fiber probe and that

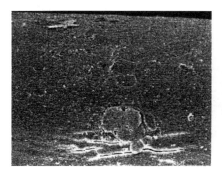 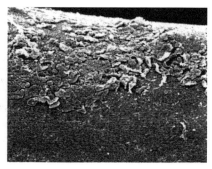

Figure 8 SEM pictures of the cellulose hollow-fiber probe coated with MGC (left) and the original cellulose hollow-fiber probe (right) after seven days of implantation in human volunteers. Original magnification was 1,000.

coated with MGC were very similar in intensity and character. Adjacent to the surface of the hollow-fiber probes, a thin layer of neutrophils, macrophages, and fibroblasts, surrounded by a thin layer of granulation tissue, had developed.

SEM pictures of the sample surface extracted from human volunteers revealed that regardless of the duration of implantation, the surface deposits of the MGC-coated hollow-fiber probes appeared smooth and even, whereas original cellulose hollow-fiber probe caused an irregular adhesion of cells, as shown in Figure 9.

TEM pictures in Figure 10 demonstrate the attachment of neutrophils and macrophages on the MPC polymer layer, but encapsulation with multilayered fibroblasts surrounding the cellulose hollow-fiber probe was found after 14 days of implantation.

In inflammatory response, polymorphonuclear leukocytes and macrophages as well as lymphocytes and fibroblasts are prominent. After 14 days, the surface of a hollow-fiber probe implanted in human subjects showed that neutrophils adhered to the MPC polymer layer but that fibroblasts encapsulated the cellulose hollow-fiber probe. Neutrophils and macrophages are expected to occur in the early stage to encapsulate a foreign material. This could be defined as a severe interaction between cellulose hollow-fiber probe and the host tissue, since the thickness of the capsule is sometimes taken as a measure of the biocompatibility. We suggested that the MPC polymer itself caused a mild inflammatory reaction. However, due to the movement of the implant inside the host tissue, the adhesion of cells mentioned earlier appeared. Conversely, the cellulose hollow-fiber probe obviously activated a different inflammatory reaction from the beginning of implantation and stimulated the process of encapsulation,

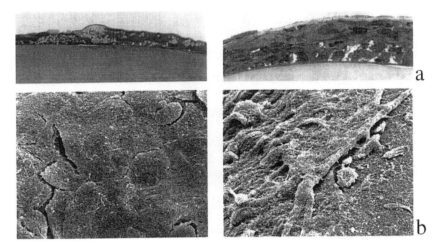

Figure 9 Microscope pictures of the cellulose hollow-fiber probe coated with MGC (left) and the original cellulose hollow-fiber prove (right) after 14 days of implantation in a human volunteer. (a): Optical microscope picture (Toluidine blue stained), original magnification was 1,000; (b): SEM picture, original magnification was 2,000.

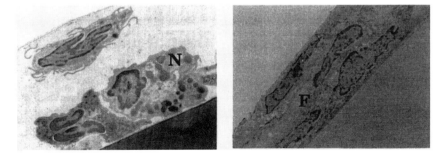

Figure 10 TEM pictures of the the cellulose hollow-fiber probe coated with MGC (left) and the original cellulose hollow-fiber prove (right) after 14 days of implantation in a human volunteer. Original magnification was 5,000. N: neutrophiles; F: fibroblasts.

which decreased the glucose penetration into the hollow-fiber probe and thus reduced the recovery rate in the dialysate.

With the MGC as a coating material, the hollow-fiber probes as part of the artificial endocrine pancreas showed high in vivo biocompatibility and stability.

IV. CONCLUSION

Water-soluble cellulose grafted with poly(MPC) is a useful material for the improvement of surface biocompatibility, such as blood compatibility and tissue compatibility of cellulose membrane. The microdialysis probe modified with the MGC can implant subcutaneously for a long period without significant inflammatory reaction. This modified microdialysis probe will be applied to diagnostic devices used in the fields of medicine, pharmaceuticals, bioengineering, and fermentation engineering.

ACKNOWLEDGMENTS

This study was supported in part by a Grant-in-Aid for Scientific Research from the MEXT Japan (09480250, 10558131). Dr. Ishihara would particularly like to express his appreciation for their support.

REFERENCES

1. T. Nishimura. Polymer materials for blood purification. In: Biomedical Applications of Polymeric Materials, T. Tsuruta, T. Hayashi, K. Kataoka, K. Ishihara, and Y. Kimura (eds.). CRC Press, Boca Raton, FL, 1993, pp. 191–218.
2. C. Woffindin and N. A. Hoenich. Blood-membrane interactions during haemodialysis with cellulose and synthetic membranes. Biomaterials 9:53–57 (1988).
3. P. R. Craddock, J. Fehr, A. P. Dalmasso, and H. S. Jacob. Hemodialysis leukopenia: pulmonary vascular leukostasis resulting from complement activation by dialyzer cellulose membranes. J. Clin. Invest. 59:879–888 (1977).
4. Y. Hashiguchi, M. Sakakida, K. Nishida, T. Uemura, K. Kajiwara, M. Shichiri. Development of a miniaturized glucose monitoring system by combining a needle-type glucose sensor with microdialysis sampling method. Diabetes Care 17:387–396 (1994).
5. M. Shichiri, M. Sakakida, K. Nishida, S. Shimoda. Enhanced simplified glucose sensors long-term clinical application of wearable artificial endocrine pancreas. Artif. Organs 22:32–42 (1998).
6. K. Ishihara, T. Ueda, N. Nakabayashi. Preparation of phospholipid polymers and their properties as hydrogel membrane. Polym. J. 22:355–360 (1990).

7. K. Ishihara, R. Aragaki, T. Ueda, A. Watanabe, N. Nakabayashi. Reduced thrombo-genicity of polymers having phospholipid polar groups. J. Biomed. Mater. Res. 24: 1069–1077 (1990).

8. K. Ishihara, N. P. Ziats, B. P. Tierney, N. Nakabayashi, J. M. Anderson. Protein adsorption from human plasma is reduced on phospholipid polymer. J. Biomed. Mater. Res. 25:1397–1407 (1991).

9. K. Ishihara, H. Oshida, Y. Endo, T. Ueda, A. Watanabe, N. Nakabayashi. Hemo-compatibility of human whole blood on polymers with a phospholipid polar group and its mechanism. J. Biomed. Mater. Res. 26:1543–1552 (1992).

10. K. Ishihara, H. Nomura, T. Mihara, K. Kurita, Y. Iwasaki, N. Nakabayashi. Why do phospholipid polymers reduce protein adsorption? J. Biomed. Mater. Res. 39: 323–330 (1998).

11. K. Ishihara, K. Fukumoto, J. Aoki, N. Nakabayashi. Improvement of blood compat-ibility on cellulose dialysis membrane. 1. Grafting of 2-methacryloyloxyethyl phos-phorylcholine onto a cellulose membrane surface. Biomaterials 13:145–149 (1992).

12. K. Fukumoto, K. Ishihara, R. Takayama, J. Aoki, N. Nakabayashi. Improvement of blood compatibility on cellulose dialysis membrane. 2. Blood compatibility of phospholipid polymer grafted cellulose membrane. Biomaterials 13:235–239 (1992).

13. K. Ishihara, H. Miyazaki, T. Kurosaki, N. Nakabayashi. Improvement of blood compatibility of cellulose dialysis membrane. 3. Synthesis and performance of wa-ter-soluble cellulose grafted with phospholipid polymer as coating materials on cel-lulose dialysis membran. J. Biomed. Mater. Res. 29(2):181–188 (1995).

14. K. Ishihara, K. Fukumoto, H. Miyazaki, N. Nakabayashi. Improvement of hemo-compatibility on a cellulose dialysis membrane with a novel biomedical polymer having a phospholipid polar group. Artif.Organs 18:559–564 (1994).

15. K. Ishihara, T. Shinozuka, Y. Hanazaki, Y. Iwasaki, N. Nakabayashi. Improvement of blood compatibility on cellulose dialysis membrane IV. Phospholipid polymer bonded to the membrane surface. J. Biomater. Sci. Polymer Edn, 10:271–282 (1999).

23

Site-Directed Immobilization of Proteins on Surfaces: Genetic Approaches

Jianquan Wang, Dibakar Bhattacharyya, and Leonidas G. Bachas
University of Kentucky, Lexington, Kentucky, U.S.A.

I. INTRODUCTION

Improving the way by which proteins are immobilized on surfaces such that they maintain their functionality is of critical importance in medical diagnostics, bioreactors, and biosensors. Depending on the intended applications, proteins can be immobilized on surfaces by different approaches [1,2]. Immobilization through physical adsorption, though simple, usually has the problem of leakage of the immobilized proteins from the support and leads to partial denaturation of the protein. This results in a short lifetime of devices based on immobilized proteins and may even cause sample contamination, which is a great concern if these devices are to be used in vivo. Chemical immobilization methods eliminate the leakage problem by covalently tethering protein molecules to supports. Different types of functional groups, such as amino, sulfhydryl, and carboxyl groups, are frequently used in chemical immobilization of proteins to the support. Since each protein molecule usually has many of these functional groups distributed on its surface, attachment through these groups inevitably leads to a different orientation of the immobilized proteins on the support (hereafter referred to as *random immobilization*). In random immobilization, the active/binding site of the protein molecule may be partially or totally blocked by neighboring protein molecules or the immobilization surface due to mixed orientation of the immobilized protein (Fig. 1A). This is one of the reasons that chemical

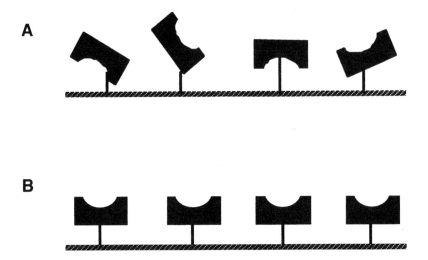

Figure 1 Immobilization of proteins on surfaces. (A) Random immobilization, where the active/binding site of the protein, shown as indentation, may be partially or totally blocked. (B) Site-directed immobilization, where all of the active/binding sites are fully accessible to the substrate.

immobilization often leads to a significant decrease in activity/binding capacity of the immobilized protein [3,4].

One way to address the issue of the orientation of immobilized proteins is to develop site-directed immobilization schemes through which proteins can be attached to surfaces in an orderly and controlled manner that allows the active/binding site to be fully accessible by its substrate (Fig. 1B). In addition, these well-defined immobilization schemes have the following advantages over random immobilization: (1) reproducible immobilization, where every protein molecule is immobilized through a unique site on the protein; (2) oriented immobilization of a protein molecule, which minimizes the conformational change usually encountered in random immobilization due to multipoint attachment on the support. Also, site-directed immobilized proteins facilitate structure/function studies of immobilized protein systems because of their uniformity; these studies are hindered in the case of randomly immobilized proteins because of the multitude of their orientations relative to the immobilization surface [5,6].

The key to achieving site-directed immobilized protein molecules on a support is to selectively attach the protein from a predetermined site on the protein surface. Several approaches have been used to accomplish site-directed immobilization of proteins, including: (1) immobilization of protein to supports through specific cysteine residues, if the protein molecule has only one cysteine residue accessible on its surface; (2) oriented immobilization of glycoproteins through their oligosaccharide residues; (3) immobilization through the biotin-(strept)avidin interaction of proteins that are site-specifically biotinylated by posttranslational modification; (4) oriented immobilization of proteins through the use of polypeptide affinity tags (for example, polyhistidine-tagged proteins can be immobilized to metal affinity chromatography supports); and (5) site-directed immobilization of antibodies through the selective binding of protein A or protein G to a specific site on the Fc region of the antibody [7,8]. The choice of immobilization approach usually depends on the protein of interest. For example, if a protein molecule has several cysteine residues accessible on its surface, the cysteine-based immobilization approach would not be applicable without additional modifications of the protein.

Of the many protein modification methods available, genetic engineering approaches provide unparalleled advantages over conventional chemical modification schemes. Not only can they be used to produce large quantities of desired proteins in organisms such as *Escherichia coli* and yeast, but they also make it possible to modify the protein of interest on the DNA molecular level in order to introduce desired properties (e.g., change in substrate specificity, improved thermostability) to the protein [9]. While native proteins are usually difficult to immobilize in an oriented fashion, genetically modified proteins can be designed in a way that allows facile site-directed immobilization.

In this study, subtilisin, alkaline phosphatase, and β-galactosidase are used as model proteins. Three different genetic engineering approaches were employed to modify the proteins in order to achieve site-directed immobilization. First, a cysteine residue was introduced to the cysteine-free subtilisin by site-directed mutagenesis, and the resultant protein was immobilized to different supports that have sulfhydryl reactive groups on their surface. Second, the octapeptide, Asp-Tyr-Lys-Asp-Asp-Asp-Asp-Lys (known as FLAG), was genetically fused to the amino terminus of alkaline phosphatase or the carboxyl terminus of subtilisin; the fused proteins were immobilized to protein A–coated surfaces through the protein A—anti-FLAG antibody—FLAG–protein interaction. Third, a posttranslational modification approach was utilized for β-galactosidase. Specifically, a peptide sequence recognized by biotin synthetase was fused to the β-galactosidase gene. After expression in *Escherichia coli*, the enzyme biotin synthetase recognizes the peptide and attaches a biotin molecule in vivo at one specific lysine residue in the recognition sequence. This site-specifically biotinylated β-galactosidase was then immobilized to avidin-coated surfaces through the biotin–avidin interaction. In all the three protein immobilization systems, site-directed immobilized proteins retained higher enzyme activity when compared to their randomly immobilized counterparts.

II. METHODOLOGY

Site-directed mutagenesis, gene fusion, and posttranslational modification are methods that can be used to modify proteins. These methods have been used previously in biochemical investigations to study structure/function relations, enhance enzyme activity, improve stability, alter substrate selectivity, etc. In our studies, these molecular biology methods are employed to modify enzymes in a way that facilitates site-directed immobilization on surfaces.

A. Site-Directed Mutagenesis

Proteins are encoded by genetic information contained in DNA segments (genes). Thus, by changing specific nucleotide(s) of a gene at the molecular level, one can site-specifically alter an amino acid residue of the protein encoded by the gene. This approach is referred to as *site-directed mutagenesis*. Although there are many different approaches to site-directed mutagenesis, in our studies we chose the one that is based on the polymerase chain reaction (PCR) [10,11]. A typical PCR reaction contains: (1) the target double-stranded DNA, (2) a set of two single-stranded oligonucleotides as primers, (3) a mixture of four deoxynucleotide triphosphates (dNTPs), and (4) DNA polymerase. Each PCR cycle goes through three different temperatures. At 94°C, the two strands of the target DNA separate from each other. When the temperature is lowered to around 50°C, the primers anneal to the separated target strands due to the complementary nucleotide base match (hydrogen bonding between adenine and thymine; guanine and cytosine). At 72°C, DNA polymerase incorporates dNTPs to the 3' end of the primer and synthesizes a copy of the target DNA. These cycles are repeated 20–30 times, so at the end of a PCR, the target DNA is amplified hundreds of thousand folds. Based on this principle, mutagenesis by PCR can be achieved simply by introducing base mismatch(es) in the primer. Once the PCR is done, the mismatched nucleotide(s) have been incorporated into the amplified DNA sequence.

Figure 2 schematically shows the steps involved in site-directed mutagenesis by overlap extension PCR. As indicated in the figure, the first two rounds of PCR are performed separately to introduce a specific base change (mutation) into the target DNA. The two PCR products overlap at one end. A third round of PCR, using these overlapping sequences as the template and primers A and D, amplifies the full-length gene with the desired mutation in the predetermined site. The mutated gene is then cloned back into a suitable vector and transformed in an appropriate host organism to express large quantities of modified proteins with desired properties.

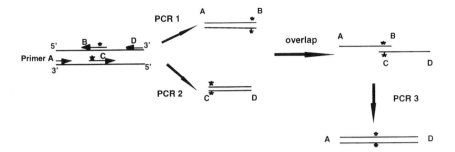

Figure 2 Site-directed mutagenesis by overlap extension polymerase chain reaction (PCR). The first two rounds of PCR (PCR 1 and PCR 2) use primer sets A, B and C, D, respectively. The third round overlap extension PCR (PCR 3) uses only the primers A and D to generate and amplify the modified full-length gene of interest. The asterisk denotes the mutated nucleotide(s).

B. Gene Fusion

Site-directed mutagenesis is not always feasible for modifying proteins for the purpose of site-directed immobilization. For example, bacterial alkaline phosphatase has more than one cysteine, lysine, and aspartic/glutamic acid residue. This makes site-directed mutagenesis impractical as a way to introduce a unique amino acid residue with a side-chain functional group for site-directed immobilization. An alternative approach to modifying such proteins is gene fusion [12–14]. In this approach, an affinity tag is fused to either terminus of the target protein through recombinant DNA technology. This is usually done by incorporating the nucleotide sequence coding for the affinity tag into oligonucleotide primers, followed by use of PCR. When the PCR is completed, the gene fusion product is cloned into a suitable vector and transformed into an appropriate host organism. After expression, the resultant tagged protein can be site-directed immobilized through the affinity tag.

C. Posttranslational Modification

After protein synthesis many proteins undergo a process termed *posttranslational modification*, in which they are modified within the cells by addition of a nonprotein moiety to form glycoproteins, lipoproteins, phosphoproteins, etc. [15,16]. Posttranslational modifications are of great importance in controlling many cellular events, such as signaling, growth, and transformation [17]. In some cases these modifications provide handles that can be used in fractionation

[18] and subsequent site-directed immobilization of proteins. For example, proteins with surface carbohydrate moieties can be separated from other proteins by binding to a column containing lectins; purified proteins can then be site-directed immobilized on lectin-coated supports.

III. RESULTS AND DISCUSSION

The enzymes subtilisin, bacterial alkaline phosphatase (BAP), and β-galactosidase were used as model proteins to demonstrate the advantages of using recombinant DNA techniques to site-specifically immobilize and orient proteins on surfaces. Subtilisin is a protease consisting of a single polypeptide, whereas BAP is a dimer, and β-galactosidase (a high-MW protein) is a tetramer. These proteins are of interest to bioanalytical and clinical chemistry and can be used for protein characterization after fragmentation (protease) [19,20] as well as in biosensors and diagnostics (alkaline phosphatase and β-galactosidase) [21,22].

Subtilisin BPN′ has several amino and carboxylic groups available on its surface, thus making it impossible to gain oriented immobilization by attaching this protein to surfaces by using these functional groups. Since subtilisin contains no cysteine residues, it is a good candidate for evaluating the use of site-directed mutagenesis to site-directly immobilize the enzyme. To achieve this, we introduced a unique cysteine residue at a predetermined position on the enzyme. After carefully examining the three-dimensional structure of subtilisin (Fig. 3),

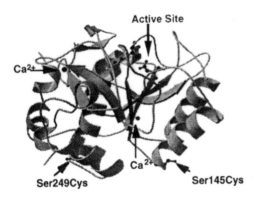

Figure 3 Structure of subtilisin BPN′. Serine-to-cysteine mutation was introduced at either position 249 or position 145, as labeled. Two calcium ions are required for stability. The graph was generated using Rasmol 2.5, Molscript, and Raster3D software. (From Refs. 23–25.)

we decided to replace serine with cysteine at either position 249 (S249C) or position 145 (S145C). These mutation sites are far away from the enzyme-active site and are exposed on the protein surface. In addition, because these mutations change only one atom (from oxygen in serine to sulfur in cysteine), either mutation should cause little conformational change to the protein.

The mutated subtilisin-(S249C) and subtilisin-(S145C) were expressed in *Bacillus subtilis*, which secretes the expressed protein outside the cells to the culture medium, thus simplifying the purification process. After expression, both the wild-type and mutant subtilisins were purified by ion-exchange chromatography using the BioCAD perfusion chromatography system. The number of sulfhydryl groups of the mutant subtilisins were determined by the Ellman's reagent and were found to correspond to one cysteine per subtilisin molecule [26]. Site-directed immobilization of the mutated subtilisin was achieved through the introduced surface cysteine residue on sulfhydro-reactive supports. Random immobilization was obtained by using a two-step glutaraldehyde reaction on amino-functionalized nonporous silica beads.

The results (see Table 1) indicate that subtilisin that was immobilized in a site-directed fashion had a k_{cat}/K_M ratio that was more than threefold the value of randomly immobilized subtilisin. Further, it was shown that the mutation site did have an effect on the overall catalytic efficiency of site-directed immobilized subtilisin. While the value of k_{cat}/K_M for immobilized subtilisin-(S249C) was $32.6 \ (\pm 3.8) \times 10^{-3} \ M^{-1} \ sec^{-1}$, the value for subtilisin-(S145C) was $42.9 \ (\pm 2.8) \times 10^{-3} \ M^{-1} \ sec^{-1}$. This can be explained by the fact that the S249C mutation is in the middle of a rigid α-helical loop; the attachment of subtilisin through this site somehow induces more conformational strain than through the more flexible hinge region of subtilisin-(S145C). It was observed that due to diffusional limitation, porous supports have a lower k_{cat}/K_M for immobilized subtilisin than non-

Table 1   Apparent Kinetic Parameters of Immobilized Subtilisin

Support	k_{cat}/K_M $(10^{-3} \ M^{-1} \ sec^{-1})$	Amount of enzyme immobilized (mg)
Immobilized subtilisin-(S249C)		
Derivatized silica (site-directed)	32.6 ± 3.8	0.54
Immobilized subtilisin-(S145C)		
Derivatized silica (site-directed)	42.9 ± 2.8	0.45
Derivatized silica (random)	12.8 ± 1.1	0.46
Activated Sepharose 4B	4.7 ± 0.6	0.46
Thiopropyl Sepharose 6B	16.1 ± 1.0	0.66

Source: Ref. 26.

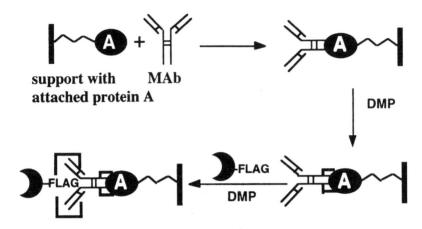

Figure 4 Schematic presentation of immobilization of the octapeptide FLAG–tagged protein onto protein A–coated surfaces through anti-FLAG monoclonal antibody (MAb) and protein A (or protein G) interaction. Dimethylpimelimidate (DMP) is used as a cross-linker to stabilize the MAb—protein A and FLAG—MAb interactions.

porous silica beads. Activated Sepharose 4B beads are more porous than thiopropyl Sepharose 6B beads. Thus, a more severe internal diffusion limitation is encountered for the former support, which can explain the corresponding lower k_{cat}/K_M value.

A gene fusion approach was used to immobilize BAP in a site-directed fashion on surfaces. Specifically, the octapeptide Asp-Tyr-Lys-Asp-Asp-Asp-Asp-Lys (FLAG) was genetically fused to the N-terminus of bacterial alkaline phosphatase [27]. The N-terminus of BAP lies geometrically at a site of the protein that is away from the active site and is solvent accessible. The FLAG peptide is recognized by a monoclonal antibody (MAb), and protein A or protein G site-specifically interacts with the Fc region of the MAb. By taking advantage of these interactions, BAP can be site-directed immobilized on protein A–(or protein G–) coated surfaces (see Fig. 4).

Table 2 compares the kinetic parameters of immobilized genetically tagged FLAG-BAP, chemically tagged FLAG-BAP, and unmodified BAP. The chemically tagged FLAG-BAP was prepared by using a carbodiimide N-hydroxysuccinimide (NHS) cross-linking chemistry, which links the FLAG through its carboxylate functional groups to the amines of lysine residues on BAP. Due to the fact that one BAP molecule may be tagged with more than one FLAG octapeptide, the immobilization of chemically tagged BAP through these FLAG residues on the protein A-MAb surface inevitably leads to multipoint attach-

Table 2 Kinetics of Bacterial Alkaline Phosphatase (BAP)-FLAG system immobilized on modified polyethersulfone (MPS) membrane

Enzyme	State	V_{max} (μmol mg^{-1} min^{-1})
BAP	Homogeneous	43.2
	Random immobilization	0.34
CC-BAP	Homogeneous	42.6
	Antibody-mediated random immobilization	0.81
SD-BAP	Homogeneous	37.2
	Antibody-mediated site-directed immobilization	31.7

BAP alone denotes native protein; CC-BAP represents chemically conjugated BAP-FLAG; SD-BAP means FLAG peptide genetically fused to the N-terminus of BAP.

ment, which is evidenced by a decreased enzyme activity. Site-directed immobilization using genetically tagged FLAG-BAP retained 85% of its homogeneous enzyme activity (compared to 1.9% for that of chemically tagged BAP). Random immobilization obtained with a glutaraldehyde reaction of unmodified BAP resulted in almost total loss of enzyme activity (only 0.8% residue activity was left after immobilization). Similar results were obtained for the immobilization of a FLAG–subtilisin BPN' fusion protein on the protein A–MAb surface in comparison to randomly immobilized subtilisin (data not shown). All these experimental results demonstrated that gene fusion technology is another way to modify a protein in order to gain favorable site-directed immobilization.

To explore the feasibility of employing recombinant DNA techniques to generate modified protein for site-directed immobilization, we selected a posttranslational modification system that site-specifically adds a biotin molecule to a biotin recognition sequence that was genetically fused to the N-terminus of β-galactosidase. Biotination of proteins by posttranslational modification has been reported as a means to label, purify, and develop competitive binding assays [28,29]. In this approach, a plasmid DNA containing the β-galactosidase gene fused to the biotin recognition sequence at its N-terminus was transformed and expressed in bacterial *Escherichia coli* cells. After expression, biotin ligase inside *E. coli* cells recognizes the biotin recognition sequence and attaches a biotin molecule to a particular lysine on the sequence. Thus, this posttranslational modification approach site-specifically attaches one biotin molecule to the N-terminal domain of each expressed β-galactosidase subunit. The expressed biotin–β-galactosidase conjugate was purified with a monomeric avidin resin, and the purified conjugate was immobilized to surfaces of a modified polyethersulfone (MPS) membrane, which was first coated with avidin [30].

Figure 5 compares the immobilization approaches of biotinylated β-galactosidase through the biotin–avidin interaction onto MPS membrane. In method A, biotinylated β-galactosidase was biotinylated by using N-hydroxysuccinimido-biotin. Since the enzyme has many lysine residues on its surface, several biotin molecules may be attached to each β-galactosidase molecule, leading to a less controlled orientation of immobilized β-galactosidase through the avidin anchor. On the contrary, the site-specifically biotinylated β-galactosidase by posttranslational modification (method B) gives rise to well-controlled and site-directed immobilization. This immobilized enzyme retains 24.9% of the corresponding homogeneous activity after immobilization, whereas immobilization by method A results in only 12.6% residual activity. Randomly immobilized β-galactosidase through its lysine residues by glutaraldehyde-mediated coupling retains even much less activity (1.7%). It should be noted that the first avidin layer on the MPS membrane is not oriented. This may be one of the reasons why the site-directed immobilized enzyme activity is about one-fourth of that of

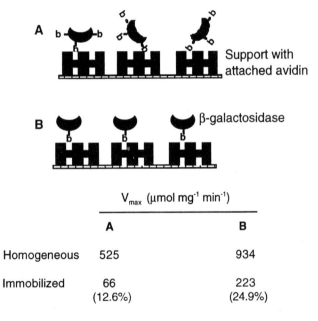

V_{max} (µmol mg^{-1} min^{-1})		
	A	B
Homogeneous	525	934
Immobilized	66	223
	(12.6%)	(24.9%)

Figure 5   Comparison of V_{max} for biotinylated β-galactosidase immobilized on surfaces of modified polyethersulfone (MPS) membrane through an avidin spacer. The symbol *b* stands for biotin. (A) Chemically conjugated biotin–β-galactosidase; (B) genetically biotinylated β-galactosidase using posttranslational modification. Numbers in parentheses are the percentage of residual activity after immobilization.

the homogeneous enzyme. These results demonstrate that well-controlled site-directed immobilized proteins retain higher activity than their randomly immobilized counterparts.

IV. CONCLUSIONS

Immobilization of proteins on surfaces is of great importance in medical diagnostics, bioreactors, and biosensor development. Both physical adsorption and conventional chemical immobilization procedures usually result in random immobilization, in which protein activity is severely reduced due to conformational change and blockage of the active/binding site of the immobilized protein. Site-directed immobilized proteins minimize these detrimental effects and thus maintain higher activity (even at higher loadings) and stability than their randomly immobilized counterparts. As demonstrated herein, recombinant DNA technology opens an avenue for genetic engineering of proteins. By employing genetically modified proteins, well-controlled and site-directed immobilization of proteins can be achieved. In addition, site-directed immobilization minimizes the impact of activity loss due to surface hydrophobicity.

ACKNOWLEDGMENTS

The authors would like to thank the National Science Foundation and NASA for financially supporting this work. We also thank Drs. W. Huang and S. Vishwanath for their contributions to this work, which are cited in Refs. 4, 26, 27, and 30.

REFERENCES

1. Bickerstaff G. F., ed. Immobilization of Enzymes and Cells, Humana Press, Totowa, NJ, 1997.
2. Rao S. V., Anderson K. W., Bachas L. G., Mikrochim. Acta 128:127–143, 1998.
3. Srere P. A., Uyeda K. Methods Enzymol. 44:11–19, 1976.
4. Vishwanath S., Wang J., Bachas L. G., Butterfield D. A., Bhattacharyya D. Biotechnol. Bioeng. 60:608–616, 1998.
5. Sota H., Hasegawa Y., Iwakura M. Anal. Chem. 70:2019–2024, 1998.
6. You H. X., Lin S., Lowe C. R. Micron 26:311–315, 1995.
7. Anderson G. P., Jacoby M. A., Ligler F. S., King K. D. Biosens. Bioelectron. 12: 329–336, 1997.
8. Lu B., Smyth M. R., O'Kennedy R. Analyst 121:29R–32R, 1996.
9. Wiseman A. J. Chem. Technol. Biotechnol. 56:3–13, 1993.

10. Newton C. R., Graham A., eds. PCR. 2nd ed. Springer, New York, 1997.
11. White B. A., ed. PCR Cloning Protocols: From Molecular Cloning to Genetic Engineering. Humana Press, Totowa, NJ, 1997.
12. LaVallie E. R., McCoy J. M. Curr. Opin. Biotechnol. 6:501–506, 1995.
13. Wang C. L., Huang M., Wesson C. A., Birdsell D. C., Trumble W. R. Protein Eng. 7:715–722, 1994.
14. Bulow L., Mosbach K. Trends Biotechnol. 9:226–231, 1991.
15. Han K. K., Martinage A. Int. J. Biochem. 24:19–28, 1992.
16. Cozzone A. J. Biochimie 80:43–48, 1998.
17. Parekh R. B., Rohlff C. Curr. Opin. Biotechnol. 8:718–723, 1997.
18. Deyl Z., Miksik I. J. Chromatogr. 699:311–345, 1997.
19. Cottrell J. S. Pept. Res. 7:115–124, 1994.
20. Gharahdaghi F., Kirchner M., Fernandez J., Mische S. M. Anal. Biochem. 233: 94–99, 1996.
21. Engblom S. O. Biosens. Bioelectron. 13:981–994, 1998.
22. Sekine Y., Hall E. A. H. Biosens. Bioelectron. 13:995–1005, 1998.
23. Kraulis P. J. J. Appl. Crystallogr. 24:946–950, 1991.
24. Merritt E. A., Murphy M. E. P. Acta Crystallogr. D50:869–873, 1994.
25. Sale R. A., Milner-White E. J. Trends Biol. Sci. 20:374–376, 1995.
26. Huang W., Wang J., Bhattacharyys D., Bachas L. G. Anal. Chem. 69:4601–4607, 1997.
27. Vishwanath S., Watson C. R., Huang W., Bachas L. G., Bhattacharyya D. J. Chem. Tech. Biotechnol. 68:294–302, 1997.
28. Cronan Jr. J. E. J. Biol. Chem. 265:10327–10333, 1990.
29. Witkowski A., Kindy M. S., Daunert S., Bachas L. G. Anal. Chem. 67:1301–1306, 1995.
30. Vishwanath S., Bhattacharyya D., Huang W., Bachas L. G. J. Membr. Sci. 108: 1–13, 1995.

24

Polymeric Microspheres and Related Materials for Medical Diagnostics

Stanislaw Slomkowski, Beata Miksa, Dorota Kowalczyk, and Teresa Basinska
Polish Academy of Sciences, Lodz, Poland

Mohamed M. Chehimi and Michel Delamar
University of Paris, Paris, France

I. INTRODUCTION

Spherical colloidal polymeric particles, often called *nanospheres* (particles with diameters from a few nanometers to 100 nm) or *microspheres* (particles with diameters larger than those of nanospheres but usually smaller than 10 μm), were found to be suitable for attachment (adsorption and/or covalent immobilization) of various proteins, nucleic acids, and their fragments, as well as larger subcellular structures (cf. examples in Ref. 1). Micro- and nanospheres, onto whose surface it was possible to attach these biocompounds in their active form, have found many applications in medical diagnostic tests. Traditional tests (called *agglutination tests*) allow for the detection and/or semiquantitative determination of chosen compounds without using any special equipment, usually within a few minutes. Agglutination tests directed toward the determination of a given antigen consist of mixing a drop of liquid to be analyzed, usually on a plastic slide, with a drop of suspension containing microspheres with attached antibodies. (Due to the similarity of the colloidal properties of suspensions of polymeric particles to the properties of natural latex from the rubber tree *Hevea brasilisensis*, the former suspensions are often also called *latexes*.) As a result of antibody–antigen interactions the microspheres form aggregates. This type of test is illustrated schematically in Figure 1.

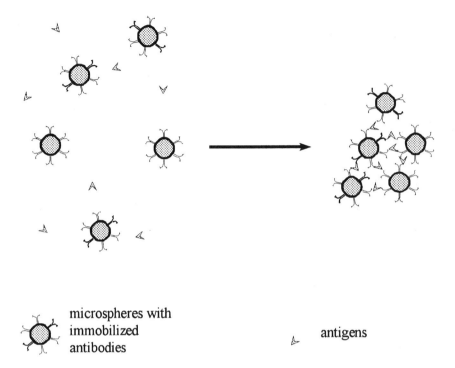

microspheres with
immobilized   antigens
antibodies

Figure 1 Schematic of aggregation test: aggregation of microspheres with antibodies resulting from antibody–antigen interactions.

In the simple latex agglutination test, aggregation is monitored with the naked eye. Such tests, usually relatively inexpensive, are often used for screening candidates for further, more detailed control. Selected examples of microsphere-based agglutination tests are given in Table 1.

Recent progress in the synthesis of various types of microspheres and the design of new microsphere-based materials opens the possibility of using them for preparation of diagnostic tests that do not require any liquid reagents (*dry tests*) and for the construction of biosensors. Therefore, synthesis of several types of microspheres, some of them developed recently, are described in this paper, together with the basic characteristics of these particles. Subsequently, procedures useful for the immobilization of proteins and data on protein concentrations on the surfaces of particle supports are also discussed. Attention is focused on various types of present and potential applications of microsphere-based materials for medical diagnostic devices.

Table 1 Examples of Microsphere-Based Agglutination Tests

Viral infections	AIDS, cytomegalovirus, enterovirus, hepatitis, *herpes simplex*
Bacterial infections	Brucella, diphtheria, leptospirosis, tuberculosis, leprosis, salmonella, *staphylococus aureus*, syphilis, tetanus toxoid, *Vibrio cholera* enterotoxin
Mycological infections	*Aspergillus fischeri, Candida albicans, Cryptococcus neoformans*
Parasitic infections	Amoebiasis, kala-azar, malaria, *Toxoplasmosa gondii, Trichinella spiralis*, trypanosoma
Autoimmune diseases	Antinuclear antibody, rheumatoid factor, thyroiditis
Hormone assays	Estrogen, human chorionic gonadotropin, human growth hormone, thyroglobulin, thyroid antibody
Drug assays	Barbiturates, cortisol, digoxin, morphine, penicillin, theophyline

II. SYNTHESIS OF MICROSPHERES

Microspheres used in diagnostic tests are synthesized in various emulsion- and/ or dispersion polymerization–related methods. Following are examples of the synthesis of microspheres useful for diagnostic purposes.

A. Polystyrene Microspheres [P(S)] by Radical, Emulsifier-Free Polymerization [2]

Monomer (10 mL of styrene purified from stabilizer) was emulsified in 70 mL of distilled water. Water solution of K_2SO_8 used as an initiator (4.4×10^{-2} g of $K_2S_2O_8$ in 30 mL) was added to this mixture. Polymerization was carried out at 65°C for 28 hr. The particles were then purified. The average diameter of these P(S) microspheres was $D_n = 0.52$ μm, and the polydispersity parameter D_v/D_n was 1.005 (D_v denotes the volume-averaged diameter). Surface concentration of $—OSO_3^-$ groups, incorporated into macromolecules of polystyrene, was found to be 3.39×10^{-6} mol/m². P(S) microspheres obtained in this process did not contain any reactive groups suitable for covalent immobilization of proteins or other bioactive macromolecules. These macromolecules could be attached to P(S) microspheres only by adsorption.

B. Polyacrolein Microspheres [P(A)] by Anionic Polymerization [3–5]

Microspheres were synthesized via the dropwise addition of 0.2 N NaOH to an aqueous solution of acrolein (5–20% wt/v) containing hydrogen sulfite–poly-(glutar aldehyde) conjugate (0.1–3% wt/v). NaOH was added until the pH was between 9 and 11.5, and then the mixture was stirred for 2 hours. This process yields microspheres with diameters from 40 nm to 8 μm, depending on the initial concentrations of acrolein and surfactant [hydrogen sulfite–polyglutar aldehyde)], and on the final pH. Aldehyde groups at the surfaces of these microspheres could be used for covalent immobilization of compounds (e.g., proteins) with primary amino groups.

C. Poly(styrene/acrolein) Microspheres [P(S/A)] by Copolymerization of Styrene and Acrolein [2]

Poly(styrene/acrolein) microspheres were synthesized from styrene and acrolein in the same manner as just described for P(S) particles. The number-average diameters of P(S/A) microspheres varied from 0.30 μm (for pure polyacrolein particles) to 0.52 μm [for pure P(S) microspheres]. The polydispersity parameter D_v/D_n for all syntheses was lower than 1.020.

D. Poly(styrene) Microspheres with Poly(ethylene oxide) Grafts [P(S)-PEO] [6]

Polystyrene microspheres with poly(ethylene oxide) grafts in the surface layer, terminated with—CH_2CH_2OH groups, were synthesized by emulsifier-free copolymerization of styrene with polyethylene oxide (PEO) macromonomers [polyethylene oxide methyl methacrylates] with chain length of PEO varying from exactly 1 to approximately 8 units. Depending on the structure of the macromonomer, its incorporation into the microspheres varied from 37% to 87%, in relation to the amount used in the monomer feed.

E. Microspheres with Thio- and/or Isothiouronium Groups (Hidden Thiol Groups) by Radical Copolymerization of Styrene and Vinylbenzylisothoiuronium Chloride (VBIC) (P(S/VBIC) Microspheres) [7,8]

Emulsion copolymerization of styrene with VBIC (cf. Scheme 1) leads to particles with isothiouronium groups at their surfaces that are easily hydrolyzed to sulfhydryl groups. [A typical synthesis is described elsewhere (see Ref. 8).]

F. Polypyrrole Core/polyacrolein Shell Microspheres [P(P/A)]

Synthesis of these microspheres was described by Miksa and Slomkowski [9]. After 24 hr of stirring the reaction mixture under nitrogen, the polypyrrole microspheres were isolated by centrifugation, washed with water, and isolated by

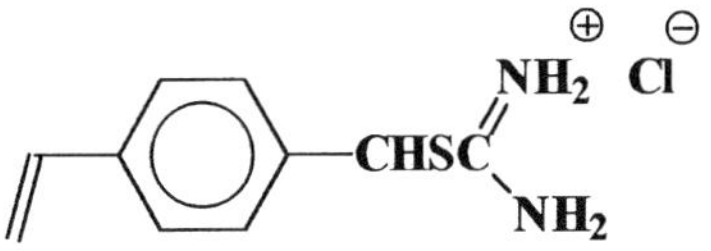

$$\text{CH}_2\text{=CH} - \text{C}_6\text{H}_4 - \text{CHSC} \overset{\overset{\oplus}{\text{NH}_2}}{\underset{\text{NH}_2}{\diagup}} \quad \overset{\ominus}{\text{Cl}}$$

VBIC

Scheme 1

centrifugation two more times. The average diameter of these particles was 124 nm. The polypyrrole microspheres (0.6 g) were resuspended in 50 mL of water solution containing 0.022 g of K_2SO_8, used as an initiator. Acrolein (0.2 mL) was added to this mixture and, after deaeration with nitrogen, polymerization of this monomer was carried out for 30 hr at 65°C. Addition of polyacrolein ad-layer resulted in an increase in the average diameter of particles to 154 nm. The P(P/A) microspheres were islolated by centrifugation and washed with fresh portions of water.

II. MICROSPHERES BY COPOLYMERIZATION OF ACRYLIC MONOMERS

A. Poly(methyl Methacrylate—Methacrylic Acid—2-hydroxyethyl Methacrylate) Microspheres (ACRYLAT) [10]

Microspheres were obtained by copolymerization of methyl methacrylate (4.56 g), methacrylic acid (0.8 g), and 2-hydroxyethyl methacrylate (HEMA) (2.4 g). Copolymerization was carried out in water (42 mL) in the presence of sodium dodecyl sulfate (0.03 g) used as surfactant. This mixture was deaerated with argon, and polymerization was initiated by raising the temperature to 70°C. After 15 min the temperature was raised to 96°C and the reaction was carried out for 2 hr with stirring (60 rev/min). Microspheres with diameter $D_n = 140$ nm and with surface concentration of carboxylic groups equal to 8.41×10^{-6} mol/m^2 were obtained.

B. Microspheres by Copolymerization of Methyl Methacrylate and 2-Hydroxypropyl Methacrylate [11]

Methacrylate (1.93 mL) and 2-hydroxypropyl methacrylate (1.13 mL) were added to 94 mL of double-distilled water preheated to 70°C (comonomer wt/wt ratio 6:4 and total monomer concentration 3% wt/v). To this mixture 3 mL of water solution containing 3×10^{-3} g of K_2SO_8 was added, and polymerization was carried out at 70°C for 8 hr. Polymerization yielded microspheres with z-averaged diameter equal to 296 nm and with zeta potential equal to -27.3 mV (at pH = 7.1). The elemental composition of the microspheres (carbon and oxygen atoms), as determined by XPS, was essentially the same as the elemental composition calculated for comonomer feed.

C. Magnetic Microspheres

There are two basic approaches used for the synthesis of magnetic microspheres. The first one, developed by Rembaum et al. [12], consists of the radical copolymerization of various acrylic comonomers (initiated by γ-radiation or by redox systems) carried out in the presence of iron oxide particles (Fe_3O_4) of nanometer size (suspensions of these particles in water are known by the name *ferrofluids*). Observations by scanning electron microscopy revealed that the diameter of these particles was 40 nm. The content of iron in the microspheres ranged from 6.2% to 28.4%.

The second method used for the preparation of magnetic microspheres was developed by Ugelstad et al. [13,14]. In this method, nanoparticles of magnetic iron oxide were prepared inside of the earlier-synthesized polymeric particles. For this purpose, the $-NO_2$ and $-ONO_2$ groups were introduced into the inner part of the parent microspheres. Then these microspheres were immersed in an aqueous solution of Fe^{2+} salts. Iron ions were transported into the inner part of the microspheres, where, after oxidation, they formed magnetic nanoparticles of iron oxides.

III. ADSORPTION AND COVALENT IMMOBILIZATION OF PROTEINS ONTO MICROSPHERES

Adsorption of proteins onto microspheres is usually very efficient in the case of hydrophobic particles, e.g., polystyrene microspheres [15–17]. This process usually comprises simple mixing of a suspension of microspheres with a protein solution in the appropriate buffer. The most effective adsorption was observed for buffers with pH close to the isoelectric point of the protein to be adsorbed. In spite of the fact that polystyrene microspheres found many applications as protein carriers used in diagnostics tests, the attachment by adsorption was often not satisfactory for the long shelf life of protein–microsphere preparations.

The aforementioned problem can be solved by covalent immobilization of proteins onto microspheres [8,18–20]. The microspheres described in the previous section are equipped with aldehyde groups (particles with polyacrolein segments) and/or carboxyl, hydroxyl, and sulfhydryl groups (microspheres from derivatives of acrylic acid and acrylates). In the simplest immobilization procedures, involving microspheres with aldehyde groups, it is sufficient to incubate a suspension of microspheres with protein solution and then to remove the unbound protein by centrifugation and eventually to wash them with buffer. During this process the reaction of aldehyde groups from the surface of the microspheres with amino groups of proteins leads to the formation of Schiff-base linkages (cf. Figure 2), which can be easily reduced to the stable form in reaction with $NaBH_3CN$.

We found that, in this way, it was possible to immobilize human serum albumin (HSA) and gamma globulins (γG) onto microspheres with aldehyde groups [9,17,20–22]. Surface concentrations of immobilized proteins (Γ) depend on the nature of the microspheres and protein. Generally, we found that for the same conditions of immobilization, the surface concentrations of immobilized γG are approximately two times higher than in the case of HSA. Moreover, the increased fraction of polyacrolein units in the surface layer of the microspheres results in lower surface concentrations of attached proteins.

For a given concentration of microspheres in suspension, the surface concentration of immobilized protein (Γ) depends on the concentration of protein in solution. In many instances, as in the case of the reversible covalent immobilization (e.g., before reduction of Schiff base with $NaBH_3CN$), it is possible to approximate this dependence by the Langmuir equation:

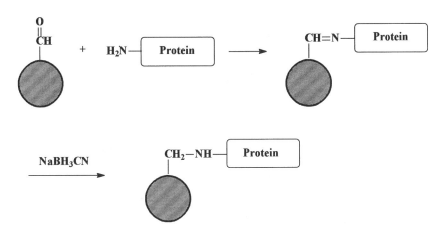

Figure 2 Schematic illustrating the covalent immobilization of proteins onto microspheres with aldehyde groups via formation of the Schiff-base linkages reduced to amine groups.

$$\frac{1}{\Gamma} = \frac{1}{\Gamma_{max}} + \frac{1}{\Gamma_{max}} K_D \frac{1}{[protein]_e} \qquad (1)$$

in which Γ_{max} denotes the maximal surface concentration of attached protein, K_D is equilibrium constant of protein attachment, and $[protein]_e$ is the concentration of protein at equilibrium. An example of such dependencies is shown in Figure 3 for HSA and human γG attached onto P(S/A) microspheres. From plots in Figure 3 it was possible to estimate the maximal surface concentrations of immobilized proteins (Γ_{max}), which were found to be 5.6 mg/m^2 and 1.1 mg/m^2 for γG and HSA, respectively.

Unfortunately, the method of immobilization by simple incubation of microspheres bearing aldehyde groups with protein solution was ineffective in the case of horseradish peroxidase (HRP) and glucose oxidase (GOD), enzymes often used in medical diagnostic assays. In the case of HRP this was due to the lack of the available —NH$_2$ groups, which are usually blocked in reaction with allylisothiocyanate present in the horseradish roots and liberated during isolation of this enzyme [23]. We solved this problem by oxidizing the sugar portion of the enzyme with NaIO$_4$ (resulting in the formation of aldehyde groups) and by treatment of P(S/A) microspheres in ethanol with an excess (100-fold with respect to the surface aldehyde groups on microspheres)

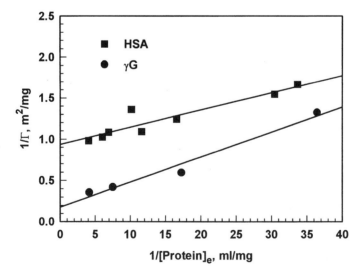

Figure 3 Dependence of $1/\Gamma$ on the reciprocal of the equilibrium protein concentration in solution. Immobilization onto P(S/A) microspheres ($D_n = 0.49$ µm, $D_v/D_n = 1.002$, surface concentration of aldehyde groups 2.28×10^{-8} mol/L).

of 1,2-ethylenediamine. This converts aldehyde groups at the surface of the microspheres into primary amino groups [24]. Eventually, we immobilized oxidized HRP with aldehyde groups (HRP–OX) onto the surface of the microspheres with amino groups. An illustration of this process is shown in Figure 4.

Oxidation of HRP was performed according to the following protocol. HRP (5 mg) was dissolved in 1 mL of water solution of $NaHCO_3$ (pH = 8.1). Then, 0.1 mL of 1% 1-fluoro-2,4-dinitrobenzene in ethanol was added to this solution. One hour later, 1.0 mL of $NaIO_4$ in water (concentration 0.06 mol/L) was added. The reaction mixture was mixed for 30 minutes and the excess $NaHCO_3$ was reduced by the addition of 1 mL of ethylene glycol solution in water (0.16 mol/L). Eventually, the modified enzyme was dialyzed against carbonate buffer (pH = 9.5), lyophilized, and stored at 4°C. The oxidized enzyme prepared and stored in this way did not change its activity after two months.

All attempts to immobilize glucose oxidase directly onto P(S/A) microspheres were unsuccessful. As one possible reason we considered the incompatibility of macromolecular chains of the surface layer of microspheres and of

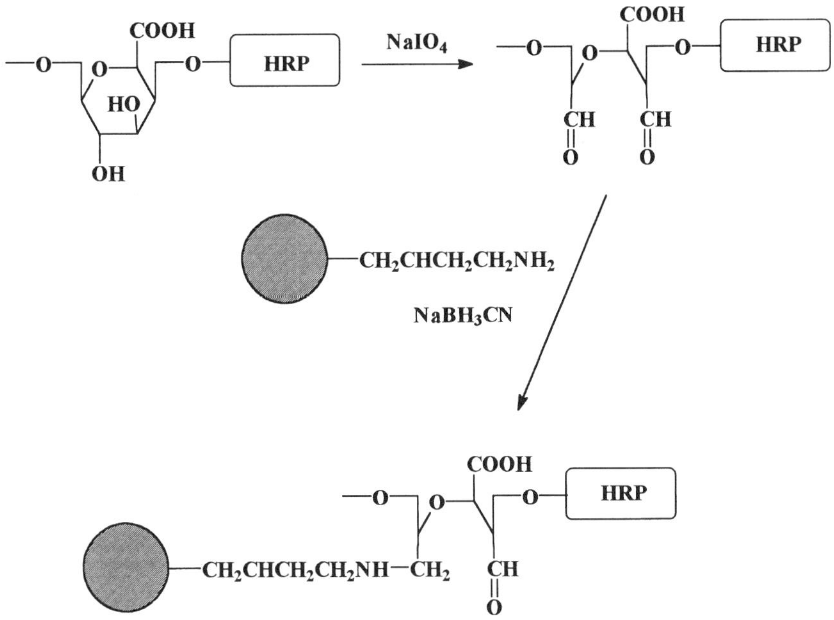

Figure 4 Scheme illustrating covalent immobilization of horseradish peroxidase onto P(S/A) microspheres modified with 1,2-ethylenediamine.

GOD. This explanation seems to be reasonable because we found that it was possible to immobilize GOD via oligo(ε-aminocaproic acid) spacers, increasing the distance between the surface of the microspheres and the molecules of the enzyme. The process of immobilization of GOD is shown schematically in Figure 5.

The first stage of this process consists of the addition of ε-aminocaproic acid linkers via aldehyde groups of microspheres. For this purpose P(S/A) microspheres (1 g), ε-aminocaproic acid (0.1 g), and 1-ethyl-3-(3-dimethylaminopropyl)carbodiimide hydrochloride (EDC) (0.25 g) were dissolved in 50 mL of phosphate-buffered saline (PBS), and this solution was slowly stirred at 4°C for 4 hr. The first stage was completed via isolation of the microspheres by centrifugation, washing them with 0.1 N NaCl and subsequently with distilled water. In the second step the modified microspheres, EDC (0.25 g), and GOD

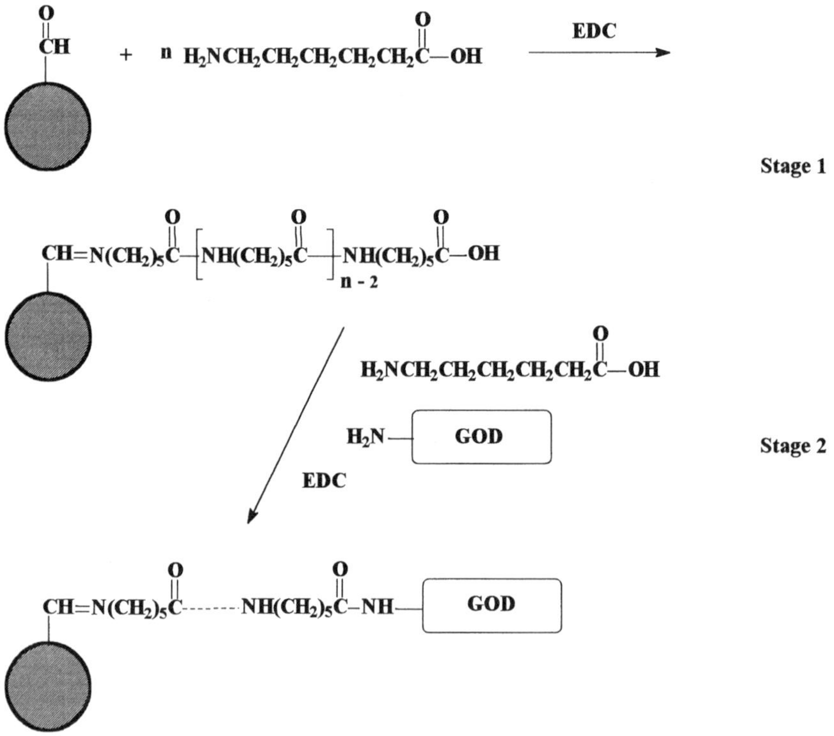

Figure 5   Scheme illustrating the covalent immobilization of GOD onto P(S/A) microspheres.

(0.19 g) were added to 50 mL of PBS and this medium was stirred for 8 hr, keeping the temperature of the mixture within the region from 0 to 4°C. Thereafter, microspheres were centrifuged and resuspended in distilled H_2O. Eventually, after fivefold repetition of the centrifugation–resuspension cycle, the purified microspheres with immobilized GOD were obtained. The surface concentration of GOD on these microspheres was $\Gamma(GOD) = 2.07 \times 10^{-3}$ g/m^2.

The foregoing carbodiimide method described above was also used for immobilization of HSA and polyclonal antiplasminogen antibodies onto the ACRYLAT microspheres with functional groups [10].

Biologically active macromolecules with amino groups can also be immobilized onto microspheres equipped with hydroxyl groups. However, prior to immobilization, hydroxyl groups have to be activated with cyanogen bromide. The corresponding processes of activation and immobilization are illustrated in Figure 6.

Following is an example illustrating immobilization of dansyl-ε-lysine onto microspheres obtained by the copolymerization of acrylic monomers [25]. CNBr (0.1 g) was added to an aqueous suspension of microspheres (ca. 0.5 g in 10 mL) with pH adjusted to 10.5. This mixture was allowed to react for 15 min at 25°C. Thereafter, the suspension was cooled down to 4°C and combined with 10 mL of sodium carbonate buffer (pH = 10) containing dansyl-ε-lysine ([dansyl-ε-lysine] = 10^{-2} mol/L). The immobilization of dansyl-ε-lysine was carried out at 4°C overnight. Eventually, the unbound dansyl-ε-lysine was removed by dialysis against an aqueous solution of NaCl (0.1 mol/L).

In principle, the same methods that are suitable for the immobilization of proteins are also used for the attachment of oligonucleotides equipped with linkers with primary amino groups [26]. Another approach was based on covalent immobilization of streptavidin onto microspheres, followed by immobilization of biotinylated DNA due to the streptavidin–biotin interactions [1].

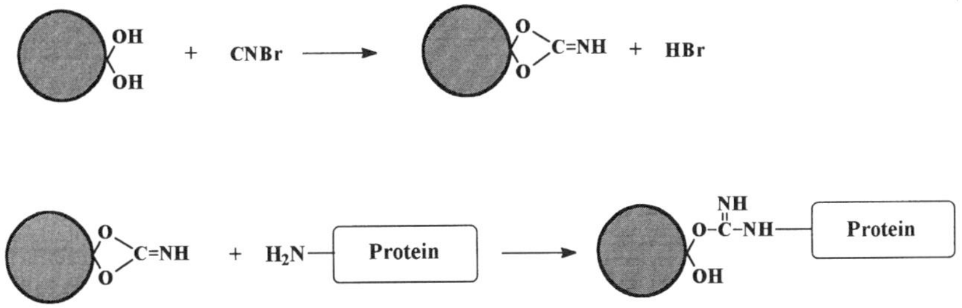

Figure 6 Scheme illustrating the immobilization of protein macromolecules onto microspheres with —OH groups activated with CNBr.

Microspheres with sulfhydryl groups [or with isothiouronium groups (hidden sulfhydryl groups)] were used for the covalent immobilization of biologically active compounds bearing sulfhydryl groups via disulfide bridges. An example of the procedure used for the immobilization of Fab fragments equipped with —SH group onto poly(S/VBIC) is given later [8]. Fab fragments $(5 \times 10^{-2}$ mol/L) in Tris buffer, pH = 9.2 (0.9 mL), were combined with 0.1 mL of a suspension of microspheres (10 w/v). Vials with this content were rotated end over end for 4 hr. Then microspheres were isolated by centrifugation and resuspended in glycine buffer $(5 \times 10^{-2}$ mol/L) containing bovine serum albumin (10 g/L) and NaCl ([NaCl] = 0.15 mol/L). Assays revealed that immobilized Fab fragments did retain, at least partially, their immunoactivity.

IV. ACTUAL AND POTENTIAL APPLICATIONS OF MICROSPHERES IN MEDICAL DIAGNOSTICS

For more than 40 years, polymeric microspheres have been used in the simple slide and/or tube agglutination tests in which the aggregation of particles with immobilized antibodies (or antigens), due to antibody–antigen interactions (cf. Fig. 1), is monitored with the naked eye. However, these tests allow only for semiquantitative determination of detected compounds, relating the maximal dilution of analyzed liquid at which aggregation still occurs to the lowest limit of analyte concentration that can be detected in a given test type.

Changes in the size and the number of the aggregates of microspheres affect the scattering of visible light. Thus, the quantitative determination of an analyte is possible in tests in which aggregation is measured nephelometrically and/or turbidimetrically. In the latter case, even a simple spectrophotometer can be used for measuring changes in the intensity of transmitted light (reduced by light scattering on microspheres and their aggregates). An example of the relation between the concentration of plasminogen in solution, in which microspheres are suspended, and the optical density at $\lambda = 600$ nm of suspension of ACRYLAT microspheres with immobilized antiplasminogen (ACRYLAT–anti-Plg), is shown in Figure 7. From Figure 7 it follows that ACRYLAT microspheres can be used for the determination of the concentration of plasminogen in the region from 1 µg/mL to ca. 100 µg/mL.

Recently, application of microspheres was proposed in so-called *dry tests* (based only on reagents in the dry state). These tests are related to paper chromatography and consist of the immobilization of antibodies (or antigens) in the required regions of blotting paper–like supports and on the placement, in the other selected regions of support, of microspheres with immobilized antibodies (or antigens) [27,28]. Black polypyrrole microspheres, easily visible on the strip, were used for this purpose. When a small amount of the analyzed liquid is

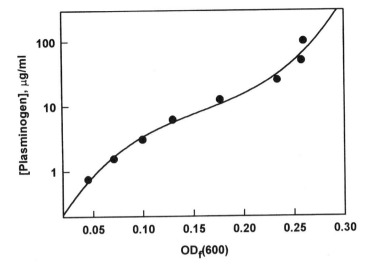

Figure 7 Relation between the concentration of plasminogen in the serum and the final optical density of ACRYLAT–anti-Plg [$OD_f(600)$] registered at 600 nm. Reference: suspension of Acrylat–anti-Plg (1.9 mg/mL) without plasminogen. (Based on data from Ref. 10.)

applied to the area in which the microspheres are present, the latter diffuse on the support and become permanently attached to the area in which antibodies (antigens) were immobilized. The corresponding antigens (antibodies) must be present in the analyzed liquid. Schematically such an assay is illustrated in Figure 8. The aforementioned dry tests based on the principle of chromatography were developed by Abbott for the detection of human chorionic gonadotropin (pregnancy test), hepatitis B surface antigen, and anti-HIV antibodies [27]. More recently, quantitative dry tests were developed (cf. Chapter 15 of this book, by Fitzpatrick and Lenda); however, in these tests colloidal gold particles were used as carriers of bioactive compounds.

   Polymeric microspheres are also potentially useful for other types of sensors. Recently we have begun to work on oximetric sensors for the determination of glucose, in which P(S/A) microspheres with immobilized GOD are used as the bioactive element. The model sensor, visualized in Figure 9, consists of the Clark-type electrode for determination of oxygen (CellOx 325, part of Oxi 330 oximeter—WTW, Weilheim, Germany) and P(S/A)-GOD microspheres confined in its vicinity.

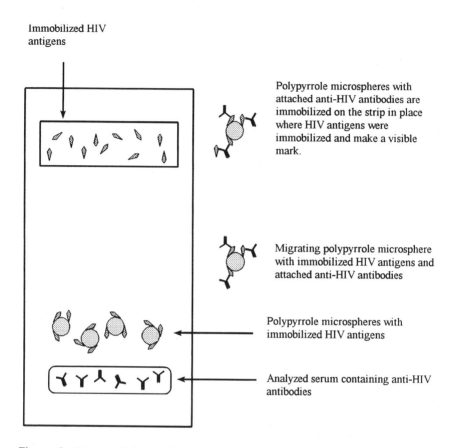

Immobilized HIV antigens

Polypyrrole microspheres with attached anti-HIV antibodies are immobilized on the strip in place where HIV antigens were immobilized and make a visible mark.

Migrating polypyrrole microsphere with immobilized HIV antigens and attached anti-HIV antibodies

Polypyrrole microspheres with immobilized HIV antigens

Analyzed serum containing anti-HIV antibodies

Figure 8 Scheme of dry test based on polypyrrole microspheres for the detection of anti-HIV antibodies.

In reaction with glucose, GOD is reduced; during subsequent oxidation of the enzyme, oxygen present in the sample is consumed (cf. Fig. 10). The plot shown in Figure 11 indicates that P(S/A) microspheres with $D_n = 0.32$ μm and with immobilized GOD (surface concentration $\Gamma(GOD) = 1.41 \times 10^{-3}$ g/m^2) can be used for determination of glucose in the region of concentrations from 10 mg/100 mL to 500 mg/100 mL.

Recently we developed methods for immobilizing microspheres covalently onto solid supports in the form of microsphere assemblies one particle thick. We hope that studies of these assemblies will open the possibility of preparing ion-selective field-effect transistor biosensors (ISFET). In this case, the bioactive compounds will be immobilized on microspheres directly

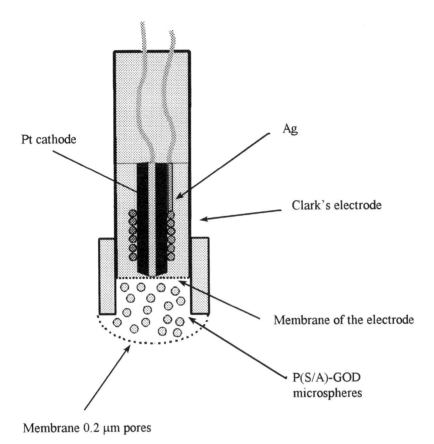

Pt cathode

Ag

Clark's electrode

Membrane of the electrode

P(S/A)-GOD
microspheres

Membrane 0.2 μm pores

Figure 9 Schematic of a biosensor based on oximetric measurements, with P(S/A)-GOD microspheres as bioactive elements.

onto the gate of the FET in a way that permits easy access of ions to this electrode. The possibility of the covalent immobilization of P(S/A) microspheres onto quartz supports was examined in a set of preliminary experiments [29].

Before the immobilization of the microspheres, the quartz plates were cleaned by dipping them in aqueous solution of KOH ([KOH] = 5 mol/L) for 15 min, washing with distilled water (10 times), and drying in the oven at 60°C. Then plates were primed for 24 hr with γ-aminopropyltriethoxysilane in toluene (concentration of the primer was varied from 2 to 12% wt/v). Effectiveness of attachment of γ-aminopropyltriethoxysilane was monitored by X-ray photoelec-

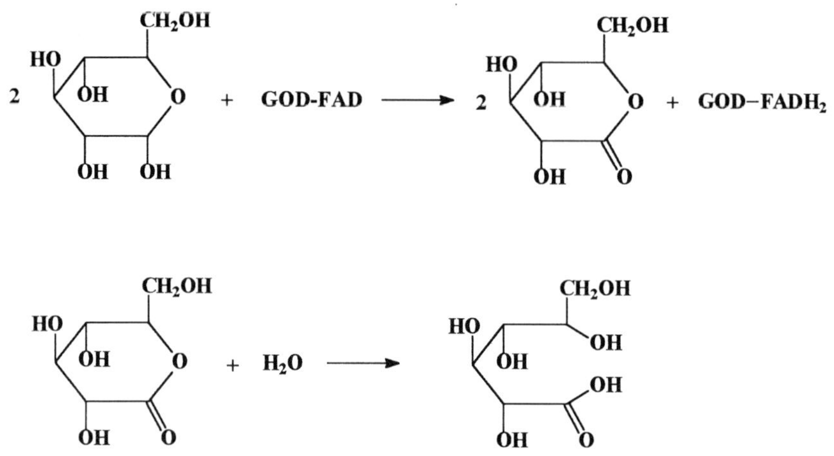

Figure 10   Redox reactions involving glucose oxidase (GOD).

tron spectroscopy (XPS) [30]. By changing the take-off angle in these measurements it was found that —NH$_2$ groups from the primer were located predominantly at the outer part of the modified surface, and thus should be easily accessible for further reactions. Plates modified with γ-aminopropyltriethoxysilane were subsequently exposed to a suspension of microspheres (0.2% wt/v) in PBS (pH = 7.4). The time of incubation was varied from 5 min to 48 hr. A scheme illustrating the covalent immobilization of microspheres is shown in Figure 12.

Analysis of scanning electron microphotographs of quartz slides revealed that the slide surfaces were covered essentially with a single layer of microspheres assembled into clusters of various sizes and orientations. We found that the degree of coverage of the surface of quartz with microspheres could be varied, depending on the concentration of microspheres in suspension and on the time of incubation, in the region from 0 to ca. 60%, leaving the remaining surface unoccupied [31]. This conforms to the theoretical analysis, which indicates that the maximal coverage in the monolayer of the rapidly and irreversibly attached particles cannot exceed 62% [32–35].

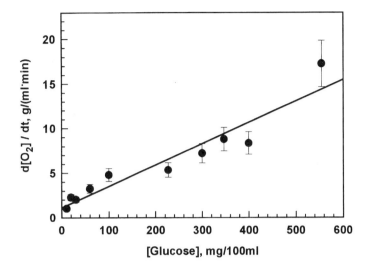

Figure 11 Dependence of the initial consumption of oxygen on the concentration of glucose. Parameters of P(S/A) microspheres: $D_n = 0.32$ μm, $D_v/D_n = 1.02$, surface concentration of aldehyde groups $\Gamma(CHO) = 1.32 \times 10^{-6}$ mol/m^2, surface concentration of immobilized GOD $\Gamma(GOD) = 1.41 \times 10^{-3}$ g/m^2, concentration of immobilized enzyme in cell compartment 2.64×10^{-4} g/mL.

It has been established that the treatment of immobilized assemblies of microspheres, containing polyacrolein units in the surface layer, with solutions of immunoglobulins yields surfaces with proteins immobilized in their active form [36]. Namely, γG anti-HSA immobilized in this way was able to recognize molecules of HSA attached to fluorescently marked microspheres and yielded fluorescent surfaces. Positive results of the foregoing experiments open the way to the design of the ISFET-based sensors with microspheres suitable for the covalent attachment of proteins, immobilized in the gate area in a manner leaving controlled, direct access of ions to the surface of the gate (depending on the degree of coverage).

V. CONCLUSIONS

Monodisperse polymeric microspheres, suitable for controlled adsorption/covalent immobilization of protein macromolecules in their active form, can be used not only for the qualitative slide agglutination tests, but also for quantitative tests (e.g,. for the determination of plasminogen) with turbidimetric detection.

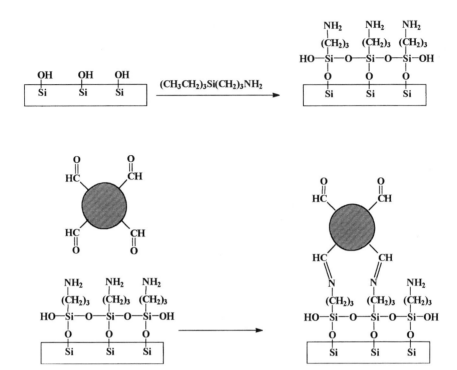

Figure 12   Scheme illustrating the priming of quartz with γ-aminopropyltriethoxysi-lane and the covalent immobilization of P(S/A) and P(P/A) microspheres.

These particles are useful also as elements of the dry assays in which the only liquid being used is the analyte. Microspheres can be used as a convenient carrier of glucose oxidase, and microsphere–GOD conjugates are suitable for oximetric assays for glucose. Preliminary experiments also indicate the usefulness of microspheres for making ISFET biosensors.

ACKNOWLEDGMENTS

This work was supported with the KBN Grant 3 T09A 033 11 and with the Polonium program promoting collaboration between Polish and French research teams.

REFERENCES

1. J. Ugelstad, A. Berge, T. Ellingsen, R. Schmid, T.-N. Nilsen, P. C. Mork, P. Stenstad, E. Hornes, O. Olsvik. Progress Polym. Sci. 17:87 (1992).
2. T. Basinska, S. Slomkowski, M. Delamar. J. Bioact. Compat. Polym. 8:205 (1993).
3. S. Margel, U. Beitler, M. Offarim. J. Cell. Sci. 56:157 (1982).
4. S. Margel. Methods Enzymol. 112:164 (1985).
5. M. Colvin, A. Smolka, A. Rembaum, M. Chang. In: A. Rebmaum, Z. A. Tökés (eds.). Microspheres: Medical and Biological Applications. CRC Press, Boca Raton, FL, 1988, p. 1.
6. F. Hoshino, M. Sakai, H. Kawaguchi, Y. Ohtsuka. Polym. J. 19:383 (1987).
7. K. Yamaguchi, S. Watanabe, S. Nakahama. Makromol. Chem. Rapid Commun. 10: 397 (1989).
8. T. Delair, C. Pichot, B. Mandrand. Colloid Polym. Sci. 272:72 (1994).
9. B. Miksa, S. Slomkowski. Colloid Polym. Sci. 272:47 (1995).
10. B. Miksa, M. Wilczynska, C. Cierniewski, T. Basinska, S. Slomkowski. J. Biomater. Sci. Polym Edn. 7:503 (1995).
11. M. C. Davies, R. A. P. Lynn, J. Hearn, A. J. Paul, J. C. Vickerman, J. F. Watts. Langmuir 11:4313 (1995).
12. A. Rembaum, S. P. S. Yen, R. S. Molday. J. Macromol. Sci.-Chem. A13:603 (1979).
13. J. Ugelstad, A. Berge, T. Ellingsen, O. Aune, L. Kilaas, T.-N. Nilsen, R. Schmid, P. Stenstad, S. Funderud, G. Kvalheim, K. Nustad, T. Lea, F. Vardtal, H. Danielsen. Makromolek. Chem. Macromolec. Symp. 17:177 (1988).
14. J. Ugelstad, P. C. Mork, R. Schmid, T. Ellingsen, A. Berge. Polymer Int. 30:157 (1993).
15. T. Basinska, S. Slomkowski. J. Biomater. Sci. Polym. Edn. 3:115 (1991).
16. W. Norde, F. G. Gonzalez, C. A. Haynes. Polym. Adv. Technol. 5:518 (1995).
17. T. Basinska, D. Kowalczyk, S. Slomkowski, F. W. Wang. In: K. S. Schmitz (ed.). Macro-Ion Characterization, from Dilute Solutions to Complex Fluids. American Chemical Society, Washington, DC, 1994, p. 449.
18. A. Rembaum, W. J. Dreyer. Science 208:364 (1980).
19. M. D. B. Oenick, A. Warshawsky. Colloid Polym. Sci. 269:139 (1991).
20. T. Basinska, D. Kowalczyk, B. Miksa, S. Slomkowski. Polym. Adv. Technol. 6: 526 (1995).
21. T. Basinska, S. Slomkowski. In: G. Guilbault, M. Mascini (eds.). Uses of Immobilized Biological Compounds. Kluwer Academic, Dordrecht, Netherlands, 1993, p. 453.
22. B. Miksa, S. Slomkowski, J. Biomater. Sci. Polym. Edn. 7:77 (1995).
23. P. K. Nakane, A. Kawaoi. J. Histochem. Cytochem. 12:1084 (1972).
24. T. Basinska, S. Slomkowski. Colloid Polym. Sci. 273:431 (1995).
25. R. W. Lim, R. W. Molday, H. V. Huand, S.-P. S. Yen. Biochim. Biophys. Acta 394:377 (1975).
26. M. T. Charreyre, O. Tcherkasskaya, M. A. Winnik, A. Hiver, P. Cros, C. Pichot, B. Mandrand. Langmuir 13:3103 (1997).

27. P. J. Tarcha, D. Misun, D. Finley, M. Wong, J. J. Donovan. In: E. S. Daniels, E. D. Sudol, M. S. El-Aasseer (eds.). Polymer Latexes: Preparation, Characterization, and Applications. American Chemical Society, Washington, DC, 1992, p. 347.
28. A. Szewczuk, M. Kuropatwa, A. Rapak. Archiv. Immun. Therapie Exp. 40:325 (1992).
29. S. Slomkowski, B. Miksa, M. Trznadel, D. Kowalczyk, F. W. Wang. ACS Polym. Prep. 37(2):747 (1996).
30. D. Kowalczyk, S. Slomkowski, M. M. Chehimi, M. Delamar. Int. J. Adhesion Adhesives 16:227 (1996).
31. B. Miksa, S. Slomkowski, M. M. Chehimi, M. Delamar, J.-P. Majoral, A.-M. Caminade. Colloid Polym. Sci. 277:58 (1999).
32. P. Schaaf, J. Talbot. J. Chem. Phys. 91:4401 (1989).
33. R. Jullien, P. Meakin. J. Phys. A25:L189 (1992).
34. Z. Adamczyk, B. Siwek, M. Zembala, P. Beloushek. Adv. Colloid Interface Sci. 48:151 (1994).
35. M. Trznadel, S. Slomkowski. Colloid Polym. Sci. 274:1109 (1996).

Index

Abell-Kendall, 328, 329
Absorbance, 64
Accu-Chek, 35
AccuChek Easy, 346
Acetaldehyde, 10
Acetate buffer, 103
Acetycholine, 10
Acid probes, 5
Acrylamide matrix, 151
Acrylic, 337, 351
Acrylodan, 247
Activity coefficients, 6
Activity concentrations, 6
Addressable high-density bead array, 134
Addressable high-density sensors, 131
Addressable transducer, 130
Adenosine, 11
Adenosine monophosphate, 11
Adhesives, 337
AEQ-biotin conjugate, 262
Aequorin, 259, 261,262, 265, 266, 268
Aequorin-bpiotin, 262
Affinity, 274

Affinity capillary electrophoresis, 222
Ag/AgCl electrode, 14, 15, 85, 98, 234
Agglutination tests, 393, 404, 409
Agricultural application, 64
Albumin, 271, 321
Alfafetoproteins, 261
Algorithm, 314, 316
Amino acid, 249, 250
Amniotic fluid, 82
Amniotic membrane, 81
Amperometric, 6, 64, 90, 95, 96, 98
    biosensors, 14
    current, 16
    detection, 95, 110
    determination, 96
    immunoassay, 96, 114, 115
    immunosensor, 100
    microcell, 82, 83, 85
    output, 103
    signal, 96
Amperometry, 13
Amplified DNA , 122
Amygdalin, 10

Anaerobic infection, 81
Analyte, 2, 3, 14, 24, 63, 93, 96, 101, 102, 106, 122, 134, 135, 139, 274, 331
Analyte capture, 3
Analyte/conjugate absorption, 98
Antisyphilis antibody, 203, 206, 210
Antibiotics, 95
Antibodies, 3, 4, 93, 94, 108, 110, 329, 332, 383, 403, 405
Antibody-antigen interactions, 21
Antibodies/antigens, 203
Antibody immobilization, 96, 208, 210
Anticoagulant, 367, 368
Anticotinine antibody, 272
Antigen recognition, 93
Antigen-antibody binding, 95
Antigen-antibody complex, 94, 105
Antigen-antibody interaction, 93
Antigens, 210, 405
Anti-HIV antibodies, 405
Apophotoproteins, 265
Apoprotein, 95, 259, 261
Arterial blood, 29, 32
Artificial cell membranes, 291
Artificial nose, 125
Artificial pancreas, 24
Aspartame, 10
Aspartic/glutamic acid, 385
Assay, 66, 109, 110, 125
Associated redox ploymers, 65
Atmospheric pollutants, 23
Atomic force micrograph, 131
Atrazine, 94
Automated DNA synthesis, 230
Avalanche photodiodes, 122
Avidin, 262, 390
Avidity, 274, 275, 277, 280, 283, 287

Bacteria, 95, 114
Bacterial cells, 111, 151
Bacterial particle, 10
Bacterial vaginosis, 81, 82
Banana electrode, 4

Beaucage's reagent, 230, 232
Beer fermentation, 129
Benzoquinone, 16
Berovin, 259
Bias, 44
Bifurcated bundles, 123
Bilirubin, 307, 346, 350
Bind antibodies, 22
Bioactive substance, 63
Bioanalytical membrane electrode, 8
Biocatalytic, 8, 10
Biochromic, 292, 293
Biocompatibility, 160, 368, 367, 374, 378
Bioelements, 3
Biohazard, 365
Biolistic delivery, 155
Biolistic embedding, 154
Biological analyte, 2
Biological recognition, 94, 127
Biological sensing, 2
Bioluminescence, 259, 261, 262, 266, 268
Biomedical diagnostic reagents, 352
Biomedical testing, 1
Biomembrane, 3
Biomolecule analyte, 262
Biomolecules, 140
Biopharmaceutical, 269
Bioreactors, 381, 391
Biorecognition mechanism, 1
Biosensor, 29, 63, 127, 140, 297, 299, 343, 345, 350, 351, 352, 381, 386, 391, 406
Biosensor coatings, 63, 67, 68, 75, 77, 79
Biosubstances, 368
Biotin, 262, 263, 264, 283, 289, 390
Biotinylated photoprotein, 262
Blood, 63, 109, 307, 332, 343, 349, 367
  analysis, 121
  cells, 30, 34, 374
  chemistry, 344
  compatibility, 368, 373, 374, 378
  glucose sensor, 16

[Blood]
glucose strips, 344
glucose, 20, 29, 63, 69, 347, 374
IgE, 96
plasma, 108
sample, 33
serum, 349
urea nitrogen, 348, 350
vessels, 21
Blue-to-red color, 292, 293, 297
Botulinum, 294, 297
Botulinum toxin, 94
Bound immunocomplex, 94
Bound immunospecies, 94
Bovine serum albumin, 83, 354
Breathe analysis, 135
Breathe vapors, 126

Calcium, 243, 350
Calcium in phagosomes, 157
Calcium sensor, 152
Calibration, 4, 14, 23, 88, 90, 108, 113, 114, 115
Calometric, 64
cAMP, 245, 246, 247, 248, 253
cAMP biosensor, 248
Cancer, 215, 345
Capillary action, 344
Capillary blood, 29, 32
Capillary channel, 30
Carbon-containing inks, 29
Carbon electrodes, 96
Carbon material electrode, 103
Carbon particle, 96, 98, 116
Cardic markers, 345
Cardiolipin, 203, 210
Cardiovascular problems, 307
Casein, 355, 357, 362, 364
Catheter, 372
Cathodic current, 103
Cathodic sweep voltammetry, 103
CCD detector, 122
Cell activity, 122
Cell culture, 370
Cell membranes, 5

Cells, 3, 148, 243, 244, 247, 304
Cellular analysis, 121
Cellular analytes, 139
Cellular communication, 291
Cellular membrane, 243
α-Cellulose, 332
Cellulose, 333
dialysis membrane, 368, 374
hollow-fiber probe, 370, 375
membrane, 367, 370, 373, 374
Charge-coupled device, 122
Chemical measurement, 29
Chemical messenger, 243
Chemical sensor, 146, 148
Chemiluminometric, 94
ChemStrip bG, 346
Cholera, 294, 297, 299, 300, 303
Choles-4en-3one, 349
Cholestech LDX analyzer, 330
Cholesterol, 93, 307, 319, 325, 330, 349, 350, 352
detection, 18
esterase, 327, 328
oxidase, 327, 328, 349
Chromatographic strip assay platform, 271
Chromophore, 259, 261, 292
Chromosome, 216
Chronoamperometry, 31
Clarke error grid, 36, 41, 319
Clytin, 259
Coagulation assays, 330
Coatings, 334, 351, 368
Coefficient of variation, 88, 89
Coelenteramide, 261
Coelenterazine, 261
Coimmobilizing, 16
Colloidal gold, 140, 146
Colorimetric assay, 82
Combinatorial drug design, 121
Comfort Curve, 30, 32, 35, 42, 44, 57, 58, 59
Complexation, 68
Conductance, 24
Conductimetric sensors, 24
Conduction band, 9

Conductometric, 6, 24, 64, 95
Continuous monitoring, 20
Contrived HCT, 35
Corona discharge, 327
Cosmic ray, 314, 319
Cotinine, 272, 277, 279, 281, 284, 286
Cottrell equation, 31
Creatine kinase, 16
Creatinine, 10, 350
Critical care, 29, 32
Cross-linked dsDNA, 219
Culture method, 113
Cyclic AMP, 243, 250
Cyclic voltammetry, 86, 231, 248
  scans, 85, 86
Cysteine, 247, 248, 383,385
Cystic fibrosis, 134, 135
Cytochrome c′, 140, 144, 145, 146, 149
  biosensors, 150
Cytokine, 244, 261

Defense application, 64
Desiccants, 338
Detection of glucose, 16
Detection limit, 2
Detection of NTA, 9
Detector pixels, 126
Dextran sulfate, 329
D-Gluconate, 10
Diabetes, 20, 121, 307, 319, 345, 368
Diagnose disease, 121
Diagnostic, 110
  coatings, 350
  polymers, 351
  reagents, 63, 343
Dialysis, 367, 370
Diamine oxidase, 82
Diaphorase, 18
Diethylaminocoumalin maleimide, 247
Differential pulse voltammetry, 231
Diffraction grating, 64
Diffusion constant, 35
Diffusion layer, 13
Diffusion with cell walls, 4
Digoxin, 95

Dimethoxytrityl nucleoside phosphoramidites, 230
Dip-coating, 23
Dip sticks, 345
Diseases, 244
Disorders, 215, 227
Disposable electrodes, 96
Disposable immunosensors, 23
DNA, 5, 226, 227, 239
  biosensors, 135
  chip, 352
  conjugates, 216
  detection, 124, 137
  macromonomer, 216, 219
  microarray, 351
  microchips, 124
  polymerase, 384
  probes, 5, 25
  sensor array, 129
  sensors, 130
  sequences, 124
  targets, 124, 134, 135
DNA-chip-based diagnostic, 351
DNA-DNA hydridization, 351
Drug screening, 253
Drugs of abuse, 345
Dry chemistry, 343, 344
Dry reagents, 331
dsDNA-vinyl polymer conjugate, 216
Dynamic fluctuations, 2

E. coli, 95, 116, 265, 297, 299, 383,
  389
E.P.T. pregnancy test, 346
Ektachem, 346
Electochemical/optical combination, 64
Electroactive interferent, 14
Electroactive products, 3
Electroactive species, 13, 65
Electrochemical assay, 96
Electrochemical:
  biosensor, 1, 64, 344, 351
  cell, 6, 98
  detection, 21
  detector, 96

[Electrochemical]
 immunosensors, 23
 measurement, 103
 oxidation, 86
 sensor, 33, 140, 151, 352
 surface, 30
 transducer, 95
Electrochemiluminescence, 64
Electrode material, 23, 96
Electrode surface, 6, 12, 23, 96
Electrolytes, 122
Electron beam (EB), 75
Electron relays, 19, 67
Electrophoresis, 216, 219, 220
Electroreduction, 103
ELISA, 112–116, 245, 280, 284, 353,
 355, 363, 364
Elite, 42, 44, 58, 59
Ellipsometry, 64
Emit format, 273
ENACT, 327, 328, 329. 346
Endocrine pancreas, 368, 378
Endogenous glucose, 35
Endonucleases, 216
Environmental application, 64
Environmental testing, 1
Enzymatic Q.E.D saliva alcohol test,
 346
Enzymatic reaction, 227
Enzyme, 3, 10, 35, 63, 140, 203, 292,
 325, 350, 351, 353
 activity, 86, 88, 89, 91
 electrode, 63
 label, 21, 96
 layer, 12
Enzyme-channel immunoassay, 23
Equilibrium constants, 6
Erythrocyte, 33, 300, 325
Ethyl cellulose membrane, 344
Ethylenediamine, 205, 207, 210
Ethylenediamine plasma, 203
Evanescent wave, 64
ExacTech, 16, 65
Exonuclease, 238
Extracellular, 139, 140

FastTake, 29, 35, 42, 44, 57, 59
Femtomolar, 228
Ferricyanide mediator, 30
Ferricyanides, 16, 58
Ferrocene, 16, 18, 58, 67
Ferrocene/ferrocenium, 16
Ferrocence-modified ODN, 228
Ferrocene-mononucleotide conjugate,
 234
Ferrocene-ODN, 228, 239
Ferrocenyl ODN, 230
Ferrocyanide, 31, 32
Fiber-based optodes, 151
Fiber optic sensors, 140, 147
Fiberless sensing, 150
Fiberless sensors, 140
Fibroblasts, 376
Field-effect transistors, 9
Film formers, 63
Finger-stick blood, 325, 329
Finger sticking, 16
Flavin adenine, 10
Flourescein, 129, 130
Flourescence, 121
 signature, 125
 spectroscopy, 139
Flourescent dye, 124, 131
Flourescent indicators, 123
Flow injection, 2, 95, 96
Flow-injection immunosensor, 98
Flow-through immunoassay, 98, 101,
 113, 116
Flow-through immunofiltration, 113
Flow-through immunosensor, 109
Fluid analysis, 131
Fluorescence, 64, 312, 317, 319
Fluorescent probe, 243
Fluorophores, 135, 245, 246
Food-borne pathogens, 113
Forssman antigen, 261
Fourth-generation biosensors, 63
Free-energy changes, 6
Free immunospecies, 94
Fresh venous blood, 32
Fructosamine, 352

Full-factorial experimental, 35
Functional materials, 341

β-Galactosidase, 383, 386, 389, 390
Gamera compact disk, 346
Ganglioside, 294, 297
Gas-sensing electrodes, 7
GDH, 30
GDH-glucose-ferricyanide reaction,
    31
Gene:
  analysis, 222
  chip technology, 65
  diagnosis, 216
  expression, 227
  fusion technology, 264
  fusion, 384, 385, 388
  gun, 154, 155
  mutation assay, 216
  mutations, 134, 135
  probe, 65, 351
  sensor, 227, 228, 234, 238, 239
  therapy, 227
  transcription, 244
GeneChip, 352
Genes, 384
Genetic analysis, 134
Genetic defects, 5, 25
Genetic disorder, 121, 126
Genetic engineering, 383
Genomics-related detection, 121
Genosensors, 351
Genotyping, 351
Gestational diabetes, 345
Glass-ceramic insulating layer, 85
Globulins, 399
Glow-discharge, 203, 205, 207,
    210
Glucometer elite, 35
Gluconic acid, 349
Glucosamine, 11
Glucose:
  dehydrogenase, 30
  electrode, 1, 14, 370
  fiber-optic, 128
  monitoring, 372

[Glucose]
  oxidase, 16, 30, 63, 67, 127, 344,
      348, 349, 400, 401
  sensor, 368
Glutamine, 11
Glutathione, 146, 148, 150
Glycemic control, 36
Glycoproteins, 385
Gold particles, 274, 275, 287
Graphite-based ink, 23
Graphite electrodes, 84
Gravimetric transducer, 94
Guanine, 11
Guanylate cyclase, 144, 145

Half-cell potential, 6
Handheld blood glucose meters, 29
Hantavirus, 110, 116
HDL, 330
HEA/acrylic acid, 76
HEMA/methacrylic acid, 76
Hemagglutinin lectin, 299
Hematocrit, 30, 32, 35, 36, 42, 44, 57,
      58, 59, 312, 319, 325
Hemodialysis, 367
  membrane, 370
  patients, 32
Hemoglobin, 95, 309, 350
Hemoprotein, 140
Heparin, 367
Hepatitis B surface antigen, 405
Herbicides, 23
Hereditary diseases, 227
Heterocyclic (N) monomers, 68
Hevea brasilisensis, 393
Hexokinase, 300, 301, 303, 304
High-density sensor, 130, 134
Highly carboxylated acrylic polymers, 76
Hitachi clinical chemistry analyzer, 36
Hollow-fiber probe, 372, 373, 376, 378
Hollow fibers, 368
Home-based diagnostic kits, 22
Hook effect, 263
Hormone regulation, 5
Hormones, 23, 93, 116, 203, 244, 265
Hot-melts, 337

Human blood, 110, 116
Human chorionic gonadotropin, 94, 287
Human cytokine mRNA, 124
Human erythrocytes, 95
Human genome, 124
Human growth hormone, 355
Human IgG, 94, 96
Human neuroblastoma, 139
Human serum albumin, 94
Human β-globin, 124
Hybridization, 227
Hydrodynamic chronoamperometry, 13
Hydrogel, 68, 216, 351
Hydrogel PEBBLEs, 153
Hydrogen peroxide, 101, 103, 104, 105
Hydroxyethyl cellulose, 351
Hydroxyethyl methacrylate copolymers, 351
Hydrozoan coelenterates, 259
Hyperglycemia, 20, 41, 372
Hypoglycemia, 20, 41, 319, 372
Hyppocampal cells, 247

IgG, 95, 116
IgM, 116
Image resolution, 126
Imaging fibers, 135
Imidazole, 78
Immobilization of an enzyme, 8
Immobilization of antibodies, 113, 114
Immobilized antibodies, 116
Immobilized enzyme, 8
Immobilized glucose oxidase, 128
Immobilized ODN, 238
Immunoagent, 113
Immunoagglomeration, 106
Immunoasays, 21, 93–96, 98, 105, 108,
    110, 113, 116, 130, 244, 261,
    273, 31, 330, 353, 363
Immunochemical, 121, 271, 323
Immunochromatographic test, 346
Immunocolumn, 98, 101, 102
Immunoconjugate, 102, 105, 106
Immunoelectrode, 98, 101, 102, 105,
    106, 110, 111
Immunogen, 280, 281, 286

Immunoglobin, 107, 108
Immunohistochemistry, 353, 363
Immunointeraction, 102, 108
Immunological measurement, 353, 354
Immunological testing, 113
Immunosensor, 22, 23, 94, 95, 98, 101,
    106, 108, 203
Immunosorbent, 96, 98, 101, 106, 110,
    113
Immunostrip, 346
Impedimetric, 64, 95
Implantable glucose, 20
Implantable sensor, 18, 367
Impregnation, 351
Indicator electrode, 6, 7
Industrial application, 64
Industrial testing, 1
Infectious disease, 345
Infectious dose, 112
Infective organism, 82
Infertility, 81
Influenza virus, 299, 300
Insulin, 344, 345
Insulin-dependent diabetes mellitus, 345
Intact bacterial particles, 9
Intensive care, 110
Interactive system, 94
Interference, 14, 65, 69, 78
Interferents, 3, 21, 148
Interferon-γ, 148
Interferon-γ1, 124
Interleukin 4, 124
Interleukin 6, 124
Internal reference electrode, 84
Intoxication, 111
Intracellular, 139
Intracellular nitric oxide, 149
Invasive monitoring, 124
Inverted flourescence microscope, 122
Ion-exchange chromatography, 387
Ion-selective electrodes, 7
ISE, 9
i-STAT, 66

Kapton (polyimide), 66
Ketones, 350

Kidney dialysis, 121
Kidney problems, 307

Label, 94, 353
Label, flourescent, 94
Labeled DNA targets, 125
Labeled immunoagent, 95
Labels, radioactive isotopes, 94
Lab-on-a-chip platform, 21
LabTab, 281, 283, 287
Lactate, 82, 350
Langmuir monolayer, 301
Langmuir-Blodgett, 292
L-Arginine, 10
Laser-scribed alumina, 83
L-Aspartate, 10
L-Cysteine, 10
LDL, 329, 330
Leaching, 18
Leukocytes, 346, 376
L-Glutamate, 11
L-Glutamic Acid, 10
L-Glutamine, 10
L-Histodine, 10
Ligation, 216
Light addressable potentiometric, 64
Linear response, 2
Lining of the intestine, 113
Lipopolysaccharide, 148
Lipoproteins, 385
Liposomal delivery, 155
Liposome, 154, 292, 294, 299, 304
Living cell, 123, 130, 135, 249, 256,
      291
Living organism, 259, 368
Local anesthesia, 372
Low redox potential, 16
L-Phenylalanine, 10
L-Pro-4-(phenylazo) phenylamide, 82
L-proline *p*-nitroanilide triflouroacetate,
      83
L-proline *p*-nitroanilide, 82, 86
L-proline β-naphylamide, 86
L-proline, 82, 83
L-prolyl β-naphylamide, 88
L-Serine, 10

L-Tyrosine, 10
Lymphocytes, 376
Lysine, 300, 385, 390

Macrophage, 139, 146, 148, 149, 158,
      376
Magnetic code, 347
Magnetic microspheres, 398
Mammalian cells, 151
Markers, 21
Mass (piezoelectric), 64
Mediator, 4, 16, 35, 65, 67, 343
Medical devices, 367
Medical diagnosis, 113
Medical diagnostic, 93, 96, 116, 134,
      215, 331, 381, 391, 393
   assays, 122, 135
   multianalyte, 135
   reagents, 344
   sensors, 121
Medical grade aliphatic polyurethane, 83
Medical/clinical application, 64
Medication, 24
MediSense glucose monitor, 65
MediSense sensors, 16
Membrane, 14, 15, 21, 332, 333, 336,
      344
Messenger, 247
Metabolite, 5, 21, 349
Methacryloyloxyethyl phosphorylcho-
      line, 355, 368
Methacryloyloxysuccinimide, 220, 225
Methotrexate, 10
Methylamine, 82
Microbead sensors, 131
Microbial diseases, 112
Microcell, 88, 89, 95
Microdialysis, 368, 370, 372, 374, 378
Microemulsion, 153
Microfabricate ISE, 65
Microfabrication, 1, 21, 82
Microporous immunosensors surface, 23
Microsensor arrays, 133, 135
Microsphere, 147, 148, 393, 395, 396,
      397, 400, 401, 402, 404, 405,
      408, 409, 410

Microsphere sensors, 134
Micro-total analysis, 21
Microwell arrays, 131
Microwells, 134
Miniature biosensor, 66, 351
Miniaturized biosensor, 9
Miniaturized sensor array, 121
Minimization, 3
Mitrocomin, 259
Mnemiopsin, 259
Modeling of the sensors response, 36
Molecular beacons, 135
Molecular imprinted polymers, 25
Molecular probe, 153
Molecular recognition, 121, 226
Monitor pH, 127
Monoclonal antibody, 5, 272
Mouse oocyte, 139, 151, 157
Multianalyte, 21, 66, 153
Multianalyte sensor, 129
Multilayered coating, 344
Multiple DNA sequences, 125
Muscle damage, 16, 18
Myocardial infraction, 18

NAD+, 10
Nanoelectronics, 121
Nanoparticles, 151
Nanosensors, 139, 393
β-Naphylamine, 83, 88
β-Naphylamide hydrochloride, 83
Neonatal, 29
Neonatal blood, 29, 32
Neonates, 41
Nernst equation, 7, 13
Neural transmission, 5
Neuroblastoma cells, 155
Neuronal cells, 247
Neuronal plasticity, 244
Neurons, 294
Neurotoxin, 294, 297, 303
Neurotransmitters, 5, 244, 265
Neutrophils, 376
NicoMeter, 277
NicoMeter strip, 281

Nicotinamide adenine dinucleotide (NAD+), 18
Nicotine metabolite, 271, 287
Nitrate, 10
Nitric oxide, 140, 141, 144
Nitric oxide sensors, 139, 149
Nitrilotriacetate acid, 9, 10
Nitrocellulose membrane, 275, 327, 332
N-Methylphenazinium, 16
Nondiffusing mediators, 18
Noninsulin-dependent diabetes mellitus, 345
Noninvasive, 139, 352
Nonlinearity, 15
Nonselective, 24
Nonwiping, 344
Normal glucose range, 41
Normalized bias, 59
n-Si semiconductors, 9
Nucleic acid ligands, 3
Nucleic acid probe, 261
Nucleic acids, 393
Nucleotide, 249, 250, 252, 253

Obelin, 259, 261, 262, 265, 266, 268
Octapeptide, 265, 266, 268
Oligodeoxynucleotide, 227, 230
Oligonucleotide, 130, 134, 215, 220, 222, 223, 224
Oligopeptide, 246, 248, 253
Oligosaccharide, 383
Oncogene, 134, 222
One-step immunosensors, 24
On-the-spot immunosensors, 24
One Touch, 345–346
Optical:
    bar codes, 131
    biosensors, 64
    bundles, 124
    detection, 21, 131
    fiber, 131, 140
    imaging, 121
    imaging fiber, 123, 126, 127, 129, 130, 131, 134
    sensor arrays, 121

[Optical]
  sensors, 122, 124, 135, 139
  transducer, 94
Optochemical, 139
  PEBBLE, 139
  sensors, 151
Organic vapor detection, 121
Organic vapors, 122, 127
Organism, 385
Os-containing redox monomers, 63, 78
Osmium-containing polymers, 67
Osmium-polypyridine, 19
Osteoporosis, 271
Ovalbumin, 355
Oxalate, 10
Oxygen, 122, 127
Oxygen electrode, 65

Palladium electrode, 30
Parathion, 94
Paratope, 272
Partial least square, 312
Particle valency, 271, 279, 283
Particle valency assays, 273, 274
Passivation of the electrode, 22
Passive adsorption of antibodies, 23
Pathogenic agents, 291, 292, 300
Pathogens, 21
Pattern recognition, 126, 135
PEBBLE sensor, 151, 153, 155, 157,
    158, 160
Pelvic inflammatory disease, 81
Penicillin, 10, 122, 127, 128, 129
Penicillin fermentation, 129
Penicillinase, 128, 129
Penicilloic acid, 129
Peptide-photoprotein conjugates, 265
Percutaneous sensors, 20
Peroxidase, 96, 105, 110, 116, 326, 348,
    349, 354, 355, 357, 400
Peroxidase label, 103
Peroxynitrite, 146, 148
Pesticides, 5
Phagocytosis, 155
Phenylazophenylamine, 82
Phenylenediamine , 85

Phosphate buffer, 85, 101
Phospholipid, 356, 367
Phospholipid polymer, 353, 359
Phosphorothioate, 232
Phosphorus, 350
Phosphorylation, 247
Photodeposited biosensors, 128
Photodeposited sensor arrays, 130
Photodeposition, 126
Photolithograpy, 91, 351
Photomultiplier tube, 122
Photopolymerize, 75
Photoprotein, 259, 261, 262, 264, 385
Physiological response, 5
Pico-injection, 156
Piezoelectric crystal, 95, 207
Piezoelectric detectors, 94
Piezoelectric immunosensor, 95, 203,
    208, 210
Piezoelectric sensors, 203
Pixel, 317, 319
Planar waveguides, 123
Plasma, 33, 328, 347, 370
  and cells, 36
  protein, 368
  technology, 207
  transport, 325
Plasmid DNA, 389
Plasminogen, 410
Platelet, 370, 374
Platelet adhesion, 368
Platinum counter electrode, 98
Platinum electrodes, 82, 85
Platinum ink, 85
Platinum working electrode, 90
Pneumonia, 111
p-nitroanaline, 82, 83
Point-of-care, 323, 345
Pollutant, 21
Poly(4-vinyl pyridine), 67
Poly(9-vinyladenine), 222
Poly(m-phenylenediamine), 85
Poly(N-isopropylacrylamide), 216
Poly(styrene) microspheres, 395, 396
Poly(styrene/acrolein) microspheres, 396
Polyacid, 75

Polyacrolein microspheres, 395
Polyacrylamide gel, 222
Polyacrylamide, 8, 215
Polyclonal antibody, 5, 287
Polydiacetylene lipids, 291
Polyelectrolyte complex, 75
Polyethylene glycol diglycidyl ether, 67
Polyethylene oxide (PEO), 35
Polymer 6/1, 67
Polymer membrane, 367
Polymer photodeposition, 129
Polymerase chain reaction, 125, 384
Polymerases, 216
Polymicrobial, 81
Polynomial regression, 42
Polypeptide, 386
Polypyrrole core/polyacrolein shell mi-
        crospheres, 396
Polysiloxanes, 67
Polyvinyl acetate, 351
Polyvinyl alcohol, 351
Polyvinyl pyrrolidone, 351
Poor stability, 341
Porex membrane, 275
Porous nylon filtration membrane, 113
Posttranslational modification, 38, 389
Potentiometric cell, 6
Potentiometric enzyme, 8
Potentiometric, 6, 95
Precision G, 35, 41, 42, 44, 58
Precision QID sensors, 16
Pregnancy test, 405
Pre-term birth, 81
Probe, 231, 234, 238
Probe DNA, 227
Profiler, 5
Proline iminopeptidase, 82, 83
Prostate-specific antigen RNA, 261
Protein, 15, 93, 94, 95, 96, 110, 116,
        301, 321, 354, 363, 365, 368,
        381, 393, 394, 398
Protein A, 111, 112, 261
Protein hormones, 5
Protein kinase, 248
Protein kinase A, 244, 245, 246, 247, 252
Protein kinase G, 252

Protein labels, 261
Protein-imprinting, 220
p-Si semiconductors, 9, 12
Putrescence oxidase, 82
Putrescine, 91
Putrescine dihydrochloride, 83
Putrescine oxidase, 82, 83, 90
Pyruvate, 10

QID glucose monitor, 65
Quantum efficiency, 309
Quantum yield, 261, 356
Quartz crystal microbalance, 203, 204
Quaternization, 68

Rabbit IgG, 105
Radioactive label, 227, 261, 265, 269
Raman signal, 317
Raman spectroscopy, 147, 307, 321
Randomly addressable bead arrays,
        135
Rat alveolar, 139
Ratiometric cytochrome c', 143
Ratiometric sensor, 140, 141, 144
Ratiometric, 146, 147, 150
Reagent matrix, 32, 33
Reagent-free immunosensors, 24
Reagentless diagnostics, 307
Receptors, 3, 292
Recognizer, 245
Recombinant antibodies, 5
Recombinant DNA, 389, 391
Recombinant hantavirus, 110
Recombinant photoproteins, 259
Red blood cells, 319, 344, 347
Redox centers, 19
Redox coatings, 72
Redox marker anion, 248
Redox polymer, 65, 67
Redox potential, 69, 234
Reference electrode, 6
Reference glucose, 36
Reference laboratories, 323
Reflectance spectroscopy, 350
Reflotron, 346, 347
Reland, 272, 279, 283

Reland technology, 271
Reland traps, 274
Remote-sensing application, 64
Respiratory disease, 110
Response, 2, 41, 44
Ringer's buffer, 146
RNA, 5
Rubber, 337
Ruthenium dye, 127, 128, 129

Salicylate, 10
Saliva strip, 281
Saliva, 287
Salmonella, 95, 116
Salmonella assay, 115
Sandwich assay, 96, 110
Sandwich scheme, 101
Saturated calomel electrode, 6
Saurerbey equation, 204, 207
Scanning tunneling microscope, 206
Scanning tunneling microscopy, 98,
    203, 207, 210
Screen printed electrode, 16, 23, 82, 83,
    86, 91
Second messenger, 243, 244, 253, 256
Selectivity, 2, 6
Semipermeable membrane, 4, 348
Semitelechelic oligomer, 219
Sensing amplification, 122
Sensing element, 98
Sensitivity, 2, 34, 35
Sensor, 133, 234
Sensor-analyte signature, 126
Sensor array, 122, 126
Sensor platform, 131
Sensor response, 108
Sensor shelf life, 131
Sensor signal, 106
Sensor technology, 121, 139
Sensors, 122, 131, 134, 291, 294, 301,
    409
Separation-free immunosensors, 23
Sepharose bead, 215, 388
Sequence-specific enzymatic reaction,
    215

Serum, 311, 319, 355
Sexually transmitted disease, 81
Shelf stability, 344
Sialic acid, 297, 299, 300
Sialidases, 82
Signal fluctuations, 15
Signal processor, 2
Signal transduction, 122, 253
Signal-to-noise, 2
Silica beads, 388
Silica gels, 215
Silica particles, 327
Silicon chips, 66
Silicone, 337
Silicon micromaching, 351
Silver electrodes, 204
Silver ink, 84
Silver-silver chloride electrode, 6
Site-directed immobilization, 381
Site-directed mutagenesis, 384
Smart materials, 291
Sodium cholate, 327
Soluble proteins, 16
Solvatochromic dye, 125
Sonic welding, 337
Spherical sensors, 153
SPR, 64
Staphylococcus aureus, 111
Sterilization, 124
Steriod drug budesonide, 96
Steroids, 5
Strep, 345
Streptavidin, 130
Stroke, 345
Styrene acrylic, 351
Styrene/maleic anhydride (SMA),
    76
Subcutaneous, 21, 372
Substrate, 8, 10
Subtilisin, 383, 386, 387
Sugar, 10
Surface energy, 326, 327
Surface-plasmon resonance, 299
Surfaces of electrode, 19
Synthetic mediators, 65

Syphilis, 208
System error, 59

Target analyte, 126
Temperature dependency, 32
Temperature-sensitive DNA conjugate, 219
Test strip, 345
Tetracyanoquinodimethane—tetrathiaful-valene, 19
Tetramethylbenzidine, 348, 349
Thalassicolin, 259
Theophylline, 95, 271, 350
Thick-film technology, 82
Thyroid-stimulating hormone, 96
Tissue, 3, 9, 11
Tissue compatibility, 375
Tissue glucose, 374
Total cholesterol, 324, 328
Total E. coli, 114
Total internal reflection, 123
Total protein, 350
Toxic shock syndrome, 111
Toxin, 5, 300, 304
Transcutaneous, 309
Transducer, 1, 6, 21, 94, 127
Transduction system, 63
Trap material, 277
Trap, 275, 277
Treponema pallidum, 208
Triglyceride, 329, 350, 352
Trypsin inhibitor, 98
Tumor necrosis factor, 261

Unlabeled DNA, 122
Unlabeled targets, 125
Urea, 8, 10, 307, 350
Urease, 8, 348

Uric acid, 10, 350
Urinalysis, 344, 345
Urine, 287, 349
Urine glucose, 344
Urine NicoMeter test strip, 279
Urine strips, 344
UV-curable dielectric, 85

Vaginal discharge, 82
Vaginal fluid, 82
Vaginal infection, 81
Valency, 275
Vascular disease, 345
Venous blood, 29, 35
Vesicles, 291
Vibrational frequency, 308
Vinyl ether/maleic anhydride, 76
Vinyl pyridine, 72, 78
Viral infection, 116
Viral neuraminidase, 300
Virus, 95, 294, 300, 303, 304
Virus liposome sensors, 300

Water soluble epoxy, 67
Waveform of the excitation, 12
Western blot, 110
Wet chemistry, 323
Whole cells, 94, 112
Wired enzyme electrodes, 19
Woodward's reagent K, 96
Working electrode, 63, 85, 86, 98, 103, 116

X-Ray diffraction, 248

Yeast, 383
YSI glucose analyzer, 65